Ethical Issues in Death and Dying

Ethical Issues
in
Death and Dying

ROBERT F. WEIR, EDITOR

New York   Columbia University Press   1977

Library of Congress Cataloging in Publication Data

Main entry under title:

Ethical issues in death and dying.

Includes bibliographies and index.
1. Terminal care—Moral and religious aspects.
2. Death—Proof and certification. 3. Euthanasia.
4. Suicide. I. Weir, Robert F., 1943–
[DNLM: 1. Ethics, Medical. 2. Death. 3. Euthanasia.
4. Suicide. 5. Attitude to Death. W50 E824]
R726.E77   174'.2   77-24707
ISBN 0-231-04306-6
ISBN 0-231-04307-4 pbk.

New York   Columbia University Press   Guildford, Surrey

Copyright © 1977 Columbia University Press
All rights reserved

Printed in the United States of America

Contents

Contributors

A. G. M. Campbell, M.D., is a member of the Department of Pediatrics, Yale University School of Medicine.

Alexander Morgan Capron is an Associate Professor of Law and Associate Professor of Human Genetics at the University of Pennsylvania.

Norman L. Cantor is a Professor of Law at the Rutgers Law School.

Robert F. Drinan was Dean of the Boston College School of Law at the time of writing the article on euthanasia; he is now a U.S. Representative from Massachusetts.

Raymond S. Duff, M.D., is an Associate Professor in the Department of Pediatrics, Yale University School of Medicine.

Arthur J. Dyck is Professor of Population Ethics in the School of Public Health and Professor of Christian Ethics in the Divinity School, Harvard University.

George P. Fletcher was an Assistant Professor of Law at the University of Washington at the time of writing the article on prolonging life; he is now a Professor of Law at UCLA.

Joseph Fletcher is Professor of Medical Ethics at the University of Virginia School of Medicine.

Stanley R. Friesen, M.D., Ph.D., is a Professor of Surgery and Lecturer in the History of Medicine at the University of Kansas Medical Center.

James M. Gustafson is University Professor of Theological Ethics at the University of Chicago.

Leon R. Kass, M.D., Ph.D., was executive secretary of the Committee on the Life Sciences and Social Policy of the National Research Council–National Academy of Sciences at the time of writing the articles on determining death; he is now Henry R. Luce Professor of the Liberal Arts of Human Biology at the University of Chicago.

William D. Kelly was a member of the Department of Surgery at the University of Minnesota Medical School at the time of writing the article with Stanley Friesen.

Richard A. McCormick is Rose Kennedy Professor of Christian Ethics at the Kennedy Center for Bioethics at Georgetown Univeristy.

Daniel Maguire is a Professor of Theology at Marquette University.

Helge Hilding Mansson was a member of the Psychology Department at the University of Hawaii when she conducted the study on euthanasia.

Bernard C. Meyer, M.D., is a practicing psychoanalyst and Clinical Professor of Psychiatry at the Mount Sinai School of Medicine in New York.

Robert S. Morison was Professor of Science and Society at Cornell University at the time of the written exchange with Leon Kass; he is now a visiting professor at the Massachusetts Institute of Technology.

Donald Oken, M.D., is a Professor and Chairman of the Department of Psychiatry at the Upstate Medical Center, the State University of New York, Syracuse.

Paul W. Pretzel was a psychologist and pastoral counselor at the Los Angeles Suicide Prevention Center at the time of his article on suicide.

Paul Ramsey is Harrington Spear Paine Professor of Religion at Princeton University.

Edwin S. Shneidman is Professor of Thanatology and Director of the Laboratory for the Study of Life-Threatening Behavior at UCLA.

Thomas S. Szasz, M.D., is a Professor of Psychiatry at the Upstate Medical Center, the State University of New York, Syracuse.

The Ad Hoc Committee of the Harvard Medical School was chaired by Henry K. Beecher, M.D., and included Raymond D. Adams, A. Clifford Barger, William J. Curran, Derek Denny-Brown, Dana L. Farnsworth, Jordi Folch-Pi, Everett I. Mendelsohn, John P. Merrill, Joseph Murray, Ralph Potter, Robert Schwab, and William Sweet.

The Task Force on Death and Dying of the Institute of Society, Ethics, and the Life Sciences was chaired at the time of this study by Eric Cassell, M.D., and Leon R. Kass, M.D., and included Marc Lappe, Henry K. Beecher, Daniel Callahan, Renee C. Fox, Michael Horowitz, Irving Ladimer, Robert Jay Lifton, William F. May, Joseph A. Mazzeo, Robert S. Morison, Paul Ramsey, Alfred Sadler, Blair Sadler, Jane Schick, Robert Stevenson, and Robert Veatch.

Introduction

DEATH is a curious phenomenon in modern society. Persons living in a scientific and secularized era regard death with the same ambivalence that has traditionally characterized attitudes toward God. As depicted most clearly by Rudolf Otto in *The Idea of the Holy*, a juxtaposition of fear and fascination lies at the center of every theistic tradition and in the lives of individual believers who are both repelled by and attracted to God. That same juxtaposition of fear/fascination is evident in the attitudes displayed by individuals when they discuss the subject of death, reflect upon their own mortality, or find themselves in the presence of a dying patient.

The element of fear can be observed in the euphemisms used for death ("departed," "passed away") and in the inability of many individuals to address themselves to the general subject of death, much less to consider seriously their own dying. A basic fear of death appears to lie behind the manifold attempts of individuals to retard the rate of aging through the use of cosmetics and surgery, to isolate the aging and dying in "rest homes" and private hospital rooms, to defer the inevitability of death by doing "whatever is necessary" to keep a patient's organs functioning artificially, and to cover up the reality of death with expensive caskets and massive displays of flowers. For many of us, the fear of death and our own dying is probably most evident on those few occasions when we have suffered through an interminable period of hesitant, irrelevant conversation and long periods of unbroken silence in the presence of a person whose death is imminent. For medically trained personnel, the fear of death is one of the motivating reasons for having selected medicine as a profession. The continuing presence of this fear among medical personnel is evident in the prevailing conception of death as an "enemy" that must be conquered by physicians, in the advice sometimes given to nurses ("Don't let the patient die on your shift"), and in the inability of many physicians to tell terminal patients the truth about their condition or to terminate treatment when further life-sustaining attempts are meaningless.

There are a number of possible explanations for the fascination with death and dying. Above all, death is a mystery which paradoxically is more mysterious in a scientific age than ever before. We are accustomed to scientific explanations for all aspects of human existence, and we would prefer that death not remain an exception to the rule. Yet in an age in which biochemists can explain the aging process, cardiologists explain what happens to the body when circulation fails, neurologists explain how the cessation of various parts of the brain affects other vital organs, and psychiatrists explain certain stages that characterize the dying pattern of most terminal patients—death still remains a mystery. A second reason for fascination with death is that dying, like human sexuality, is an inescapable part of human existence, yet until recently has been a forbidden topic of conversation and an unimportant area of research. Just as a dying person is taboo in primitive societies (as are persons having any contact with the dead), so in our enlightened society the reality of death and dying has been studiously avoided. As a result, many young people are fascinated by the subject of death, partly because it has been forbidden, and partly because they have been reared in an environment that sheltered them from dying animals and dying relatives. A third reason for fascination with death is that some persons among us are apparently motivated by a martyr complex that occasionally manifests itself in the form of a "death wish." As a result, a physician's decision relating to allowing a patient to die or to committing an act of euthanasia is made much more difficult by the knowledge that some individuals want to die "before their time" in order to redeem their lives with a last noble gesture, or to save their families large medical bills, or simply to cut short their own existence. For the physician, it is one thing to consider an act of "mercy killing" to relieve a patient from what appears to be unbearable suffering; it is another thing to realize that he may be assisting a patient who wants to die for psychosocial reasons, perhaps more than for physiological ones.

The articles collected in this volume are intended to show that, while physicians and patients may approach death and dying with a mixture of fear and fascination, neither of these attitudes is helpful in working through the complex ethical issues that must frequently be confronted by a dying patient, an attending physician, and/or members of the patient's family. Rather than facilitating decision making in the face of these issues, the attitudes of fear and fascination may inhibit decision making to the point where a physician cannot terminate useless life-sustaining treatment out of fear of losing another battle to the "enemy," and a patient cannot ask the physician to terminate treatment because he is fearful of dying and/or fascinated by his physician's role as a combatant against death.

The articles are also intended to show the interface of three professions as they deal with the subject of death and, more particularly, with the treatment of persons near death. Many persons trained in medicine, law, and/or ethics have important contributions to make to the analysis of the issues discussed in this book. Rather than regarding the issues as belonging exclusively to one of these domains, physicians, attorneys, and ethicists are increasingly recognizing that these issues of life and death cut across traditional disciplinary and professional lines.

The issues are ethical in nature—with obvious medical and legal dimensions—in that they call for critical, systematic reflection upon moral conduct in a variety of situations involving life-and-death decisions. Questions about truthtelling with terminal patients, the appropriate care and treatment of patients known to be dying, the meaning of death, the permissibility of withholding life-sustaining procedures in the face of death, and the justifiability of euthanasia and suicide are not merely procedural (to be decided by physicians) or technical (to be decided by attorneys and judges). They are, in addition, questions about the decisions and conduct in the face of death which can be justified on moral grounds.

The medical and legal dimensions to these issues are obvious. All of the issues arise in a hospital context and/or involve decisions made by individuals with medical training. Physicians clearly bear significant moral responsibility as they attempt to determine the right course of action to follow with patients who indicate they want to die or who, despite modern medical technology, are known to be irreversibly dying. But members of the medical profession are not alone in their concern over the proper treatment of persons who either want to die but cannot in a hospital context, or do not want to die but cannot avoid it even in a hospital context. Questions regarding the treatment of defective infants, the refusal of life-prolonging procedures by adult patients, the withdrawal of life-support systems by physicians, and the termination of human lives (inside or outside a hospital setting) are not only medical matters, but are of substantial interest to attorneys and judges as well.

The need for interdisciplinary analysis of these issues has become clear in recent years as the field of biomedical ethics has increased in popularity and courts have with some frequency intervened in decisions traditionally left in the hands of patients and physicians. As illustrated by the *Tucker* and *Quinlan* cases in this volume, some judicial decisions have recently addressed the jurisdictional problems of medicine vis-à-vis law: are decisions of life and death to be decided by the medical profession or the courts? Other court decisions have reflected significantly different views on how such decisions should be made. The first court case involving Karen Quinlan, for example, was determined in large measure by the judge's view that permitting her to die by withdrawing medical treatment was "a medical decision, not a judicial one." When the Quinlan case was appealed to the Supreme Court of New Jersey, the justices ruled that the decision was not a medical one only, but involved the patient's right of self-determination and the deliberations of a hospital ethics committee as well.

The articles are organized into five parts, each addressing a particular ethical issue connected with death and dying. The issues can and should at times be considered independently, but connections among them will be discernible as the reader proceeds through the volume.

Part One—Truthtelling

Surely the most recurrent ethical issue connected with death and dying is the classic problem of truthtelling. In his "On the Supposed Right to Lie from Altruistic Motives" (*Critique of Practical Reason*), Kant dealt with the problem of truthtelling in a straightforward manner: a moral agent is obligated to tell the truth even if undesirable consequences follow from that act. The contributors to this volume, however, see the issue as a complex moral problem of modern medicine: depression, despair, rapid physical deterioration, and suicidal behavior can result when patients cannot cope with the prognosis that they are irretrievably dying.

The articles in this section present striking contrasts. The survey by William Kelly and Stanley Friesen indicates that a large majority of patients prefer to be told the truth about their condition, whereas the later survey by Donald Oken suggests that most physicians prefer to deceive terminal patients by misrepresenting their illness or withholding information from them. The article by Joseph Fletcher argues that a physician has a moral obligation to tell a terminal patient the truth about his condition because that truth belongs to the patient. Bernard Meyer, in contrast, is convinced that truthtelling may occasionally need to be compromised in order not to harm the patient.

Part Two—Determining Death

A crucial ethical issue in modern medicine is the determination of death. Clearly, medical technology can, when needed or desirable, circumvent the traditional interpretation of death as the irreversible cessation of spontaneous respiration and heartbeat. With intravenous nourishment, heart-lung machines, artificial respirators, and the possibility of a totally implantable artificial heart, medical technology has advanced far beyond the time not long ago when the use of a mirror or feather was recommended to determine if an individual was exhaling and thus still alive.

The advent of sophisticated life-prolonging techniques has given rise to numerous questions related to the dying patient. What is the meaning of death? Is a new definition of death necessary? By what criteria is a physician to determine that death has occurred? How does brain activity figure in the determination of death? Are we at the point where some patients can die only when artificial, organ-sustaining machines are turned off?

The articles in this section are addressed to the issue of how death is to be determined—and by whom. The Robert Morison-Leon Kass exchange sets the stage by showing that the determination of when a human being is dead is integrally related to the conception of death as either a process or an identifiable moment. The next article presents the four criteria suggested by the Ad Hoc Committee of the Harvard Medical School for determining that a patient is dead. The fourth article contains an assessment of the Harvard criteria and a discussion of their implications by the Task Force on Death and Dying of the Institute of Society, Ethics, and the Life Sciences. The article by Alexander Capron and Leon Kass discusses the Kansas statute on death and proposes that a unified, legislative standard for determining death will remove much of the ambiguity in this vital area of decision making. The Capron-Kass article also contains comments about the *Tucker* case, a judicial decision in Virginia which was the first major court case dealing with the concept of brain death and its relation to organ transplantation.

Part Three—Allowing to Die

A closely related ethical issue is deciding when it is justifiable to withhold or withdraw treatment in order that a patient may be allowed to die. However this question is answered, it needs to be distinguished from two other issues taken up in this volume. It is important to point out that the issue of allowing to die is not the same as the issue of determining that death has occurred. The question of "When may a patient be permitted to die?" must not be confused with the question of "When is a patient to be declared dead?" Likewise, the issue of allowing to die is not the same as the issue of euthanasia. The question of "When may a patient be permitted to die?" must not be confused with the question of "When may a physician intervene directly to terminate the life of a patient?"

The articles in this section are divided into two parts because the issue of allowing to die is present in two significantly different situations in modern medicine: infants who may be permitted to die because they have severe congenital disorders, and adults who may be permitted to die because further life-sustaining procedures are judged useless. The first of these situations represents a new moral dilemma, at least as far as public awareness of the situation is concerned. Although infanticide (the direct killing of an infant) has been practiced in numerous societies over the years (especially in societies placing little value on female infants), allowing an infant to die because he or she has a serious genetic disease represents an unprecedented moral dilemma because few such infants survived prior to the advent of modern special-care nurseries.

The issue of allowing infants to die is handled in different ways by the contributors to this volume. Raymond Duff and A. G. M. Campbell argue that withholding treatment is justifiable when the infant has a genetic condition that offers it an extremely poor chance for "meaningful life." James Gustafson provides an ethical analysis of the decision to permit a genetically defective infant to die at the Johns Hopkins Hospital; he concludes that the decision was wrong because "a mongoloid infant is human" and should have all ordinary means used to save its life, including corrective surgical procedures. Richard McCormick analyzes several cases involving infants and suggests that an infant's "potential for human relationships" could function as a guideline in determining which defective infants are to be saved and which are to be permitted to die. One of the cases mentioned in McCormick's article is the "Baby Boy Houle" case in which a genetically defective infant died even though court-ordered surgery had been performed to keep him alive.

The second situation has received considerable attention in the literature of biomedical ethics. Here the issue is whether and under what conditions it is morally permissible to withhold or withdraw treatment from a dying adult patient in order that he or she may die more quickly, with less suffering, and in a more dignified manner. Roman Catholic theologians have traditionally distinguished between "ordinary" and "extraordinary" means of prolonging life. Even though it is readily apparent that this distinction is a relative one (relative both to the status of medical technology and to the circumstances surrounding each particular dying patient), it is important to emphasize that most writers on this subject at some point distinguish between life-sustaining measures that are morally obligatory because they offer "a reasonable hope of benefit" to the patient, and life-sustaining measures judged to be "extraordinary" or "heroic" because they are useless to the particular patient for whom they are being employed.

The issue of permitting adult patients to die by withholding or withdrawing life-sustaining treatment has in recent years often moved out of the hospitals into the courtrooms and legislative chambers of this country. The widely publicized case of Karen Quinlan is the most obvious example. The Superior Court of New Jersey first refused permission, and the Supreme Court of New Jersey later granted permission to remove her from the life-sustaining equipment to which she had been attached for a year. Less publicized, but equally important, have been the attempts to pass legislative bills (proposed in 17 statehouses in 1976) which would grant adults the legal right to have life-prolonging treatment stopped. One of these bills, which has become law in California, grants an adult the right to make "a written directive instructing his physician to withhold or withdraw life-sustaining procedures in the event of a terminal condition."

The articles by Paul Ramsey, George Fletcher, and Norman Cantor provide a helpful analysis of this type of medical situation and how it can be interpreted in terms of ethics and the law. Ramsey provides a clear, thorough argument for the justifiability of allowing an adult patient to die, while rejecting the alternatives of using all available life-prolonging procedures or intervening directly to end the life of a terminal patient. George Fletcher distinguishes between permitting harm to occur and causing harm to occur, and then discusses the legal implications of the medical decision to permit some terminal patients to die. Cantor discusses the right of a patient to refuse life-prolonging treatment and analyzes the competing individual and societal interests at stake in such a decision. The section ends with excerpts from the two court decisions in the Quinlan case.

Part Four—Euthanasia

Euthanasia is probably the most widely discussed issue covered in this volume. The moral dimension of euthanasia can be seen in several distinctions frequently made by ethicists who write on this subject. First, there is the moral distinction between acts of omission and acts of commission. Whereas allowing a patient to die involves the omission of certain life-prolonging procedures (the physician stands aside and permits death to occur), euthanasia, as the word is now generally used, involves the commission of an act that terminates the patient's life (the physician causes death to occur). Rather than merely withholding or withdrawing now-useless medical treatment (e.g., unplugging a respirator), a physician who commits euthanasia administers a death-dealing agent (such as potassium chloride) that kills the patient. The morally relevant difference between permitting a patient to die and killing a patient is sufficient to lead some ethicists to conclude that euthanasia is never justifiable.

Second, there is the moral distinction between indirect and direct termination of life. This distinction is unfortunately blurred by some persons who either misunderstand or intend to revise the traditional moral rule of "double effect." Based on a distinction between a moral agent's foresight and intention, and a second distinction between two or more effects ensuing from that moral agent's act, the traditional rule of double effect applies to the termination of life in cases where a physician administers pain-relieving drugs (one effect) which may also debilitate a patient's strength and hasten his death (the second effect). The moral difference between a "double effect" case and euthanasia is that a patient's death in the former case is unintended but foreseen as a possible consequence and indirectly but unavoidably caused by the act of administering the pain-relieving drug. Euthanasia, in contrast, is an act involving the direct, intentional termination of a patient's life. This difference is sufficient for some persons to judge that the indirect termination of life can be morally justifiable, whereas the direct termination of life through an act of euthanasia must always be prohibited.

Third, there is the distinction between voluntary and involuntary euthanasia. In the case of a patient who consciously decides that he prefers a merciful death to the torture of unbearable suffering, the central moral problem is that of informed consent: is an individual racked with pain or in a drugged stupor actually capable of giving voluntary, informed consent to his own death? As far as involuntary euthanasia is concerned, anyone attempting to justify the decision of a physician directly to terminate the life of a hopelessly comatose patient is immediately confronted with the specter of compulsory euthanasia programs for the mentally and physically "unfit" members of society. That prospect, for most writers on the subject, is sufficient to restrict any consideration of the justifiability of euthanasia to cases involving a voluntary request by a patient seeking relief from unmitigatable suffering.

Some of the articles in this section address the legal dimension of euthanasia. Even if euthanasia can be justified on moral grounds, the legalization of euthanasia is another matter entirely. Thus far, attempts to make voluntary euthanasia a legal option have met with failure: the 1969 British Voluntary Euthanasia Act was defeated, and an earlier legislative bill presented to the New York General Assembly was defeated in 1947 even though the bill was signed by more than 1,000 New York physicians. Proposals to legalize euthanasia are currently before several state legislatures, but none has been enacted into law. Under American criminal law at the present time, therefore, any physician who commits an act of euthanasia can be convicted of first-degree murder. As a matter of fact, however, only a very few American physicians have been prosecuted for committing euthanasia, and they have been acquitted (the most famous case involving Dr. Herman Sander in 1950, the most recent being that of Dr. Vincent Montemarano in 1974).

The articles on euthanasia provide diverse and conflicting points of view. Arthur Dyck maintains that euthanasia is never a permissible moral option because human life does not belong to individual human beings who may dispose of it when and as they desire. Robert Drinan defends the traditional Roman Catholic prohibition of euthanasia and argues that the legalization of euthanasia ("mercy murder") is problematic because of the difficulties connected with securing the voluntary consent of a dying patient to have his life ended. Helge Mansson's article, a representative of the "wedge" argument often present in euthanasia debates, explores the receptivity of certain groups to the possibility of compulsory euthanasia programs established to alleviate problems of overpopulation. Daniel Maguire counters by examining several of the objections to voluntary euthanasia and arguing that "death by choice" is a permissible moral option. Joseph Fletcher concludes the section by maintaining that euthanasia is morally justifiable in a number of situations because it is a compassionate way of hastening the death of a suffering patient.

Part Five—Suicide

Like truthtelling, suicide has been debated through the centuries. Some philosophers (e.g., Seneca, David Hume) have regarded suicide as a justifiable act on the grounds of the right of self-determination. Theologians in the Christian tradition (e.g., Augustine, Thomas Aquinas) have generally held self-destruction to be an intrinsically wrong act because it denies that life is to be valued as a gift of God, it inflicts harm upon the relatives and friends of the individual who commits the act of self-destruction, and it runs counter to the biblical injunction against killing (in fact, Exodus 20:13 forbids murder, not other forms of killing). Yet the double suicide of Dr. and Mrs. Henry van Dusen in 1975 indicates that some persons within the Christian tradition occasionally conclude that suicide is a justifiable course of action.

Although it is a classical problem, suicide has in recent years taken on significance as an issue in modern medicine because of its connection with voluntary euthanasia and because it is frequently interpreted as a manifestation of mental illness. The relationship between voluntary euthanasia and suicide needs more analysis, but it is clear that a patient requesting euthanasia is engaging in some type of suicidal action and a physician who fulfills that request is assisting a suicide. Less clear is the classification by psychiatrists of all persons who contemplate self-destruction as emotionally disturbed individuals who may require psychiatric treatment. In either case, whether the suicidal individual is living with intractable pain in a hospital or considering self-destruction in a nonmedical setting, physicians who encounter that person in a responsible way are confronted with the alternatives of acting to prevent the suicide, refusing to intervene in any way, or assisting the person's self-destruction.

Previously mentioned articles by Cantor, Drinan, Dyck, and Joseph Fletcher address the relationship between voluntary euthanasia and suicide. The articles in this section deal with the morality of suicide and suicide prevention. Edwin Shneidman is convinced that suicide is self-evidently wrong and that all members of a society are morally obligated to prevent others from taking their own lives. Thomas Szasz disagrees, maintaining that suicide falls within the right of self-determination and that suicide prevention centers frequently infringe upon a rational expression of human freedom. Paul Pretzel concludes the section by exploring the polarity set up by Shneidman and Szasz between a society's normative standard of behavior and the right of self-determination.

Ethical Issues in Death and Dying

ONE
Truthtelling

Do Cancer Patients Want to Be Told?

WILLIAM D. KELLY AND STANLEY R. FRIESEN

THE PROBLEM of whether or not to tell a patient that he has cancer is an old one that must be met from day to day by the practicing physician. It frequently involves philosophic and psychologic considerations of extreme complexity. As may be expected, there are many viewpoints on this subject, varying from one extreme to the other.

Cancer is a disease which formerly by its very name carried the knell of doom to the victim. This dates from earlier days when there was little in the way of treatment to offer the victims of this disease. Now with the tremendous advances in diagnosis and treatment the situation is far from hopeless in many instances and does not justify the feeling of doom it formerly engendered.

Extensive efforts are being made to educate the public both in regard to the early recognition of the disease and to the benefits of timely treatment. These efforts are being expanded constantly so that more and more people are being made aware of the symptoms as well as the likely treatment of cancer. In view of this, it is difficult to believe that many people are not aware of the presence of cancer following the extensive examinations and treatment they receive. . . .

How does the patient feel about this problem? In an effort to obtain information on this point, a survey which was essentially an opinion poll was set

Reprinted from *Surgery* 27 (June 1950): 822–26, with the permission of the publisher. Copyright © 1950 by the C. V. Mosby Company.

up. Two groups of patients were surveyed, each group composed of 100 cases. One group consisted of patients in whom the diagnosis of cancer had been established. The other group was constituted of patients without known cancer. All of these patients were seen in the outpatient departments of the University Hospitals. The patients in the cancer group were all personally interviewed and their opinions recorded on the sheets prepared for the study. This group included both patients with operable and patients with inoperable or recurrent lesions, although the former were in the majority. The patients in the noncancer group were interviewed personally in some cases, and in others were simply asked to fill in the questions on the sheet handed them, although they usually were queried as to whether or not they understood what was asked when the forms were collected. In the latter group it was made clear this was merely an opinion poll and did not imply that they had cancer.

The following questions were asked of those patients in the cancer group. The method of querying in Question 1 was indirect at first, and as tactful as possible.

1. Is this the first time you knew about having cancer? Yes——— No———.
2. If you knew previously, when and how did you learn?
3. Doctors and patients' relatives are occasionally inclined to believe they are protecting patients from worry by not telling them they have cancer. Do you agree? Yes——— No———.
4. Patients with cancer are frequently cured by treatment but never find out they had cancer. It would probably help in the fight against cancer if these people knew their condition and could help to alert others to the possibility of cancer as well as offer encouragement about having it cured. Do you agree? Yes——— No———.

The noncancer patients were asked two questions:

1. If our examinations should disclose that you have a cancer, would you want to know about it? Yes——— No———.
2. Patients with cancer are frequently cured by treatment but never find out they had cancer. It would probably help in the fight against cancer if these people knew their condition and could help to alert others to the possibility of cancer as well as offer encouragement about having it cured. Do you agree? Yes——— No———.

Answers Obtained

In answering Question 3 of the cancer group queries, almost all the patients answered in the affirmative or negative and went on to say that they did or did not want to be told about having cancer. In addition, many of them tended to make a distinction between their own feelings on the matter and what they thought people in general would feel. In those who did not make this division spontaneously, specific questions were asked to elicit their opinion.

Cancer Group

QUESTION 1.
   85—Had previous knowledge of cancer.
   15—Did not.
QUESTION 2.
   40—Were told by local physician.
   33—Were told at the University Hospitals.
   5—Were told accidentally by friends, etc.
   7—Were told at another hospital.
QUESTION 3. (A) In regard to self:
   89—Preferred to know about having cancer.
   6—Rather not.
   5—Indefinite.
      (B) In regard to telling people in general:
   73—Think people should be told.
   4—Think people should not be told.
   3—Indefinite.
   20—Believe it is an individual matter.
QUESTION 4.
   94—Agree.
   3—Disagree.
   3—Indefinite.

Noncancer Group

QUESTION 1.
   82—Want to be told.
   14—Do not want to be told.
   4—Indefinite.

QUESTION 2.
88—Agree.
3—Disagree.
9—Indefinite.

Another group, consisting of patients being examined in the Cancer Detection Center at the University Hospitals, has been given the same questionnaire as was given to the noncancer group in this study. These patients were individuals over 45 years of age who were apparently well and on whom yearly complete physical examinations are being carried out in an effort to detect malignancies in an early stage.

To date, 740 opinions have been obtained in this group. The results are as follows:

QUESTION 1.
729—(98.5%)—Want to be told.
7—Do not want to be told.
4—Indefinite.
QUESTION 2.
737—Agree.
0—Disagree.
3—Indefinite.

Of the seven patients who answered no to Question 1, six of these specified that this was in the event that their condition was hopeless. It is probably to be expected that this group would be strongly in favor of being told about the presence of cancer, as cancer detection is the object of their undergoing yearly examinations on a voluntary basis.

Discussion

It is interesting to note that whereas 89 percent of the cancer patients said they preferred knowing their condition, of this same group only 73 percent thought that people in general should be uniformly told. This would seem to imply that they feel others somewhat less capable of bearing the truth or more prone to emotional shock than themselves. Another interesting point is in regard to the wording of Question 3 in the cancer patients' form, which would tend to suggest a yes answer to the patient, whereas the answers obtained were almost overwhelmingly no.

In addition, 24 patients in the cancer group were asked if the knowledge that they had cancer had in any way altered their routine of existence or style of living outside of any physical disability. The answer was no in all cases.

Many of the patients remarked that they would be more willing and careful to follow directions in regard to necessary follow-up examinations if they knew they had cancer. Moreover, many of them stated that they worried more about the unknown and felt they preferred to know they had cancer, even if it was bad news, because it removed the indefiniteness of the situation. Some were indignant that they had not been informed sooner than they were. Of the 15 patients who said they had not been previously told, most of these added that they had suspected their condition to be cancer. The fact that the remaining 85 patients in the cancer group already knew they had cancer would indicate that many physicians, both here in the hospital and in the local communities, are following the policy of informing the patients when they have cancer. The last question in both groups tends somewhat to confirm the answers given to the previous question as to whether or not the patient thought people should be told they have cancer. In addition, it indicates that they believe in educating people in general to the possibility of cancer.

In an effort to see whether the opinions given by the patients have changed with the passage of time (approximately one year since the original study), we recently sent out letters to 41 of the patients in the cancer group, asking them if their feelings were still the same in regard to whether or not they wanted to know about the presence of cancer. Answers were obtained in 31 cases. Two of the patients had expired in the interim. The remaining 29 all replied essentially in the same way as they had on the first querying. This group included both those patients who originally stated they would rather not know about the presence of cancer as well as those who wanted to know.

Obviously the significance or validity of the replies obtained can be debated at great length. However, it would seem to indicate that patients want to be informed of the nature of their illness perhaps to a far greater extent than the average physician would anticipate.

Summary

Two groups, each containing 100 individuals, were polled regarding the question of whether or not they would want to be told about having cancer and their answers were recorded. One group contained patients with known cancer and the other consisted of patients not known to have cancer.

The answers obtained would indicate that the great majority in both groups want to be told about the presence of cancer.

What to Tell Cancer Patients:
A Study of Medical Attitudes

Donald Oken

NO PROBLEM is more vexing than the decision about what to tell the cancer patient. (Although the word "cancer" is neither a medical term nor a specific entity, commonsense considerations provide a basis for use of this general term. As used in the present work, the term should be understood *to apply to all malignant neoplasms of characteristically grave prognosis.*) The situation is an ever-recurring one and the questions involved are knotty. What should the patient be told? How and when should this be done? The manner in which such questions are handled is crucial for the patient and may determine his emotional status and capacity for function from that time on. It is easy enough to decide to follow a course which will "do least harm," but it is far from simple to determine just what course that is. The issues involved are complex factors which are difficult to assess, weigh, and place in proper perspective.

In his attempt to work out some solution, the doctor needs all the help he can get. The issues are a favorite and often heated topic of "corridor consultations." Often the opinion of a psychiatrist is sought: but psychiatric knowledge provides no clear and unequivocal answers. A considerable number of authors have attempted to provide assistance by describing their own views

Reprinted from the *Journal of the American Medical Association* 175 (April 1, 1961): 86–94, with the permission of the author and publisher. Copyright © 1961 by the American Medical Association.

and approach. These writers, often wise and distinguished teachers drawing on long experience, offer solutions based on that experience. This too proves of insufficient help. Though many issues have become clarified, these experts differ widely about what to do. Opinions vary from one extreme to the other. A careful review of this literature discloses a further lack: the almost complete absence of systematic research. There is a plethora of opinion but a minimum of dependable fact. This is a curious situation in an area of so great importance. The present paper represents an initial attempt to provide some research data which bear on this situation and on the general issue of "telling."

The Present Research

The research on which this report is based represents a further attempt to study physicians' approaches to the problem of what to tell cancer patients. The aim here has been not merely to learn what is done but, more importantly, to understand the attitudes which are underlying determinants of these strategies. Initially, a detailed questionnaire was sent to all of the 219 members of the staff of the departments of internal medicine, obstetrics-gynecology, and surgery (including thoracic, genito-urinary and neuro-surgery, and orthopedics) of the Michael Reese Hospital, a private nonprofit teaching hospital in Chicago. This questionnaire included items concerned with (1) the policy with regard to "telling"; (2) factors involved in making a decision with an individual patient; (3) the sources from which the policy had been acquired; (4) the role of personal emotional factors; (5) changes from a previous different policy and the possibility of future change; (6) attitudes about the research; and (7) personal choice, i.e., "if you were the patient, do you think you would want to be told?" A personal interview of 30 minutes' duration was held subsequently with 62 (30 percent) of the respondents, devoted to the intensive exploration of these and related areas and designed especially to elicit attitudes about cancer and its treatability. No attempt was made to probe for unconscious material. Interviews were unstructured and neutral in tone, but opposing arguments were raised to points of view expressed, in order to clarify the nature and intensity of determining attitudes. Interviewees were selected to represent a cross-section of each staff level within each specialty with regard to the policy about telling espoused on the questionnaire.

It is necessary to describe some of the characteristics of the group studied since these may bear on the findings. The great bulk of these physicians are in active private practice, in addition to taking a regular part in the teaching program. Most hold faculty positions at one or more medical schools. Though they are deeply involved in "academic medicine," for them the problem of dealing with the cancer patient is no academic matter; it is an everyday reality. Interest and cooperation was high, so that a 95 percent return of questionnaires was achieved, a level rarely attained. A group of general practitioners were included in the study, for a moderate number are members of the staff in the Department of Medicine, largely with "courtesy" (nonteaching) status. These, however, are probably the least representative group, for they are primarily older men. The remainder of the sample seems fairly typical of the larger specialty groups which are represented. The sample has, however, certain definite characteristics. The average age is 50. All practice in Chicago or surrounding suburban communities. Three-quarters received their medical education in Illinois. All but six are male. Almost all are Jewish; their private practices, correspondingly, include a predominance of middle-class Jewish patients. Balancing this is their wide experience, in this and other hospitals, working with ward service patients, the majority of whom are non-Jewish.

Questionnaire

The following questions apply to your policy about telling patients they have cancer. For the purpose of this questionnaire, assume that the diagnosis is certain and that though treatment may be possible the eventual prognosis is grave.

1. What is your usual policy about telling patients?
   (check one) A. Tell—— B. Don't tell——
2. How often do you make exceptions to your rule?
   (check one) A. Never—— B. Very rarely——
3. The following is a list of factors pertaining to the patient which may be relevant in your decision about telling a particular patient.
   Check *every* item which you would include in making your decision.
   a. Age
   b. Sex
   c. Religion

d. Intelligence
e. State of personal affairs
f. Community standing
g. Medical sophistication
h. Patient a physician
i. Length of expected survival
j. Acceptance of recommended therapy
k. Patient asking no questions
l. Patient's expressed wish to be told
m. Relatives' wish (about telling patient)
n. Emotional stability
o. Other personality factors
p. Other factors (specify)

4. Circle any item about which you feel is of *special* importance.
5. For each item check in 3, briefly explain how and in which direction it applies.
6. When you do not tell a patient, do you always tell a relative? (Yes or No)———
7. How did you acquire your policy? (check *every* item which applies)
A. Taught you in med. school——— B. taught you during clinical training——— C. Clinical experience——— D. Nonprofessional experience with ill friends, family, etc.——— E. Other (specify)———
8. Which of these was the single most important source?———
9. Were you ever specifically taught some policy? (not necessarily your current one) (Yes or No)———
10. A. Apart from your training, experience, etc., do you think that your *personal* attitudes about cancer, life illness, etc., are determinants of your policy? (Yes or No)———
B. Do you think that such personal factors are more———or less——— important than the others in determining your policy? (check one)
11. How likely do you think it is that your policy will change? (check one)
A. No possibility——— B. Very unlikely——— C. Unlikely——— D. Probably——— E. Certainly———
12. A. Has your policy changed in the past? (Yes or No)———
B. If yes, how would you have previously answered Question 1——— Question 2———
13. How do you think most surgeons would answer Question 1——— Question 2———
14. How do you think most psychiatrists would answer Question 1——— Question 2———

15. Would your present policy be swayed by the results of research on this problem? (Yes or No)——
16. Do you think research in this area should be done? (Yes or No)——
17. Do you find it more difficult to tell a cancer patient than other patients who have another disease but the *same* prognosis? (Yes or No)——
18. If you were the patient, do you think you would want to be told? (Yes or No)——

COMMENTS: (Any comments you can make on any question above, or related issues will be appreciated. If you can amplify or describe your personal policy or the reasons behind it this will be especially useful.)

BIOGRAPHICAL DATA: 1. Age—— 2. Specialty or Subspecialty—— 3. Name of Medical School——————————— 4. Year graduated—— 5. Board Certified (fields (s) and year)———————

A few comments regarding statistics are in order. All questionnaire results were subjected to analysis by standard procedures: chi square, analysis of variance, student's "t" test, and the sign test. For simplicity of presentation the details of each procedure and probability levels are not reported here. No finding reported fails to reach at least the generally accepted criterion ($p < .05$), unless specifically noted. Small discrepancies between the total figures reported for different items reflect variations in the numbers of subjects who failed to answer some questions.

"Telling"

The initial undertaking in this research was the determination of whether or not physicians tell their patients they have cancer. It is evident, as seen in Table 2.1, that there is a strong and general tendency to *withhold* this information. Almost 90 percent of the group is within this half of the scale. Indeed, a majority tell only very rarely, if ever. No one reported a policy of informing every patient. . . . No difference between specialities was uncovered; the small differences seen in Table 2.1, or involving the smaller groups of surgical subspecialties not detailed there, are far from significant statistically. (This lack of specialty differences was a consistent finding for all questionnaire items. Differences when present were small and offset by wider divergencies within each specialty.) These findings also cut across the hospital staff rank and age. Younger and less experienced men did not have any greater inclination to tell than their seniors.

Table 2.1 Physicians' Policies about "Telling" Cancer Patient

Usual Policy	Exceptions Made	Internists		Surgeons [a]		Generalists		Total Group	
		No.	%	No.	%	No.	%	No.	%
Do not tell	Never	7	8	7	8	4	15	18	9
	Very rarely	36	43	44	53	10	37	90	47
	Occasionally	28	34	21	25	7	26	56	29
	Often	4	5	1	1	0	0	5	3
Subtotal		75	90	73	87	21	78	169	88
Tell	Often	3	4	4	5	1	4	8	4
	Occasionally	4	5	4	5	2	7	10	5
	Very rarely	1	1	2	2	3	11	6	3
	Never	0	0	0	0	0	0	0	0
Subtotal		8	10	10	12	7	22	24	12
Total		83	100	83	100 [b]	27	100	193	100

[a] Includes gynecologists and thoracic, genitourinary, orthopedic, and neurosurgeons as well as general surgeons.
[b] Sum appears to equal 99 percent because of rounding to nearest percentage.

Use of a questionnaire, of course, forces answers into an artificially rigid mold. But information derived from the interviews strengthens the finding. Answers indicating that patients are told often turned out to mean telling the patient that he had a "tumor," with strict avoidance of the terms cancer, malignancy, and the like. These more specific words were almost never used unless the patient's explicit and insistent questioning pushed the doctor's back to the wall.

Euphemisms are the general rule. These may extend from the vaguest of words ("lesion," "mass"); to terms giving a general indication that the process is neoplastic ("growth," "tumor," "hyperplastic tissue")—often tempered by a false explicit statement that the process is benign; to a somewhat more suggestive expression (a "suspicious" or "degenerated" tumor). Where major surgical or radiation therapy is involved, especially if the patient is hesitant about proceeding, recourse may be had to such terms as "precancerous," or a tumor "in the early curable stage." Some physicians avoid even the slightest suggestion of neoplasia and quite specifically substitute another diagnosis. Almost every one reported resorting to such falsification on at least a few occasions, most notably when the patient was in a far-advanced stage of illness at the time he was seen.

It is impossible to convey all the flavor of the diverse individual approaches. No two men use exactly the same technique. Each has his preferred plan, his select euphemisms, his favored tactics, and his own views about the optimal time for discussion and the degree of directness to be used. Some have a set pattern, while others vary their approach. But the general trend is consistent.

The modal policy is to tell as little as possible in the most general terms consistent with maintaining cooperation in treatment. Exceptions are made most commonly when the patient is in a position of financial responsibility which carries the necessity for planning. Questioning by the patient almost invariably is disregarded and considered a plea for reassurance unless persistent, and intuitively perceived as "a real wish to know." Even then it may be ignored. The vast majority of these doctors feel that almost all patients really do not want to know regardless of what people say. They approach the issue with the view that disclosure should be avoided unless there are positive indications, rather than the reverse. Intelligence and emotional stability are considered prerequisites for greater disclosure only if other "realistic" factors provide a basis for doing so. For the fewer physicians who tell with some frequency, these two factors assume more primary importance.

A few additional consistent themes emerge. Agreement was essentially unanimous that some family member must be informed if the patient is not made aware of the diagnosis. Legal and ethical considerations are by no means the only points of relevance here. Repeated instances were reported of patients who, dissatisfied with the progression of their disease in the face of treatment and desperate for help, were dissuaded from fruitless and unwise shifts to a new physician (or quack) only by the cooperation of an informed relative. Beyond this is the need to have someone to share the awful burden of knowledge. As one man put it, "I just can't carry the load alone." Few responsibilities are as heavy as knowing that someone is going to die; dividing it makes it easier to bear.

Variations in approach also converge to a single major goal: maintenance of hope. No inference was necessary to elicit this finding. Every single physician interviewed spontaneously emphasized this point and indicated his resolute and determined purpose is to sustain and bolster the patient's hope.

Each in his own way communicates the possibility, even the likelihood, of recovery. Differences revolve about the range of belief about just how much information is compatible with the maintenance of hope. While some doctors believe "cancer means certain death and no normal person wants to die," others hold that "knowledge is power": power which can conquer fear. The crux of the divergence centers on two issues: whether cancer connotes certain death, and whether the expectation of death insurmountably deprives the patient of hope. The data indicate that an impressively large number of physicians would answer affirmatively to both.

Acquisition

The approach used by a physician may derive from many sources. Perhaps he acquired it as a result of teaching in medical school or while a house officer; maybe it grows out of his own clinical experience or is a result of personal experiences with afflicted friends and family; it may arise as a result of reading; or perhaps it is a personal conviction which stems from the deeper influences of his personality and individual philosophy. Information about this was specifically requested on the questionnaire. These results are available in Table 2.2.

Clinical experience would seem to be of overwhelming importance. Only 6 percent (12 of 203) failed to list this as a factor. Other sources are reported with far less frequency, and if reported at all, usually in addition to clinical experience, which is the factor accorded primary importance by more than three-quarters of the group. Medical school teaching apparently plays a

Table 2.2 Sources from Which Policies Were Acquired

	Contributing Source		Major Source	
	No.	%	No.	%
Medical school teaching	14	7	0	0
Hospital training	72	35	10	5
Clinical experience	191	77	146	77
Illness in friends, family, etc.	61	30	15	8
Other	24	12	17	9
	362[a]	–	188	100[b]

[a] More than one answer can be given by a respondent.
[b] Sum appears to equal 99 percent because of rounding to nearest percentage.

minimal role. Internship and residency training is somewhat more often listed. Yet, only about one-third of the group did include this (and it was infrequently felt to be salient) when it might seem that the subject could not have failed to arise during training. The interviews confirmed this. Few people could remember hearing about the subject during their training. When someone did, usually there was no recall of anything specific said, other than the emphasis of the need of the physician to deal with the problem. This silence, like the lack of research, is striking. It is possible, of course, that what is reflected here is as much a failure of recall as the absence of teaching. Still, if this is true it requires explanation and points to some deficiency in the teaching process.

Personal factors are reported by only a moderate number of the group. The experience of seeing a close relative (most commonly a parent) die of cancer, was a decisive occurrence for some. This experience, however, did not lead to any difference in policy between these physicians and the group as a whole; they were neither more nor less likely to tell. Less concretely derived personal feelings were reported by a small group. These responses, comprising all but two of those listed as "other," were described in such terms as "my philosophy of life," "my personal conviction," or "projecting myself into the patient's situation." Interestingly, if such a feeling was reported at all, there was a strong likelihood that it was considered the determining factor.

Experience versus Emotion

Results like these might seem to be anticipated. After all, why should we not expect clinical experience to provide the basis for action, and personal factors to play only a secondary role? Sound practice grows from experience. But is this actually the case here? Is this an area in which reason really prevails? There is much further data from the present research which suggests quite the opposite.

To begin with, experience can be acquired only over a span of time. A young group, whose graduation from medical school has taken place not many years earlier, might be expected to report that their policy stems largely from other sources. At least they should cite experience less often than their seniors. This is not the case. The group under 45 years of age, or those in the lower staff ranks, are just as likely to list experience as a factor as their older colleagues. Indeed, they are no less likely to cite it as the major determinant. The mean age and the staff level of those who reportedly based their policy on experience does not differ from those who do not. Nor do the policies of the two groups differ.

Experience, moreover, implies a state of knowledge based upon a range of earlier observation, with the opportunity to become familiar with the outcomes of various alternatives. Occasions for some such experience, of course, have been available to all these physicians. Yet only 27 (14 percent) have had the opportunity for firsthand knowledge based on their own trial of any policy different from their current one. More detailed exploration in the interviews cast a great deal of further doubt about the role of experience. It was the exception when a physician could report known examples of the unfavorable consequences of an approach which differed from his own. It was more common to get reports of instances in which different approaches had turned out satisfactorily. Most of the instances in which unhappy results were reported to follow a differing policy turned out to be vague accounts from which no reliable inference could be drawn.

Instead of logic and rational decision based on critical observation, what is found is opinion, belief, and conviction, heavily weighted with emotional justification. As one internist said: "I can't give a good reason except that I've always done it." Explanations are begun characteristically with such phrases as "I feel . . ." or "It is my opinion. . . ." Personal convictions were stated flatly and dogmatically as if they were facts. Thus, "Most people do not want to know," "It is my firm belief that they always know anyway," or "No one can be told without giving up and losing all hope." Highly charged emotional terms and vivid expressions were the rule, indicating the intensity and nature of feelings present. Knowledge of cancer is "a death sentence," "a Buchenwald," and "torture." Telling is "the cruelest thing in the world," "awful," and "hitting the patient with a baseball bat." It is not necessary even to read the words on the questionnaires. Heavy underlinings and a peppering of exclamation points tell the story. These are hardly cool scientific judgments. It would appear that personal conviction is the decisive factor.

There is direct confirmation of this point. *Subsequent* to the general inquiry: "How did you acquire your policy?," it was specifically asked if personal issues were determinants. Nearly three-fourths (98 of 138) reported that personal elements were involved, in contrast to the much smaller number who listed this originally. These 98 were about equally divided as to whether these factors were the most important.

Inflexibility and Emotion

Attitudes to which much emotion is bound are characteristically modified only with great difficulty. Data has been presented indicating that little past change has occurred. What about the future? Here we can look at the question about the likelihood of policy change. Of five alternatives offered, "no possibility" was indicated by a small group (6 percent). The response of these 11 is understandable since they are an older group (mean age 65.2). The remainder of the respondents showed a similar trend. The largest segment (78, 40 percent) felt that change was "very unlikely" and an additional third (70) "unlikely." Only a total of one-fifth felt that change was either "probable" (39) or "certain" (7). This group showed a significant tendency to be the same people who had reported earlier change. Apparently, there is a minority who tend to be generally flexible. Again, this was not a younger group.

Strong resistance to change is also evident in the responses to questions about research. Thirty of the group (16 percent) indicated that their policy would not be swayed by research. An additional 54 respondents (29 percent) felt sufficiently doubtful so that they were unable to answer yes or no, as requested (the only item in which this difficulty arose), and instead wrote in "perhaps" or "maybe." While this leaves a majority who answered yes, these negative answers are noteworthy. These are physicians who read assiduously and themselves conduct research. In what other area would they fail to be swayed by research? Many comments were made that "I wouldn't believe it" or "it couldn't be true," if research suggested a policy different from their own. Still more striking is the finding that 10 percent (19) of the group felt that research in this area should not be done at all! Small wonder so little has appeared.

Another relevant finding is the doctor's wish to be told if he were the patient. As expected, those who tend to tell their patients wished to be told, themselves, more often than those who do not tell. But the total number of those who said they wished to be told (73 of 122) is far greater than those who tend to tell their patients. The explanation usually given was that, "I am one of those who can take it" or "I have responsibilities." That they did not feel this to be true for all physicians, however, is attested to by their treatment of other doctor-patients. Most of the group said they were neither more nor less likely to tell physicians than other patients. Of the group who did modify their policy, it was just as likely to find that they were *less* prone to tell doctors. It is impossible to draw any precise conclusion from this type of hypothetical question about oneself. But the inconsistency is characteristic of emotionally determined attitudes.

Depression and Suicide

The pros and cons of telling have been discussed so often that there is little point in doing so again. Whatever the reasons for telling, the argument against doing so centers on the anticipation of profoundly disturbing psychological effects. There is no doubt that this disclosure has a profound and potentially dangerous impact. Questions do arise about the capacity of human beings to make a satisfactory adaptation to the expectation of death. Can anyone successfully handle such news without paying a price which mitigates whatever value this knowledge brings? If so, how widespread is the ability to call forth the necessary psychological defenses? What about time: does this readjustment take place within some reasonable span? Can the emotional cost of such a shattering experience, or of the effort required for mastering it, be weighed and predicted? The truth is that we know very little about these matters.

It has been repeatedly asserted that disclosure is followed by fear and despondency which may progress into overt depressive illness or culminate in suicide. This was the opinion of the physicians in the present study. Quite representative was the surgeon who stated, "I would be afraid to tell and have the patient in a room with a window." When it comes to actually documenting the prevalence of such untoward reactions, it becomes difficult to find reliable evidence. Instances of depression and profound upsets came quickly to mind when the subject was raised, but no one could report more than a case or two, or a handful at most. This may merely follow from the rarity with which patients are told. Such an explanation must be reconciled with the fact that these same doctors could remember many instances in which the patient was told and seemed to do well. It may also reflect the selection of those told. Or perhaps the knowledge produces covert psychological changes which are no less malignant for their sublety. But actually, the incidence and severity of depression and other psychological reactions in cancer patients, and their relation to being told, is not known.

The same situation holds with regard to suicide. Only six doctors could report definite known cases of suicide (two of these reported two cases and one "several"), although about one-third of the group had "heard of" suicides after being told. Further investigation indicated that at least two of these patients had never been told. (And it is not altogether inconceivable that they would have felt better, not worse, had this been done.) Actually, the circumstances surrounding all but one or two of these cases are quite vague; it is impossible to feel any certainty about what lay behind the suicide. . . .

The group who tell are equally vague in documenting that their patients do well. We simply do not have adequate data about the consequences of telling. As in any dreaded situation, emotion fills a vacuum with rumor, pseudofact, and projected fears. It is noteworthy that the question is posed: "can a patient stand being told," whereas "can the patient stand not being told" is almost never heard, although it is equally valid from the scientific viewpoint.

A physician who tells some of his patients uses certain rules of thumb to guide his decisions. It is striking how inconsistently these guides vary from one physician to another. Thus, some are more likely to tell the very aged while others especially avoid telling this group. Some are inclined to tell patients with a better prognosis and others only when the prognosis is poor. The disagreement about doctor-patients has already been noted. Such discrepancies may portray quite accurately chance differences in experience. More intriguing is the possibility that they reflect the doctor's personality. In any event they are typical of *a priori* judgments unsubstantiated by facts.

Pessimism

Cancer has many unconscious meanings and fantasies associated with it. Whatever the unconscious feelings which it stirs, typically it is feared consciously as a process equated with suffering and certain death. There was good general agreement among the physicians interviewed that these are what patients primarily fear. Other connotations (for example, that cancer is dirty or shameful) were far less prevalent. Many patients mouth statements about curability, and "know" neither suffering nor death are inevitable. But the physicians here report that this knowledge is only skin deep. People continue to think of cancer as "the killer."

What is impressive is that the doctors themselves feel very much the same way. It was not patients who described the diagnosis as a "death warrant" or "a date of execution." The internist who referred to cancer as an "incurable disease with an inevitable demise" expressed a view which was not atypical. The extent and intensity of this underlying pessimism stands out. The general feeling was that we can do very little to save lives and not a great deal to prevent suffering. Sighs and shrugging of the shoulders were the almost usual accompaniment of discussion in this area. Not that these men give up where the individual patient is concerned; on the contrary they fight ceaselessly and without compromise. But just below the surface is the feeling: "To me, it's like a stone wall—no prospects."

Early diagnosis is viewed with a not much more sanguine eye. Nearly all could remember a few cases, at least, where early diagnosis seemed of critical importance. (Breast and bowel lesions were signaled out for special mention.) But a common feeling was that usually this makes no difference: "What's the use? You make an early diagnosis, the patient goes through a horrible operation and suffers, and two years later he's dead anyway." They are not convinced that it helps more than a handful.

"Death Shall Have No Dominion"

Among the motivations for entering medicine, the wish to conquer suffering and death stands high on the list. Practicing physicians are not the kind of persons who can sit quietly by while nature pursues its course. One of the hardest things for a fledgling medical student to learn is watchful waiting. Few situations are as frustrating as sitting by impotently and "helplessly" in the face of illness. Fatal illness is felt as a major defeat. It is not uncommon to know at a glance that a colleague has recently lost a patient: it leaves its mark. . . .

Situations of this kind, associated with intense charges of unpleasant emotions, call forth a variety of psychological defenses which reduce the intensity of feelings to manageable proportions. Among such defenses are those which involve the avoidance, negation, or denial of the existence of some unpleasant fact, and acting as if it were not real. These can be economical and effective mechanisms which find particular usefulness in dealing with situations in which no appropriate action is open. Unless they are given up at that point where something realistic and practical can be done, however, they become dangerous blocks to effective action.

Such mechanisms play a prominent role in the attitudes reported here. There is a strong tendency to avoid looking at the subject of cancer and the facts related to it. There is an avoidance of research and teaching, opposition to potential research, resistance to personal experimentation and change, and the projection of strongly held rationalizations into the vacuum of knowledge. To some extent, we do not *want* to know about what we are doing or why, because the subject is so upsetting. Unfortunately, in our denial we go beyond the limits of usefulness. By blocking off access to new knowledge, we cut ourselves off from the acquisition of facts which could be of real help.

The behavior of members of our own profession who develop cancer amply demonstrates the prevalence of these ostrichlike denial mechanisms. It is common to see colleagues with malignancies cling to an alternative diagnosis when their condition is obvious even to the untutored eye. (The tendency for physicians to ignore their illness of all types is also common knowledge.) Delay in the diagnosis of their own cancers by physicians is well documented. Not only do physicians postpone seeking medical care, but their doctors delay further, perhaps because the diagnostician must especially avoid recognition of cancer in a patient so like himself.

Withholding the diagnosis seems to represent a further manifestation of denial. . . . If a physician wishes to avoid being confronted by his troubled feelings under ordinary circumstances, he will certainly not want to have these feelings stimulated when he is in the actual presence of a cancer patient. A fractured limb is kept splinted. Thus, the subject is not broached or is minimized and pushed aside from consideration. Failure of the patient to ask for his diagnosis under these circumstances is no corroboration that the doctor's avoidance is logically grounded. With his own tendencies to deny what he must greatly fear, the patient may take his cue from the doctor's silence as confirmation that the situation is hopeless and therefore better shunned. Tactful wishes to spare his distraught physician even may play a part.

Although avoidance of telling reflects the psychological problems of the doctor, this by no means implies that such a policy is therapeutically incorrect. It would be entirely erroneous if this study were interpreted to mean that patients should be told. This must be emphasized. Telling the patient may have no less emotional basis as a "counterphobic" denial that cancer is a terribly serious disease. The data indicate that equally irrational and affect-laden attitudes lie behind *both* tendencies. . . .

Delay in Diagnosis

Cancer authorities have been greatly concerned with the problem of delay in diagnosis and treatment. Much of the delay is due to patients themselves, but many studies have revealed a significant proportion which is ascribable to physicians. A recently published critical survey of this literature documents the importance of attitudinal factors such as pessimism and insensitivity (low index of suspicion).

The American Cancer Society has devoted vast effort and sums of money to public information campaigns. Publicity about the "danger signals" of cancer has led to howls of protest by some physicians who feel that such campaigns stimulate cancerophobia. Leaving aside any possible correctness of such contentions, why has the issue been so heated? Perhaps we have here another manifestation of the wish to keep cancer out of sight and mind. For the most part, officials of the Society have responded to such complaints with defensive statements that the majority of the medical profession agrees that their approach has merit which exceeds the harm. The interviews here tend to support this view, although agreement was usually lukewarm. Reservations centered less on the problem of cancerophobia than on the positive value of public education. Part of this reflects the pessimism already described, but more is involved. The view expressed was that patients who respond to publicity are usually complaint- (and cancer-) free, while those with symptoms requiring attention are dominated by their irrational fears and are unaffected. The general conclusion was that education utilizing only a rational appeal is insufficient. New techniques must be developed which will modify emotional attitudes.

The same conclusion can be drawn about the education programs directed towards physicians. Cancer authorities cannot be lulled into complacency by the overt agreement of the profession with their goals or by their successes in providing technical information. Much more ingenuity and effort will be required to alter and surmount the formidable psychological barriers of physicians' covert attitudes. The medical profession plays a pivotal role in cancer control far beyond its direct functions in diagnosis and treatment. When doctors lose hope their patients know it. If doctors communicate the feeling that cancer is dreadful and irremediable, how can patients fail to despair? And frightened and despairing, how can they deal with the possibility that they have cancer? Their only recourse is to keep the possibility hidden—from themselves as well as their doctors. Thus, they court the very fate which they most fear. No physician, no matter how skillful, can treat the patient who stays away. Unwittingly, our own feelings reinforce the anxieties which keep them away, the very opposite of our intent. Perhaps the doctor, more than the patient, should be a target for emotional reeducation.

Summary and Conclusions

Medicine is a difficult and exacting profession, making heavy psychological as well as physical demands. Our personalities, feelings, and attitudes play a major role in determining the manner in which we communicate with and treat patients. They can constitute a tool of incalculable value: the art of medicine. But they can also interfere. No area in which we work makes heavier claims than the treatment of cancer patients, with the suffering, pain, and death which are its frequent attendants. Pressed by these demands, we turn away in order to blunt their awful impact. In doing so, we sap the strength of our most potent asset, the ability to concentrate the full force of our reason. We fail to apply our scientific skills or to do adequate research. Thus we block our own efforts. Only by conquering our irrational attitudes, proceeding to acquire knowledge, and acting on the basis of reason can we advance. Awareness of these attitudes is the first step. Knowing of our deep pessimism about cancer and of our avoidance of research and teaching regarding communications with the cancer patient, we can advance to develop new knowledge of more sensitive and skilled approaches. We will know then how to be *truly* kind to our patients.

3

Medical Diagnosis:
Our Right to Know the Truth

JOSEPH FLETCHER

The Truth Can Hurt

"A GENTLEMAN," said Dr. John M. Birnie (1931) in the *New England Journal of Medicine*, "is one who has more regard for the rights of others than for his own feelings, and for the feelings of others than for his own rights." Disraeli, bemused by the troublesome problem of truthtelling, put it this way: "A gentleman is one who knows when to tell the truth, and when not to." His diplomatic impulses served him better than the cynic's who observed that "a gentleman is one who never unintentionally hurts the feelings of others." But Dr. Birnie meant, presumably, that the gentle person is one who avoids saying anything that *needlessly* hurts a person's feelings.

The issue over truthtelling in medical diagnosis and advice raises the question, therefore, whether doctors can be "gentlemen" and at the same time meet their obligations to the patients under their care. What, to be quite to the point about it, is the duty of the physician in sharing his diagnosis and prognosis? Is he under any obligation morally to reveal his findings to his patient, even if it hurts to know them? Has the patient, in his turn, a right to expect the truth? Or are we to accept the bold claim by

Reprinted from *Morals and Medicine*, pp. 34–41, 45–56, and 60–64, with the permission of Princeton University Press. Copyright ©1954 by Princeton University Press. Some footnotes omitted.

Dumas' heroine in *Camille* who declared, "When God said that lying was a sin, he made an exception for doctors, and he gave them permission to lie as many times a day as they saw patients"? It is an old and perennial problem, giving cause in every age to complaints against doctors as masters of equivocation, complaints sometimes made with great hilarity by a Gregory Glyster. This is the kind of question in people's minds which popular interpreters never undertake to clarify.

We have already set forward the premise that moral status (our ethical integrity) depends upon two things at least: first, freedom of choice, and, second, knowledge of the facts and of the courses between which we may choose. In the absence of either or both of these things we are, in the forum of conscience, more like puppets than persons. Lacking freedom and knowledge, we are not responsible; we are not moral agents or personal beings. We have pointed out, furthermore, that mankind is constantly growing and gaining ground both in knowledge of life and health and in human control over them. This is, indeed, the same as saying that the *means* to heightened moral stature are available. The appeal of moral idealism is that we take advantage of every opportunity to grow in wisdom and stature, that we *assume* our responsibility; in short, that we act like human beings. As far as medical care is concerned we can only repeat what we said above: "Without their freedom to choose and their right to know the truth, patients are only puppets. And there is no moral quality in a Punch and Judy show; at least, there is none in Punch or Judy!"

Dr. Birnie's dilemma was a real one. Sometimes the doctor's discoveries are appalling. To whom, then, shall he give his findings? As a gentleman he hates to hurt his patients' feelings, to depress them, or possibly to drive them to despair. When the truth about our health is a bitter pill to swallow, known as yet only to the physician and perhaps not even suspected by those who put themselves in his hands, he will of course have compassionate regard for their feelings. For this reason—a perfectly understandable one—Dr. Birnie concluded that "in hopeless cases, it is cruel and harmful to tell the patient the truth," and even if the doctor tells some member of the family it will be necessary for both "to lie like gentlemen." It is a hoary old problem of conscience in medical care. For our purposes we may attempt to explore it by posing two questions between which to shuttle back and forth. They are really obverse sides of the same coin, but they represent two distinguishable issues involved. First, has the patient a *right* to know the truth about himself? Next, has the doctor an *obligation* to tell it? Most of us upon occasion are patients, but only a few are physicians. The discussion, therefore, will naturally and properly tend to emphasize the first viewpoint and its question, namely, the *patient's right*.

If the doctor is thus obliged to tell the truth, what difference would it make if the patient is not sure he wants to know it, or if he actually does not want to know it? This question raises a matter of almost crucial importance for psychotherapy, and even for the less pathological areas of clinical counseling. And (most difficult of all) what if the doctor cannot know whether the patient wants to know? Is there a valid principle of therapeutic reservation when it comes to truthtelling in medical diagnosis? Very good reason would have to be found—better, at least than has ever been brought forward—to justify us in avoiding the answer that follows from the premise that our moral stature is proportionate to our responsibility and that we cannot act responsibly without the fullest possible knowledge. The patient *has* a right to know the truth. We are morally obligated to pay others the rights due them. Therefore a doctor is obligated to tell the truth to his patient. He *owes* the patient the truth as fully and as honestly as he owes him his skill and care and technical powers.

We have already expressed the view that "a person-centered approach to illness is superior to the problem-centered approach." To support it we quoted Dr. Francis Peabody's thesis (1928) that "one of the essential qualities of the clinician is interest in humanity, for the secret of the care of the patient is caring *for* the patient." What does it mean to care *for* somebody? The mere business of taking care *of* a person may be entirely a matter of efficiency, and quite impersonal, as many of us have discovered by watching the ministrations of a very young or very bored nurse (or waiter, clerk in a store, barber, or dentist). Caring *for* a person, on the other hand, is a decidedly moral relationship. The phrase "care for" has even come in popular speech to mean love or highly affectionate regard. It means, of course, that we have a care, a sense of concern. A man is said to care for his wife, and that means vastly more than providing for her physical needs; it means a lot more than offering fuel, shelter, food, and clothing. It means, indeed, that he has an attitude of respect and solicitude toward her in all things. So should the doctor's attitude be toward his patient. The sufferer is not just a case of pneumonia or pyloric stenosis or peptic ulcer; the patient is a person, with feelings of hope or despair, of purpose or defeat, of loneliness or fraternity. The patient is not a problem; he is a person with a problem.

From the point of view of morality, we might look at this question as it would be seen by Martin Buber, philosopher at the University of Jerusalem. There is, as Buber (1937) points out, a radical difference in a man's attitude to other men and his attitude to things. In the one case we are related to other persons, like ourselves, to another subject, a *thou*. In the other case we are related to objects, to things, to *its*. These are the two attitudes with which we relate ourselves to what is other than ourselves. A doctor's patient is a person, a *thou*, someone with an integrity and a moral quality of his own. Relationship to persons is a moral experience because persons are responsible (they can *respond*). Unlike things, they can say "yes" or "no." They have rights, especially the right to say "yes" or "no" in response (in being responsible), the right to self-determination, the right to be themselves, to choose; in short, to be a *thou* and not an *it*, a subject and not an object.

The ethical importance of this distinction is plain enough. We have reasoned thus far that the moral stature of men and women is directly proportionate to the freedom they enjoy, that their freedom to choose is, in its turn, proportionate to the control they have gained over their alternatives of action and to *the knowledge they possess of the alternatives open to them.* If a patient is simply an object of medical treatment, who submits without any knowledge of his condition and its prognosis, that patient has ceased to be a *thou*, has become an *it*. He is being manipulated as a thing, not met and accredited as a person. He has lost his place in the forum of conscience; he is deprived of responsibility and therefore of moral status. This is the ethical implication of the belief that physicians ought to serve according to the demands of a person-centered rather than a problem-centered approach to the patient's suffering. Something of this philosophy of practice is surely working like a leaven in the medical schools and in the profession itself. It was a common feature of the work of the old country doctor, even though his role has been somewhat romantically colored from time to time. When medical technology and urbanism had not yet outmoded the practice of medicine out of a little black bag, it was psychologically easier to maintain a strong personal factor in the physician-patient relationship. The dangers of specialism, in this regard, have stimulated efforts to recover the human values of general practice, as we may see in the experiments of the Peter Bent Brigham Hospital and the Harvard Medical School in teaching "integrated medicine."

"What Is Truth?"

To say, however, that the doctor owes the truth to his patient does not altogether cover the ground of conscience involved. First of all, we ought to recognize that this right to know the truth does not apply to all truths. There are secrets of others, for example, to which few if any of us have any right at all. Furthermore, the classic question put by Pilate to Jesus, "What is truth?" can be applied to the problem of medical diagnosis and truthtelling. As Pilate's question seems to have been intended to suggest, none of us has perfect knowledge; also, the human intelligence with which we try to make sense of what knowledge we have is not infallible. Given a doctor's willingness and desire to respect the patient's right to know the truth, how shall he convey it? How can he be *sure?* In the tradition of ethics and moral theology in Western Christendom it has generally been said that truth is of two kinds, logical truth and moral truth. This distinction appears to have considerable bearing upon the problem of truthtelling as between physician and patient. Logical truth (or accuracy) is the correspondence of outward or verbal expressions to or with the matter which is the subject of the expression. Moral truth (or veracity) is the correspondence of the outward expression given to our thought, with the thought itself. Accuracy, in other words, is telling the truth as it actually is, at least as far as our knowledge of it goes; veracity is telling the truth honestly and not withholding or changing or obscuring a part of what we believe to be true.

When it comes to telling the truth, we can never be sure that we know it, nor can we always be sure that we convey it as we *do* know it or believe it to be. Our modern sociology of knowledge, and psychology with its new understanding of the subtleties of communication and the role of the unconscious, have humbled us a great deal about our capacity either to grasp or to convey the truth. But these considerations are only cautionary; they have to do only with the negative defects of truth, due to human limitations, not with positive injuries to the truth, due to willful distortion and suppression. Problems of morality or of conscience in connection with truthtelling arise only in the case of moral truth (veracity), not with logical truth (accuracy).

It is presumed that inaccuracy or error, in the case of medical advice or in any other area, is unintentional and therefore by definition entirely outside the forum of conscience. In short, as far as morality is concerned (although not so far as science is concerned) what is at stake in telling the truth is, precisely, honesty. Dr. John Homans (1934) once protested, "There can be no universal rule to tell the brutal truth. And the first and best reason for not telling the truth is the impossibility of being certain what the truth is." But this admitted fact is too often a red herring, drawn across the trail to confuse conscience, since it bears only upon the problem of accuracy, not upon the problem of honesty. Indeed, a part of the truth which the doctor owes the patient is just that: that the doctor cannot be absolutely correct. After all, doctors, like their patients, have to be prepared to meet frustration through knowledge. Their very science often gives them an insight into bitter realities which would leave the primitive medicine-man, who could not know, reasonably hopeful. To take refuge in finitude to avoid reality is only a sophisticated form of escapism, when it is used as an excuse for departing from honesty. No: the question before us really is: : *are we obliged to tell the truth as we see it according to our best knowledge?* For this very reason it is a matter of simple justice that the law does not require a physician to be responsible for errors in judgment, or to possess any unusual skill beyond the average. This is the principle of law under which every issue of professional responsibility is adjudicated. Indefectibility of the person—whether in knowledge, skill, or strength—is assumed to be out of the question. Therefore, to deny the obligation of truthtelling by pointing to human limitations is neither here nor there. . . .

Is Ignorance Bliss?

There are many ways by which a physician can deceive his patient, either by misrepresenting the facts as he sees them or by withholding them. Our opinion is that in either case such deceptions are morally speaking unlawful, being acts of theft because they keep from the patient what is rightfully his (the truth about himself), or acts of injustice because they deny to another what is his due as a free and responsible person. The most dramatic case of conscience in medical diagnosis and truthtelling has to do, of course, with the patient who is found to be the victim of a possibly or probably fatal disease, or one for whom no hope at all can be held out. In medical practice, as a matter of fact, there are many other diagnoses that entail sadness equal to or greater than the sadness that is caused by the malignant neoplasms; there are such conditions as brain damage in babies, leading to spastic paralysis, cardiovascular diseases with poor prognosis, and the like. Yet even in terminal diseases the reaction of patients to the truth is varied and unpredictable. . . . Experienced pastors can tell of episodes wherein their own faith has been deepened by the faith and assurance and joy with which terminal patients faced death, sometimes over a long period, and in some cases *not until* they were made fully aware of the truth. But fear of the truth is very strong in many people, including physicians, and this fear accounts for the fact that from ancient to modern times no universal or local code of medical ethics has ever attempted to regulate the doctor's conscience in matters of truthtelling. The first code on the tablets of Hammurabi, 2080 B.C., said nothing about it; the confessors' manuals of the Middle Ages dealing with the rules of shriving surgeons and leechers said nothing; the latest code of the American Medical Association, by its silence or equivocation, leaves the whole thing up to the individual practitioner.

Suppose we turn for a moment to the opinion set forth by Dr. Richard C. Cabot, who was for so many years a physician and teacher at the Massachusetts General Hospital. As Professor of Social Ethics at Harvard University and Lecturer in Pastoral Care at Andover-Newton Theological School and at the Episcopal Theological School, Dr. Cabot followed his art and his conscience wherever they took him, into hospitals, laboratories, social agencies, and into the labyrinth of morals. In the last of his books to be published (*Honesty*, in 1939) he included an enlightening chapter on "Honesty and Dishonesty in Medicine." After a long life of medical service and the most constant moral concern, he wrote: "As a young physician I tried the usual system of benevolent lying from 1893 to 1902. About that time a bitter experience convinced me that I could not be an amateur liar, an occasional, philanthropic liar in medicine or in any part of life. I swore off and have been on the water wagon of medical honesty ever since."

In another work, written some years earlier (*The Meaning of Right and Wrong*), Dr. Cabot put the matter along these lines:

How can we ever be sure where a conscientious liar will draw the line? It appears to me, therefore, that the doctrine that it is sometimes right to lie can never be effectively asserted. For our hearers take notice, and so make ineffective our subsequent attempts to lie. I recall a sick man who ordered his physician never to tell him the truth in case he should be seriously ill. Picture the state of that sick man's mind when later he hears his physician's reassurances. "Perhaps he really doesn't consider this sickness a serious one. Then he will be telling me the truth!" How can the sick man know? If he asks the doctor whether he considers the disease serious and gets a negative answer, how is he to interpret that answer? If the doctor did consider the disease serious he would also have to say "No." His words have become mere wind. No one can interpret them. His reassuring manner, his smiles, his cheering tones may be true or they may be lies. Who can say? . . .

A good example of the dilemma here is to be found in the newspapers of February 1923. The prize fighter J. J. Corbett had died of cancer, and the *New York Times* ran the story with this headline: "Ex-Champion Succumbs Here to Cancer. He Believed He Had Heart Disease." Such was the conscientious lie with which Gentleman Jim's doctor had let him live out his last days. However, other doctors soon began violently to protest the open publication of the deception in a news story, one physician complaining to the editor that several of his own patients with heart diseases were wild with fear that they too really had cancer of the liver. . . . We can be thankful that great strides have been made in the past century toward humanizing the sickroom and the hospital, but there will always be an element of degradation in it as long as sensitive and self-respecting patients have reason to suspect that they are being lied to by their medical servants, no matter how kindly the motives may be. Truthtelling is essential to any personal, thou-thou, relationship; just as essential as love, *agape*, solicitude. The two go together, trust and truth; they require and presuppose each other. Paul's phrase (Ephesians 4:15), "speaking the truth in love," applies not only to our growth in Christ but to our growth in all relationships higher than *I-it*. On a broader scale in the body politic, it is vital to our whole democratic ideal. Government of, by, and for the people is only a myth unless it adheres to the principle that human beings act and respond on the basis of what they know, not on what is concealed from them. There is no responsibility once knowledge is denied or subject to cheating.

There is inescapably a subversive result of occasional lying. It makes no real difference whether it is perpetrated by a direct commission of an untruth, or indirectly through the omission of a truth. Lying troubles the waters of human relations and takes away the one element of mutual trust without much medical practice becomes a manipulation of bodies rather than the care of and for persons. The assumption made by the physician, when he has the *presumption* to withhold the truth, is that the patient is really no longer an adult, but rather either a child or an idiot, more an *it* than a *thou*. In this connection we should note that medical experience by no means lends support to the idea that telling the patient ominous truths will aggravate a serious condition. Some years ago (1936) the Division of Cancer in the Massachusetts Department of Public Health issued a bulletin in which it was said, "The fallacious argument [that lies are necessary] may be answered as follows. . . . [We find that] those physicians and hospitals making a practice of telling the patients frankly when they have the disease, report only the fullest cooperation of the patient in his treatment. But the physician who lies to his patient denies him a chance to show his common sense and helps him one step nearer to the undertaker."

Dr. Cabot, as we have seen, put forward a number of good reasons for truthtelling in medical care. In much of what he had to say he was answering a statement by Dr. Joseph Collins, who had defended medical falsehoods in *Harper's* Magazine for August 1927 in an article entitled "Should Doctors Tell the Truth?" Dr. Cabot pointed out, among other things, that without the truth patients will often object to decisive and costly forms of treatment, surgical or otherwise, since their urgency will not be apparent while the cost will be. If the patient is not told of approaching death, or at least of its grave possibility, he may fail to make proper preparation for his death in wills and testaments, or in reparations and restorations of one kind or another, or in reconciliations with God and/or men. Respect for the *rights* of a man whose time is running out is the real meaning of that famous petition in the Anglican litany: "From lightning and tempest . . . [plus a long list of other calamities] and from *sudden death*, good Lord, deliver me." It is not death itself that is the calamity, but its sudden coming. Sudden death is the extreme fatality, and (as we have already observed) fatality is the denial and negation of morality. In the ethical perspective, fatality is nothing more or less than willy-nilly helplessness, being pushed around by circumstances in ignorance.

Furthermore, only a little experience with doctors, patients' families, and ministers of religion as they deal with terminal diseases or some other condition threatening death or helplessness is enough to show that a great deal of the time their evasion of the plain truth is a protective mechanism for themselves, a rationalization of their own embarrassment and dis-ease. Much of our human behavior, even among doctors, is aimed at satisfying our own needs, emotional and otherwise, not the needs of others. It is a fact to be faced that reservation or corruption of the truth is not always based on a genuine and maturely weighed decision that the patient "is just as well off if he (or she) doesn't know." Fear, we repeat, leads to lies. Fear and lies tend to require and presuppose each other, as do love and truth. Perhaps we need not feel so threatened emotionally by the truth. Dr. Walter Alvarez of the Mayo Clinic says, "Often it is the relatives who have fear and mental pain. . . . In forth-odd years of practice I cannot remember anyone's committing suicide because I told him the hopeless truth. Instead hundreds of persons thanked me from their hearts and told me I had relieved their minds." Who are we to choose ignorance for others? We *have* to make the choice for animals, because they are animals, incapable of receiving or making creative use of such knowledge. But *ought* we to make it for men?

These considerations apply with just as much force to illnesses of the kind that are far from fatal. Even in imaginary illnesses of a neurasthenic nature, the common practice of the medical lie called "placebo" or the bread pill, the "pink water" or the "water subcut" (a pretended hypodermic), can be shown to undermine a truly moral relationship between physician and patient. A false pill of sugar, or something of the sort to deceive the patient into thinking he receives treatment or medication, is a self-defeating practice. In the first place, it *is* a deception, however well-meant. In the second place, it is amazing how few good liars (to use a curious and contradictory phrase) there are, especially in such intimate relationships as illness and medical care. A good many doctors would be well advised, in the light of what we know nowadays about the dynamics of personal relationships, to rely instead, for supportive therapy and encouragement, upon a confident and genuine empathy. In the third place, these practices encourage the idea among neurotic patients that drugs will cure most ailments, and thus serve to extend the patient-medicine evil.

It may be pointed out, of course, that phychiatrists *on principle* do not in all cases share their diagnoses with the patient. Sometimes ignorance is bliss in correcting mental and emotional disorders. It might be claimed that something of the same therapeutic principle may apply to the general practitioner in his work. But for one thing we can answer that the cases are not parallel, inasmuch as the psychiatrist withholds his knowledge precisely because he may prevent the patient's recovery by revealing it, at least if he does so too soon. It is by no means evident that the same is true if the truth has to do with a pink pill for an imaginary illness, or with a diagnosis of cancer disguised to the patient as a tumor, or a heart disease camouflaged as overweight or indigestion. And in any case, the psychiatrist's ministrations are not even relevant in cases where imminent death or its probability is a chief reality factor, or in cases of primarily physical pathology, surgery, and the like.

There is no good reason, merely out of rigid adherence to abstract principle, to be hard or brutally logical about the morality of truthtelling in illness and dying. On the other hand it seems fair to say that the right of the patient to know the truth is clear on moral grounds, and this is true whether or not our ultimate sanction for loyalty to truth and to personal rights is religious. . . . Any sensitive person can sympathize with Dr. Alfred Worcester (1929), who showed in the following plaintive remark that he recognized his duty to tell the truth yet disliked it:

> Devotion to the truth does not always require the physician to voice his fears or tell his patient all he knows. But, after he had decided that the process of dying has actually begun, only in exceptional circumstances would a physician be justified in keeping to himself his opinion. In such cases his only question should be whether to tell the patient or the family, and, when both are to be told, which to tell first.

Dr. Worcester's surrender to conscience is questionable only insofar as, like St. Paul, who "kicked against the pricks," he tried to transfer his debt to his patient by farming it out to the family as middlemen or brokers.

The Medical Code on Lying

The AMA *Code of Ethics*, 1940, says: "A physician should give timely notice of dangerous manifestations of the disease to the friends of the patient." Not, we should notice, to the patient himself! The Code goes on to say, still with patent uncertainty, that the doctor should "assure himself that the patient *or* his friends have such knowledge of the patient's condition as will serve the best interests of the patient and his family." It should be obvious that this is assuming much more knowledge of a family's affairs than medical care, as such, would normally provide. And again, how often the family's and the patient's idea of the best interests at stake are not the same! How often by keeping the patient in ignorance precisely the opposite of what the patient would want has in fact come about, perhaps through a consequent failure to change a will, or to add a codicil, or to make some explanation to a loved one—all of these being things which only the patient could have done had he known the true state of affairs. It is also ironical to observe how often doctors and families are mistaken in supposing that the patient can be fooled by evasion and suppression of the truth. Dr. William H. Robey, in the George Washington Gay lecture of 1936, asserted that "the family is not to be fooled by any dissimulation." Why, then, imagine that the patient is any easier to fool? Patients may sometimes be at a very low ebb and still show an almost preternatural awareness. If any self-possession at all remains, they are still persons with a person's right to know the truth. It is cruel and inhuman to leave them in doubt, suspicious and confused. Furthermore, it is an insult to be babied whether big or little issues are concerned. . . .

A strange inconsistency is also to be found in the *Code of Ethics.* Following the equivocation we have already noted, it declares that in cases of medical consultation "all the physicians interested in the case should be frank and candid with the patient and his family." It is not at all clear why a medical consultant should thus be directly charged to be candid with the patient when the physician in charge is not. Yet even here the Code qualifies itself by remarking at another point that the consultant should "state the result of his study to the patient *or* his next friend in the presence of the physician in charge." And after all this temporizing about the doctor's obligation to tell the patient the truth, the Code ends with a Golden Rule of medicine, that the physician should "constantly behave towards others as he desires them to deal with him." But can it really be that doctors who practice professional deception would, if the roles were reversed, want to be coddled or deceived? . . .

The tradition in Western civilization allows for what the law calls "privileged communications" between patient and physician, as between people and pastor. This, indeed, is one of the few priestly aspects of the doctor's role left over from the ancient times. What we tell our doctors and our clergymen is private, personal, our own; and in that sense, secret. Now, as it bears upon truthtelling, the significant thing is that this ethical principle of the professional secret rests upon the conviction that knowledge of a person's private life gained in the course of professional services is a *trust,* the stewardly possession by a professional servant of what belongs to another. The secrets of the confessional box and pastor's study, and of the consulting room and clinic, *belong* to the person served, not to the priest or to the physician. They therefore have no *right* to pass them on to others *without the owner's consent*. By the nature of his office the priest has only that knowledge of a penitent's life which is already known to the penitent and shared by him with the priest. In the case of medicine, however, the physician, the diagnostician, gains knowledge of the patient which (in the nature of the case) the patient does not yet have. But it is still the patient's knowledge and information; it is his life and health which are at stake. The patient has "opened his books" to the doctor on the reasonable assumption that what is found there will be turned over to him, just as a business firm has a right to expect no deception or suppression from an auditor. In spite of all this, some doctors assume the godlike power to ignore the propriety or proper ownership of the secret. On their own behalf they will insist upon the rule of privileged communication, espressing righteous indignation when others attempt to pry or extort information from them; at the same time, however, what they have refused others as not rightfully theirs to give, they will also deny to the patient himself, the rightful owner! Or, with a strange further confusion of ethical reasoning, they will deny the patient the truth which belongs to him, and then proceed to give it to his family or friends, regardless of the principle of professional secrecy. . . .

Do People Want the Truth?

By way of summary, we may say that in general we can validly assert our right as patients to know the medical facts about ourselves. Several reasons have been given for it, but perhaps the four fundamental ones are: first, that as persons our human, moral quality is taken away from us if we are denied whatever knowledge is available; second, that the doctor is *entrusted* by us with what he learns, but the facts are ours, not his, and to deny them to us is to steal from us what is our own, not his; third, that the highest conception of the physician-patient relationship is a personalistic one, in the light of which we see that the fullest possibilities of medical treatment and cure in themselves depend upon mutual respect and confidence, as well as upon technical skill; and, fourth, that to deny a patient knowledge of the facts as to life and death is to assume responsibilities which cannot be carried out by anyone but the patient, with his own knowledge of his own affairs. On the negative side, we have reasoned that the common excuse given for deceiving the patient—"after all the doctors are fallible and make mistakes"—is not a valid excuse. In the first place, physicians are in conscience bound to indicate that they find pathological conditions and advise treatment only to the best of their knowledge and judgment, not with absolute certainty. In the second place, while the admission of human fallibility always qualifies any claims a doctor might make as to accuracy, *it does not qualify and cannot disqualify the obligation to be honest.* And, finally, we have rejected any distinction between lies (positive injuries to the truth) and concealment (merely negative failure to convey what is foreseen as prognosis and discovered by diagnosis). When moralists such as K. E. Kirk offer this distinction, condemning the former and justifying the latter, they have failed completely to grasp the foundation principles of the ethics of communication. We have argued, instead, that commission of untruth and suppression of truth are alike deprivations of a patient's right; and therefore theft, therefore unjust, therefore immoral.

The only remaining question is: what if the patient does not ask for the truth? This problem may arise either because he does not *want* the truth (perhaps out of fear, being threatened by what he suspects, or for some other reason), or because he does not realize that there is a truth not known to him but now discovered by the doctor. This problem, surely, cannot be regarded as a very difficult one in conscience. In the first case, when the patient has no desire to know the truth and the doctor has good reason to believe that the patient does not want to know it, the doctor should respect his wishes, even though it might well be a proper part of his role to help his patient to want the truth and to become able to accept it. It is no part of a doctor's duty to impose his diagnosis upon a patient or flout his wishes, unless, of course, he has reason to believe that he could not continue to treat the patient properly, according to the demands of the best medical care, without telling him. In such a case, surely, he should explain why he needs to tell (or at least that he feels obliged to tell), and if the patient still refuses to hear, then ask leave to withdraw from the case, urging that another physician be called in his place. In the second case, when the patient is too ignorant to ask for the information acquired by the doctor, it is clearly the doctor's moral obligation to supply it, together with an explanation of its meaning and importance. A person cannot refuse to return his neighbor's watch if he finds it, or at least to tell him where it is lying in the garden, merely because his neighbor does not know that he has lost it and has not asked the doctor if he found it or knows where it is.

Throughout this discussion of medical truthtelling our frame of reference has been physical rather than psychological diagnosis. A great many people naturally raise the question whether the reasoning here would be or could be applied equally to psychotherapy. In all probability it would not, and could not be without upsetting well-tested principles of therapy. In the first place, genuinely psychotic patients fall into Jeremy Taylor's category of "children and idiots," as far as competence to seek or to receive the truth is concerned. If it is judged to be in their best interests, surely the truth about them ("their" truth) can be withheld in the same way that a minor's or dependent's property can be withheld and rationed by a parent or guardian. Yet, even in the case of people who are far from psychotic, suffering some much less pathological disorder such as emotional or personality problems, there is a further consideration that makes a great difference between the right to know the truth in their case, and a patient's who has come, for example, for advice in internal medicine. In the latter case the doctor discovers a truth which is factually perceived. But in the case of psychiatric medicine and clinical psychology, apart from a physical analysis which may be related to it, the diagnosis is one of *evaluative judgment* about the patient's behavior and sentiments. However sound and wise the professional expert's diagnosis of behavior and motives and drives may be, it is, as far as honesty is at stake, in the area of *opinion*. Here, surely, the expert's obligation to tell the patient or client what is in or on his mind (i.e., the doctor's) is not as certain or compelling. He has formed an estimate of the patient and his problems; he has not learned a truth about him. The "truth" of his estimate still remains to be established, and probably cannot be established by any means other than exploratory and tentative therapy. Until it is established it is not a truth owed to the patient, as knowledge of glandular imbalance or low blood pressure would be. Speaking of the psychological forms of illness and diagnosis, we may say with Carl R. Rogers (1951), "In a very meaningful and accurate sense, therapy *is* diagnosis, and this diagnosis is a process which goes on in the experience of the client, rather than in the intellect of the clinician."

Neither the spirit of rigorism nor of laxism has dominated our discussion. It seems difficult, in the extreme, to imagine how a conference of medical men could take serious exception to it. If a seminar of physicians were to discuss, just for example, Immanuel Kant's ethical tract *On a Supposed Right to Tell Lies from Benevolent Motives*, and apply its reasoning to morals and medical care, we could fairly confidently expect them to come to much the same conclusion as we have. We have looked into a subject too much avoided, using applications and reasons of our own, but the conclusion reached is by no means a new one, any more than the problem itself is new.

References

Birnie, John M. "Ethics for the Doctor." *New England Journal of Medicine* 205 (November 19, 1931): 1026.

Buber, Martin. *I and Thou*. Edinburgh: R. & R. Clark, 1937.

Cabot, Richard C. *The Meaning of Right and Wrong*. New York: Macmillan, 1936.

—— *Honesty*. New York: Macmillan, 1938.

Homans, John. *The Care of the Patient from the Surgeon's Standpoint*. Boston, 1934.

Peabody, Francis. *The Care of the Patient*. Cambridge, Mass.: Harvard University Press, 1928.

Worcester, Alfred. *Physician and Patient*. Cambridge, 1929.

4

Truth and the Physician

Bernard C. Meyer

Truth does not do so much good in this world as the semblance of it does harm.
(*La Rouchefoucauld*)

AMONG the reminiscences of his Alsatian boyhood, my father related the story of the local functionary who was berated for the crude and blunt manner in which he went from house to house announcing to wives and mothers news of battle casualties befalling men from the village. On the next occasion, mindful of the injunctions to be more tactful and to soften the impact of his doleful message, he rapped gently on the door, and, when it opened, inquired, "Is the widow Schmidt at home?"

Insofar as this essay is concerned with the subject of truth it is only proper to add that when I told this story to a colleague, he already knew it and claimed that it concerned a woman named Braun who lived in a small town in Austria. By this time it would not surprise me to learn that the episode is a well-known vignette in the folklore of Tennessee where it is attributed to a woman named Smith or Brown whose husband was killed at the battle of Shiloh. Ultimately, we may find that all three versions are plagiarized accounts of an occurrence during the Trojan War.

Reprinted from E. Fuller Torrey, ed., *Ethical Issues in Medicine*, pp. 161–77, with the permission of the author and editor. Copyright © 1968 by Little, Brown and Company, Inc.

Communication between Physician and Patient

Apocryphal or not, the story illustrates a few of the vexing aspects of the problem of conveying unpalatable news, notably the difficulty of doing so in a manner that causes a minimum amount of pain, and also the realization that not everyone is capable of learning how to do it. Both aspects find their application in the field of medicine where the imparting of the grim facts of diagnosis and prognosis is a constant and recurring issue. Nor does it seem likely that for all our learning we doctors are particularly endowed with superior talents and techniques for coping with these problems. On the contrary, for reasons to be given later, there is cause to believe that in not a few instances, elements in his own psychological makeup may cause the physician to be singularly ill-equipped to be the bearer of bad tidings. It should be observed, moreover, that until comparatively recent times, the subject of communication between physician and patient received little attention in medical curriculum and medical literature.

Within the past decade or so, coincident with an expanded recognition of the significance of emotional factors in all medical practice, an impressive number of books and articles by physicians, paramedical personnel, and others have been published, attesting to both the growing awareness of the importance of the subject and an apparent willingness to face it. An especially noteworthy example of this trend was provided by a three-day meeting in February 1967, sponsored by the New York Academy of Sciences, on the subject of *The Care of Patients with Fatal Illness.* The problem of communicating with such patients and their families was a recurring theme in most of the papers presented.

Both at this conference and in the literature, particular emphasis has been focused on the patient with cancer, which is hardly surprising in light of its frequency and of the extraordinary emotional reactions that it unleashes not only in the patient and in his kinsmen but in the physician himself. At the same time, it should be noted that the accent on the cancer patient or the dying patient may foster the impression that in less grave conditions this dialogue between patient and physician hardly warrants much concern or discussion. Such a view is unfounded, however, and could only be espoused by someone who has had the good fortune to escape the experience of being ill and hospitalized. Those less fortunate will recall the emotional stresses induced by hospitalization, even when the condition requiring it is relatively banal.

A striking example of such stress may sometimes be seen when the patient who is hospitalized, say, for repair of an inguinal hernia, happens to be a physician. All the usual anxieties confronting a prospective surgical subject tend to become greatly amplified and garnished with a generous sprinkling of hypochondriasis in physician-turned-patient. Wavering unsteadily between these two roles, he conjures up visions of all the complications of anesthesia, of wound dehiscence or infection, of embolization, cardiac arrest, and whatnot that he has ever heard or read about. To him, lying between hospital sheets, clad in impersonal hospital clothes, divested of his watch and the keys to his car, the hospital suddenly takes on a different appearance from the place he may have known in a professional capacity. Even his colleagues—the anesthetist who will put him to sleep or cause a temporary motor and sensory paralysis of the lower half of his body, and the surgeon who will incise it—appear different. He would like to have a little talk with them, a very professional talk to be sure, although in his heart he may know that the talk will also be different. And if they are in tune with the situation, they too know that it will be different, that beneath the restrained tones of sober and factual conversation is the thumping anxiety of a man who seeks words of reassurance. With some embarrassment he may introduce his anxieties with the phrase, "I suppose this is going to seem a little silly, but . . ."; and from this point on he may sound like any other individual confronted by the ordeal of surgical experience. Indeed, it would appear that under these circumstances, to say nothing of more ominous ones, most people, regardless of their experience, knowledge, maturity or sophistication, are assailed by more or less similar psychological pressures, from which they seek relief not through pharmacological sedation, but through the more calming influence of the spoken word.

Seen in this light the question of what to tell the patient about his illness is but one facet of the practice of medicine as an art, a particular example of that spoken and mute dialogue between patient and physician which has always been and will always be an indispensable ingredient in the therapeutic process. How to carry on this dialogue, what to say and when to say it, and what not to say, are questions not unlike those posed by an awkward suitor; like him, those not naturally versed in this art may find themselves discomfited and needful of the promptings of some Cyrano who will whisper those words and phrases that ultimately will wing their way to soothe an anguished heart.

Emotional Reactions of Physicians

The difficulties besetting the physician under these circumstances, however, cannot be ascribed simply to his mere lack of experience or innate eloquence. For like the stammering suitor, the doctor seeking to communicate with his patient may have an emotional stake in his message. When that message contains an ominous significance, he may find himself too troubled to use words wisely, too ridden with anxiety to be kind, and too depressed to convey hope. An understanding of such reactions touches upon a recognition of some of the several psychological motivations that have led some individuals to choose a medical career. There is evidence that at times that choice has been dictated by what might be viewed as counterphobic forces. Having in childhood experienced recurring brushes with illness and having encountered a deep and abiding fear of death and dying, such persons may embrace a medical career as if it will confer upon them a magical immunity from a repetition of those dreaded eventualities; for them the letters M.D. constitute a talisman bestowing upon the wearer a sense of invulnerability and a pass of safe conduct through the perilous frontiers of life. There are others for whom the choice of a career dedicated to helping and healing appears to have arisen as a reaction formation against earlier impulses to wound and to destroy. For still others among us, the practice of medicine serves as the professional enactment of a long-standing rescue fantasy.

It is readily apparent in these examples (which by no means exhaust the catalogue of motives leading to the choice of a medical career) that confrontation by the failure of one's efforts and by the need to announce it may unloose a variety of inner psychological disturbances: faced by the gravely ill or dying patient the "counterphobic" doctor may feel personally vulnerable again; the "reaction-formation" doctor, evil and guilty; and the "rescuer," worthless and impotent. For such as these, words cannot come readily in their discourse with the seriously or perilously ill. Indeed, they may curtail their communications; and, what is no less meaningful to their patients, withdraw their physical presence. Thus the patient with inoperable cancer and his family may discover that the physician, who at a more hopeful moment in the course of the illness had been both articulate and supportive, has become remote both in his speech and in his behavior. Nor is the patient uncomprehending of the significance of the change in his doctor's attitude. Observers have recorded the verbal expressions of patients who sensed the feelings of futility and depression in their physicians. Seeking to account for their own reluctance to ask questions (a reluctance based partly upon their own disinclination to face a grim reality), one such patient said, "He looked so tired." Another stated, "I don't want to upset him because he has tried so hard to help me"; and another, "I know he feels so badly already and is doing his best" (Abrams 1966). To paraphrase a celebrated utterance, one might suppose that these remarks were dictated by the maxim: "Ask not what your doctor can do for you; ask what you can do for your doctor."

Adherence to a Formula

In the dilemma created both by a natural disinclination to be a bearer of bad news and by those other considerations already cited, many a physician is tempted to abandon personal judgment and authorship in his discourse with his patients, and to rely instead upon a set formula which he employs with dogged and indiscriminate consistency. Thus, in determining what to say to patients with cancer, there are exponents of standard policies that are applied routinely in seeming disregard of the overall clinical picture and of the personality or psychological makeup of the patient. In general, two such schools of thought prevail; i.e., those that always tell and those that never do. Each of these is amply supplied with statistical anecdotal evidence proving the correctness of the policy. Yet even if the figures were accurate—and not infrequently they are obtained via a questionnaire, itself a rather opaque window to the human mind—all they demonstrate is that more rather than less of a given proportion of the cancer population profited by the policy employed. This would provide small comfort, one might suppose, to the patients and their families that constitute the minority of the sample.

Truth as Abstract Principle

At times adherence to such a rigid formula is dressed up in the vestments of slick and facile morality. Thus a theologian (Fletcher 1954) has insisted that the physician has a moral obligation to tell the truth and that his withholding it constitutes a deprivation of the patient's right; therefore it is "theft, therefore unjust, therefore immoral." "Can it be," he asks, "that doctors who practice professional deception would, if the roles were reversed, want to be coddled or deceived?" To which, as many physicians can assert, the answer is distinctly *yes*. Indeed so adamant is this writer upon the right of the patient to know the facts of his illness that in the event he refuses to hear what the doctor is trying to say, the latter should "ask leave to withdraw from the case, urging that another physician be called in his place." (Once there were three boy scouts who were sent away from a campfire and told not to return until each had done his good turn for the day. In 20 minutes all three had returned, and curiously each one reported that he had helped a little old lady to cross a street. The scoutmaster's surprise was even greater when he learned that in each case it was the same little old lady, prompting him to inquire why it took the three of them to perform this one simple good deed. "Well sir," replied one of the boys, "you see she really didn't want to cross the street at all.")

In this casuistry wherein so much attention is focused upon abstract principle and so little upon humanity, one is reminded of the no less specious arguments of those who assert that the thwarting of suicide and the involuntary hospitalization of the mentally deranged constitute violations of personal freedom and human right. It is surely irregular for a fire engine to travel in the wrong direction on a one-way street, but if one is not averse to putting out fires and saving lives, the traffic violation looms as a conspicuous irrelevancy. No less irrelevant is the obsessional concern with meticulous definitions of truth in an enterprise where kindness, charity, and the relief of human suffering are the essential verities. "The letter killeth," say the Scriptures, "but the spirit giveth life."

Problem of Definition

Nor should it be forgotten that in the healing arts, the matter of truth is not always susceptible to easy definition. Consider for a moment the question of the hopeless diagnosis. It was not so long ago that such a designation was appropriate for subacute bacterial endocarditis, pneumococcal meningitis, pernicious anemia, and a number of other conditions which today are no longer incurable, while those diseases which today are deemed hopeless may cease to be so by tomorrow. Experience has proved, too, the unreliability of obdurate opinions concerning prognosis even in those conditions where all the clinical evidence and the known behavior of a given disease should leave no room for doubt. To paraphrase Clemenceau, to insist that a patient is hopelessly ill may at times be worse than a crime; it may be a mistake.

Problem of Determining Patient's Desires

There are other pitfalls, moreover, that complicate the problem of telling patients the truth about their illness. There is the naive notion, for example, that when the patient asserts that what he is seeking is the plain truth he means just that. But as more than one observer has noted, this is sometimes the last thing the patient really wants. Such assertions may be voiced with particular emphasis by patients who happen to be physicians and who strive to display a professional or scientifically objective attitude toward their own condition. Yet to accept such assertions at their face value may sometimes lead to tragic consequences, as in the following incident.

A distinguished urological surgeon was hospitalized for a hypernephroma, which diagnosis had been withheld from him. One day he summoned the intern into his room, and after appealing to the latter on the basis of we're-both-doctors-and-grown-up-men, succeeded in getting the unwary younger man to divulge the facts. Not long afterward, while the nurse was momentarily absent from the room, the patient opened a window and leaped to his death.

Role of Secrecy in Creating Anxiety

Another common error is the assumption that until someone has been formally told the truth he doesn't know it. Such self-deception is often present when parents feel moved to supply their pubertal children with the sexual facts of life. With much embarrassment and a good deal of backing and filling on the subjects of eggs, bees, and babies, sexual information is imparted to a child who often not only already knows it but is uncomfortable in hearing it from that particular source. There is indeed a general tendency to underestimate the perceptiveness of children not only about such matters but where graver issues, notably illness and death, are concerned. As a consequence, attitudes of secrecy and overprotection designed to shield children from painful realities may result paradoxically in creating an atmosphere that is saturated with suspicion, distrust, perplexity, and intolerable anxiety. Caught between trust in their own intuitive perceptions and the deceptions practiced by the adults about them, such children may suffer greatly from a lack of opportunity of coming to terms emotionally with some of the vicissitudes of existence that in the end are inescapable. A refreshing contrast to this approach has been presented in a paper entitled "Who's Afraid of Death on a Leukemia Ward" (Vernick and Karon 1965). Recognizing that most of the children afflicted with this disease had some knowledge of its seriousness, and that all were worried about it, the hospital staff abandoned the traditional custom of protection and secrecy, providing instead an atmosphere in which the children could feel free to express their fears and their concerns and could openly acknowledge the act of death when one of the group passed away. The result of this measure was immensely salutary.

Similar miscalculations of the accuracy of inner perceptions may be noted in dealing with adults. Thus, in a study entitled "Mongolism: When Should Parents Be Told?" (Drillion and Wilkinson 1964), it was found that in nearly half the cases the mothers declared they had realized before being told that something was seriously wrong with the child's development, a figure which obviously excludes the mothers who refused consciously to acknowledge their suspicions. On the basis of their findings the authors concluded that a full explanation given in the early months, coupled with regular support thereafter, appeared to facilitate the mother's acceptance of and adjustment to her child's handicap.

A pointless and sometimes deleterious withholding of truth is a common practice in dealing with elderly people. "Don't tell Mother" often seems to be an almost reflex maxim among some adults in the face of any misfortune, large or small. Here, too, elaborate efforts at camouflage may backfire, for, sensing that he is being shielded from some ostensibly intolerable secret, not only is the elderly one deprived of the opportunity of reacting appropriately to it, but he is being tacitly encouraged to conjure up something in his imagination that may be infinitely worse.

Discussion of Known Truth

Still another misconception is the belief that if it is certain that the truth is known it is all right to discuss it. How mistaken such an assumption may be was illustrated by the violent rage which a recent widow continued to harbor toward a friend for having alluded to cancer in the presence of her late husband. Hearing her outburst one would have concluded that until the ominous word had been uttered, her husband had been ignorant of the nature of his condition. The facts, however, were different, as the unhappy woman knew, for it had been her husband who originally had told the friend what the diagnosis was.

Denial and Repression

The psychological devices that make such seeming inconsistencies of thought and knowledge possible are the mechanisms of repression and denial. It is indeed the remarkable capacity to bury or conceal more or less transparent truth that makes the problem of telling it so sticky and difficult a matter, and one that is so unsusceptible to simple rule-of-thumb formulas. For while in some instances the maintenance of denial may lead to severe emotional distress, in others it may serve as a merciful shield. For example,

> A physician with a reputation for considerable diagnostic acumen developed a painless jaundice. When, not surprisingly, a laparotomy revealed a carcinoma of the head of the pancreas, the surgeon relocated the biliary outflow so that postoperatively the jaundice subsided. This seeming improvement was consistent with the surgeon's explanation to the patient that the operation had revealed a hepatitis. Immensely relieved, the patient chided himself for not having anticipated the "correct" diagnosis. "What a fool I was!" he declared, obviously alluding to an earlier, albeit unspoken, fear of cancer.

Among less sophisticated persons the play of denial may assume a more primitive expression. Thus a woman who had ignored the growth of a breast cancer to a point where it had produced spinal metastases and paraplegia, attributed the latter to "arthritis" and asked whether the breast would grow back again. The same mental mechanism allowed another woman to ignore dangerous rectal bleeding by ascribing it to menstruation, although she was well beyond the menopause.

In contrast to these examples is a case reported by Winkelstein and Blacher (1967) of a man who, awaiting the report of a cervical node biopsy, asserted that if it showed cancer he wouldn't want to live, and that if it didn't he wouldn't believe it. Yet despite this seemingly unambiguous willingness to deal with raw reality, when the chips were down, as will be described later, this man too was able to protect himself through the use of denial.

From the foregoing it should be self-evident that what is imparted to a patient about his illness should be planned with the same care and executed with the same skill that are demanded by any potentially therapeutic measure. Like the transfusion of blood, the dispensing of certain information must be distinctly indicated, the amount given consonant with the needs of the recipient, and the type chosen with the view of avoiding untoward reactions. This means that only in selected instances is there any justification for telling a patient the precise figures of his blood pressure, and that the question of revealing interesting but asymptomatic congenital anomalies should be considered in light of the possibility of evoking either hypochondriacal ruminations or narcissistic gratification.

Under graver circumstances the choices confronting the physician rest upon more crucial psychological issues. In principle, we should strive to make the patient sufficiently aware of the facts of his condition to facilitate his participation in the treatment without at the same time giving him cause to believe that such participation is futile. "The indispensable ingredient of this therapeutic approach," write Stehlin and Beach (1966), "is free communication between [physician] and patient, in which the latter is sustained by hope within a framework of reality." What this may mean in many instances is neither outright truth nor outright falsehood but a carefully modulated formulation that neither overtaxes human credulity nor invites despair. Thus a sophisticated woman might be expected to reject with complete disbelief the notion that she has had to undergo mastectomy for a benign cyst, but she may at the same time accept postoperative radiation as a prophylactic measure rather than as evidence of metastasis.

> A doctor's wife was found to have ovarian carcinoma with widespread metastases. Although the surgeon was convinced she would not survive for more than three or four months, he wished to try the effects of radiotherapy and chemotherapy. After some discussion of the problem with a psychiatrist, he addressed himself to the patient as follows: to his surprise, when examined under the microscope the tumor in her abdomen proved to be cancerous; he fully believed he had removed it entirely; to feel perfectly safe, however, he intended to give her radiation and chemical therapies over an indeterminate period of time. The patient was highly gratified by his frankness and proceeded to live for nearly three more years, during which time she enjoyed an active and a productive life.

A rather similar approach was utilized in the case of Winkelstein and Blacher previously mentioned.

> In the presence of his wife the patient was told by the resident surgeon, upon the advice of the psychiatrist, that the biopsy of the cervical node showed cancer; that he had a cancerous growth in the abdomen; that it was the type of cancer that responds well to chemotherapy; that if the latter produced any discomfort he would receive medication for its relief; and finally that the doctors were very hopeful for a successful outcome. The pa-

tient, who, it will be recalled, had declared he wouldn't want to live if the doctors found cancer, was obviously gratified. Immediately he telephoned members of his family to tell them the news, gratuitously adding that the tumor was of low-grade malignancy. That night he slept well for the first time since entering the hospital and he continued to do so during the balance of his stay. Just before leaving he confessed that he had known all along about the existence of the abdominal mass but that he had concealed his knowledge to see what the doctors would tell him. Upon arriving home he wrote a warm letter of thanks and admiration to the resident surgeon.

It should be emphasized that although in both of these instances the advice of a psychiatrist was instrumental in formulating the discussion of the facts of the illness, it was the surgeon, not the psychiatrist, who did the talking. The importance of this point cannot be exaggerated, for since it is the surgeon who plays the central and crucial role in such cases, it is to him, and not to some substitute mouthpiece, that the patient looks for enlightenment and for hope. As noted earlier, it is not every surgeon who can bring himself to speak in this fashion to his patient; and for some there may be a strong temptation to take refuge in a stereotyped formula, or to pass the buck altogether. The surgical resident, in the last case cited, for example, was both appalled and distressed when he was advised what to do. Yet he steeled himself, looked the patient straight in the eye, and spoke with conviction. When he saw the result, he was both relieved and gratified. Indeed, he emerged from the experience a far wiser man and a better physician.

The Dying Patient

The general point of view expressed in the foregoing pages has been espoused by others in considering the problem of communicating with the dying patient. Aldrich (1963) stresses the importance of providing such persons with an appropriately timed opportunity of selecting acceptance or denial of the truth in their efforts to cope with their plight. Weisman and Hackett (1961) believe that for the majority of patients it is likely that there is neither complete acceptance nor total repudiation of the imminence of death. "To deny this 'middle knowledge' of approaching death," they assert, ". . . is to deny the responsiveness of the mind to both internal perceptions and external information. There is always a psychological stream; fever, weakness, anorexia, weight loss, and pain are subjective counterparts of homeostatic alteration. . . . If to this are added changes in those close to the patient, the knowledge of approaching death is confirmed."

Other observers agree that a patient who is sick enough to die often knows it without being told, and that what he seeks from his physician are no longer statements concerning diagnosis and prognosis, but earnest manifestations of his unwavering concern and devotion. As noted earlier, it is at such times that for reason of their own psychological makeup some physicians become deeply troubled and are most prone to drift away, thereby adding, to the dying patient's physical suffering, the suffering that is caused by a sense of abandonment, isolation, and emotional deprivation.

In contrast, it should be stressed that no less potent than morphine nor less effective than an array of tranquilizers is the steadfast and serious concern of the physician for those often numerous and relatively minor complaints of the dying patient. To this beneficent manifestation of psychological denial, which may at times attain hypochondriacal proportions, the physician ideally should respond in kind, shifting his gaze from the lethal process he is now helpless to arrest to the living being whose discomfort and distress he is still able to assuage. In these, the final measures of the dance of life, it may then appear as if both partners had reached a tacit and a mutual understanding, an unspoken pledge to ignore the dark shadow of impending death and to resume those turns and rhythms that were familiar figures in a more felicitous past. If in this he is possessed of enough grace and elegance to play his part the doctor may well succeed in fulfilling the assertion of Oliver Wendell Holmes that if one of the functions of the physician is to assist at the coming in, another is to assist at the going out.

If what has been set down here should prove uncongenial to some strict moralists, one can only observe that there is a hierarchy of morality, and that ours is a profession which traditionally has been guided by a precept that transcends the virtue of uttering truth for truth's sake; that is, "So far as possible, do no harm." Where it concerns the communication between the physician and his patient, the attainment of this goal demands an ear that is sensitive to both what is said and what is not said, a mind that is capable of understanding what has been heard, and a heart that can respond to what has been understood. Here, as in many difficult human enterprises, it may prove easier to learn the words than to sing the tune.

We did not dare to breathe a prayer
Or give our anguish scope!
Something was dead in each of us,
And what was dead was Hope!

OSCAR WILDE, *The Ballad of Reading Gaol*

References

Abrams, R. C. "The Patient with Cancer—His Changing Pattern of Communication." *New England Journal of Medicine* 274 (1966): 317–22.

Aldrich, C. K. "The Dying Patient's Grief." *Journal of the American Medical Association* 184 (May 1963): 329–31.

Drillien, C. M. "Mongolism: When Should Parents Be Told?" *British Medical Journal* 2 (1964): 1306.

Fletcher, Joseph. *Morals and Medicine*. Princeton, N.J.: Princeton University Press, 1954.

Stehlin, J. S. and K. A. Beach. "Psychological Aspects of Cancer Therapy." *Journal of the American Medical Association* 197 (July 1966): 100–4.

Vernick, Joel and Myron Karon. "Who's Afraid of Death on a Leukemia Ward?" *American Journal of Diseases of Children* 109 (May 1965): 393.

Weisman, Avery D. and Thomas Hackett. "Predilection to Death: Death and Dying as a Psychiatric Problem." *Psychosomatic Medicine* 23 (June 1961): 232–56.

Winkelstein, C. and R. Blacher. Personal communication. 1967.

TWO
Determining Death

Death: Process or Event?

ROBERT S. MORISON

MOST discussions of death and dying shift uneasily, and often more or less unconsciously, from one point of view to another. On the one hand, the common noun "death" is thought of as standing for a clearly defined event, a step function that puts a sharp end to life. On the other, dying is seen as a long-drawn-out process that begins when life itself begins and is not completed in any given organism until the last cell ceases to convert energy.

The first view is certainly the more traditional one. Indeed, it is so deeply embedded, not only in literature and art, but also in the law, that it is hard to free ourselves from it and from various associated attitudes that greatly influence our behavior. This article analyzes how the traditional or literary conception of death may have originated and how this conception is influencing the way in which we deal with the problem of dying under modern conditions. In part, I contend that some of our uses of the term "death" fall close to, if not actually within, the definition of what Whitehead (1967) called the "fallacy of misplaced concreteness." As he warned, "This fallacy is the occasion of great confusion in philosophy," and it may also confuse our handling of various important practical matters.

Nevertheless, there is evidence that the fallacy may be welcomed by some physicians because it frees them from the necessity of looking certain unsettling facts in the face.

Reprinted from *Science* 173 (August 20, 1971): 694–98, with the permission of the author and publisher. Copyright 1971 by the American Association for the Advancement of Science.

In its simplest terms, the fallacy of misplaced concreteness consists in regarding or using an abstraction as if it were a thing, or, as Whitehead puts it, as a "simple instantaneous material configuration." Examples of a relatively simple kind can be found throughout science to illustrate the kinds of confusion to which the fallacy leads. Thus, our ancestors who observed the behavior of bodies at different temperatures found it convenient to explain some of their observations by inventing an abstraction they called heat. All too quickly the abstract concept turned into an actual fluid that flowed from one body to another. No doubt these conceptions helped to develop the early stages of thermodynamics. On the other hand, the satisfaction these conceptions gave their inventors may also have slowed down the development of the more sophisticated kinetic theory.

It should be quite clear that, just as we do not observe a fluid heat, but only differences in temperature, we do not observe "life" as such. Life is not a thing or a fluid any more than heat is. What we observe are some unusual sets of objects separated from the rest of the world by certain peculiar properties such as growth, reproduction, and special ways of handling energy. These objects we elect to call "living things." From here, it is but a short step to the invention of a hypothetical entity that is possessed by all living things and that is supposed to account for the difference between living and nonliving things. We might call this entity "livingness," following the usual rule for making abstract nouns out of participles and adjectives. This sounds rather awkward, so we use the word "life" instead. This apparently tiny change in the shape of the noun helps us on our way to philosophical error. The very cumbersomeness of the word "livingness" reminds us that we have abstracted the quality for which it stands from an array of living things. The word "life," however, seems much more substantial in its own right. Indeed, it is all too easy to believe that the word, like so many other nouns, stands for something that must have an existence of its own and must be definable in general terms, quite apart from the particular objects it characterizes. Men thus find themselves thinking more and more about life as a thing in itself, capable of entering inanimate aggregations of material and turning them into living things. It is then but a short step to believing that, once life is there, it can leave or be destroyed, thereby turning living things into dead things.

Now that we have brought ourselves to mention dead things, we can observe that we have invented the abstract idea of death by observing dead things, in just the same way that we have invented the idea of life by observing living things. Again, in the same way that we come to regard life as a thing, capable of entering and leaving bodies, we come to regard death as a thing, capable of moving about on its own in order to take away life. Thus, we have become accustomed to hearing that "death comes for the archbishop," or, alternatively, that one may meet death by "appointment in Samarra." Only a very few, very sophisticated old generals simply fade away.

In many cases then, Death is not only reified, it is personified, and graduates from a mere thing to a jostling woman in the marketplace of Baghdad or an old man, complete with beard, scythe, and hourglass, ready to mow down those whose time has come. In pointing to some of the dangers of personification, it is not my purpose to abolish poetry. Figures of speech certainly have their place in the enrichment of esthetic experience, perhaps even as means for justifying the ways of God to man. Nevertheless, reification and personification of abstractions do tend to make it more difficult to think clearly about important problems.

Abstractions Can
Lead to Artificial Discontinuity

A particularly frequent hazard is the use of abstractions to introduce artificial discontinuities into what are essentially continuous processes. For example, although it is convenient to think of human development as a series of stages, such periods as childhood and adolescence are not discontinuous, sharply identifiable "instantaneous configurations" that impose totally different types of behavior on persons of different ages. The infant does not suddenly leave off "mewling and puking" to pick up a satchel and go to school. Nor at the other end of life does "the justice, . . . with eyes severe and beard of formal cut" instantly turn into "the lean and slipper'd pantaloon." The changes are gradual; finally, the pantaloon slips through second childishness into "mere oblivion, sans teeth, sans eyes, sans taste, sans everything" (Shakespeare). Clearly we are dealing here with a continuous process of growth and decay. There is no magic moment at which "everything" disappears. Death is no more a single, clearly delimited, momentary phenomenon than is infancy, adolescence, or middle age. The gradualness of the process of dying is even clearer than it was in Shakespeare's time, for we now know that various parts of the body can go on living for months after its central organization has disintegrated. Some cell lines, in fact, can be continued indefinitely.

The difficulty of identifying a moment of death has always been recognized when dealing with primitive organisms, and the conventional concept has usually not been applied to organisms that reproduce themselves by simple fission. Death as we know it, so to speak, is characteristic only of differentiated and integrated organisms, and is most typically observed in the land-living vertebrates in which everything that makes life worth living depends on continuous respiratory movements. These, in turn, depend on an intact brain, which itself is dependent on the continuing circulation of properly aerated blood. Under natural conditions, this tripartite, interdependent system fails essentially at one and the same time. Indeed, the moment of failure seems often to be dramatically marked by a singularly violent last gasping breath. Observers of such a climactic agony have found it easy to believe that a special event of some consequence has taken place, that indeed Death has come and Life has gone away. Possibly even some spirit or essence associated with Life has left the body and gone to a better world. In the circumstances surrounding the traditional deathbed, it is scarcely to be wondered at that many of the observers found comfort in personifying the dying process in this way, nor can it be said that the consequences were in any way unfortunate.

Now, however, the constant tinkering of man with his own machinery has made it obvious that death is not really a very easily identifiable event or "configuration." The integrated physiological system does not inevitably fail all at once. Substitutes can be devised for each of the major components, and the necessary integration can be provided by a computer. All the traditional vital signs are still there—provided in large part by the machines. Death does not come by inevitable appointment, in Samarra or anywhere else. He must sit patiently in the waiting room until summoned by the doctor or nurse.

Perhaps we should pause before being completely carried away by the metaphor. Has death really been kept waiting by the machines? If so, the doctor must be actively causing death when he turns the machines off. Some doctors, at least, would prefer to avoid the responsibility, and they have therefore proposed a different view of the process (Beecher 1968). They would like to believe that Death has already come for the patient whose vital signs are maintained by machine and that the doctor merely reveals the results of his visit. But if Death has already come, he has certainly come without making his presence known in the usual way. None of the outward and visible signs have occurred—no last gasp, no stopping of the heart, no cooling and stiffening of the limbs. On the other hand, it seems fairly obvious to most people that life under the conditions described (if it really is life) falls seriously short of being worth living.

Is a "Redefinition" of Death Enough?

We must now ask ourselves how much sense it makes to try to deal with this complex set of physiological, social, and ethical variables simply by "redefining" death or by developing new criteria for pronouncing an organism dead. Aside from the esoteric philosophical concerns discussed so far, it must be recognized that practical matters of great moment are at stake. Fewer and fewer people die quietly in their beds while relatives and friends live on, unable to stay the inevitable course. More and more patients are subject to long, continued intervention; antibiotics, intravenous feeding, artificial respiration, and even artificially induced heartbeats sustain an increasingly fictional existence. All this costs money—so much money, in fact, that the retirement income of a surviving spouse may disappear in a few months. There are other costs, less tangible but perhaps more important—for example, the diversion of scarce medical resources from younger people temporarily threatened by acute but potentially curable illnesses. Worst of all is the strain on a family that may have to live for years in close association with a mute, but apparently living, corpse.

An even more disturbing parameter has recently been added to the equation. It appears that parts of the dying body may acquire values greater than the whole. A heart, a kidney, someday even a lung or a liver, can mean all of life for some much younger, more potentially vigorous and happy "donee."

Indeed, it appears that it is primarily this latter set of facts which has led to recent proposals for redefining death. The most prominent proposals place more emphasis on the information-processing capacity of the brain and rather less on the purely mechanical and metabolic activities of the body as a whole than do the present practices. The great practical merit of these proposals is that they place the moment of death somewhat earlier in the continuum of life than the earlier definition did. By so doing, they make it easier for the physician to discontinue therapy while some of what used to be considered "signs of life" are still present, thus sparing relatives, friends, and professional attendants the anguish and the effort of caring for a "person" who has lost most of the attributes of personality. Furthermore, parts of the body which survive death, as newly defined, may be put to other, presumably more important uses, since procedures such as autopsies or removal of organs can be undertaken without being regarded as assaults.

In considering the propriety of developing these new criteria, one may begin by admitting that there is nothing particularly unusual about redefining either a material fact or a nebulous abstraction. Physical scientists are almost continuously engaged in redefining facts by making more and more precise measurements. Taxonomists spend much of their time redefining abstract categories, such as "species," in order to take into account new data or new prejudices. At somewhat rarer intervals, even such great concepts as force, mass, honor, and justice may come up for review.

Nevertheless, in spite of the obvious practical advantages and certain theoretical justifications, redefinition of abstractions can raise some very serious doubts. In the present instance, for example, we are brought face to face with the paradox that the new definitions of death are proposed, at least in part, because they provide that certain parts of the newly defined dead body will be *less dead* than they would have been if the conventional definition were still used. Looked at in this light, the proposed procedure raises serious ethical questions (Ramsey 1969; Jonas 1970). The supporters of the new proposal are, however, confronted every day by the even more serious practical problems raised by trying to make old rules fit new situations. Faced with a dilemma, they find it easier to urge a redefinition of death than to recognize that life may reach a state such that there is no longer an ethical imperative to preserve it. While one may give his support to the first of these alternatives as a temporary path through a frightening and increasingly complicated wilderness, it might be wise not to congratulate ourselves prematurely.

As our skill in simulating the physiological processes underlying life continues to increase in disproportion to our capacity to maintain its psychological, emotional, or spiritual quality, the difficulty of regarding death as a single, more or less coherent event, resulting in the instantaneous dissolution of the organism as a whole, is likely to become more and more apparent. It may not be premature, therefore, to anticipate some of the questions that will then increasingly press upon us. Some of the consequences of adopting the attitude that death is part of a continuous process that is coextensive (almost) with living may be tentatively outlined as follows.

An unprejudiced look at the biological facts suggests, indeed, that the "life" of a complex vertebrate like man is not a clearly defined entity with sharp discontinuities at both ends. On the contrary, the living human being starts inconspicuously, unconsciously, and at an unknown time, with the conjugation of two haploid cells. In a matter of some hours, this new cell begins to divide. The net number of living cells in the organism continues to increase for perhaps 20 years, then begins slowly to decrease. Looked at in this way, life is certainly not an all-or-none phenomenon. Clearly the amount of living matter follows a long trajectory of growth and decline with no very clear beginning and a notably indeterminate end. A similar trajectory can be traced for total energy turnover.

A human life is, of course, far more than a metabolizing mass of organic matter, slavishly obeying the laws of conservation of mass and energy. Particularly interesting are the complex interactions among the individual cells and between the totality and the environment. It is, in fact, this complexity of interaction that gives rise to the concept of human personality or soul.

Whatever metaphors are used to describe the situation, it is clear that it is the complex interactions that make the characteristic human being. The appropriate integration of these interactions is only loosely coupled to the physiological functions of circulation and respiration. The latter continue for a long time after the integrated "personality" has disappeared. Conversely, the natural rhythms of heart and respiration can fail, while the personality remains intact. The complex human organism does not often fail as a unit. The nervous system is, of course, more closely coupled to personality than are the heart and lungs (a fact that is utilized in developing the new definitions of death), but there is clearly something arbitrary in tying the sanctity of life to our ability to detect the electrical potential charges that managed to traverse the impedance of the skull.

If there is no infallible physiological index to what we value about human personality, are we not ultimately forced to make judgments about the intactness and value of the complex interactions themselves?

"Value" of a Life Changes with Value of Complex Interactions

As the complexity and richness of the interactions of an individual human being wax and wane, his "value" can be seen to change in relation to other values. For various reasons it is easier to recognize the process at the beginning than at the end of life. The growing fetus is said to become steadily more valuable with the passage of time (Callahan 1970): its organization becomes increasingly complex and its potential for continued life increases. Furthermore, its mother invests more in it every day and becomes increasingly aware of and pleased by its presence. Simultaneous with these increases in "value" is the increased "cost" of terminating the existence of the fetus. As a corollary, the longer a pregnancy proceeds, the more reasons are required to justify its termination. Although it may be possible to admire the intellectual ingenuity of Saint Thomas and others who sought to break this continuous process with a series of discontinuous stages and to identify the moment at which the fetus becomes a human being, modern knowledge of the biological process involved renders all such efforts simply picturesque. The essential novelty resides in the formation of the chromosomal pattern— the rest of the development is best regarded as the working out of a complicated tautology.

At the other end of life the process is reversed: the life of the dying patient becomes steadily less complicated and rich, and, as a result, less worth living or preserving. The pain and suffering involved in maintaining what is left are inexorably mounting, while the benefits enjoyed by the patient himself, or that he can in any way confer on those around him, are just as inexorably declining. As the costs mount higher and higher and the benefits become smaller and smaller, one may well begin to wonder what the point of it all is. These are the unhappy facts of the matter, and we will have to face them sooner or later. Indeed, attempts to face the facts are already being made, but usually in a gingerly and incomplete fashion. As we have seen, one way to protect ourselves is to introduce imaginary discontinuities into what are, in fact, continuous processes.

A similar kind of self-deception may be involved in attempts to find some crucial differences among the three following possibilities that are open to the physician attending the manifestly dying patient.

1. Use all possible means (including the "extraordinary measures" noted by the Pope) to keep the patient alive.
2. Discontinue the extraordinary measures but continue "ordinary therapy."
3. Take some "positive" step to hasten the termination of life or speed its downward trajectory.

Almost everyone now admits that there comes a time when it is proper to abandon procedure 1 and shift to procedure 2, although there is a good deal of disagreement about determining the moment itself. There is much less agreement about moving to procedure 3, although the weight of opinion seems to be against ever doing so.

The more one thinks of actual situations, however, the more one wonders if there is a valid distinction between allowing a person to die and hastening the downward course of life. Sometimes the words "positive" and "negative" are used, with the implication that it is all right to take away from the patient something that would help him to live but wrong to give him something that will help him to die.

The intent appears to be the same in the two cases, and it is the intent that would seem to be significant. Furthermore, one wonders if the dividing point between positive and negative in this domain is any more significant than the position of zero on the Fahrenheit scale. In practice, a physician may find it easier not to turn on a respirator or a cardiac pacemaker than to turn them off once they have been connected, but both the intents and the results are identical in the two cases. To use an analogy with mathematics, subtracting one from one would seem to be the same as not adding one to zero.

Squirm as we may to avoid the inevitable, it seems time to admit to ourselves that there is simply no hiding place and that we must shoulder the responsibility of deciding to act in such a way as to hasten the declining trajectories of some lives, while doing our best to slow down the decline of others. And we have to do this on the basis of some judgment on the quality of the lives in question.

Clearly the calculations cannot be made exclusively or even primarily on crude monetary or economic criteria. Substantial value must be put on intangibles of various kinds—the love, affection, and respect of those who once knew the fully living individual will bulk large in the equation. Another significant parameter will be the sanctity accorded to any human life, however attenuated and degraded it may have become. Respect for human life as such is fundamental to our society, and this respect must be preserved. But this respect need not be based on some concept of absolute value. Just as we recognize that an individual human life is not infinite in duration, we should now face the fact that its value varies with time and circumstance. It is a heavy responsibility that our advancing command over life has placed on us.

It has already been noted that in many nations, and increasingly in the United States, men and women have shouldered much the same kind of responsibility—but apparently with considerably less horror and dismay—at the beginning of the life span. In spite of some theological misgivings and medical scruples, most societies now condone the destruction of a living fetus in order to protect the life of the mother. Recent developments have greatly broadened the "indications" to include what is essentially the convenience of the mother and the protection of society against the dangers of overpopulation.

A relatively new, but very interesting, development is basing the decision of whether or not to abort purely on an assessment of the quality of the life likely to be lived by the human organism in question. This development has been greatly enhanced by advances in the technique of amniocentesis, with its associated methods for determining the chromosomal pattern and biochemical competence of the unborn baby. Decisions made on such grounds are difficult, if not impossible, to differentiate, in principle, from decisions made by the Spartans and other earlier societies to expose to nature those infants born with manifest anatomical defects. We are being driven toward the ethics of an earlier period by the inexorable logic of the situation, and it may only increase our discomfort without changing our views to reflect that historians (Lecky 1870) and moralists (Sidgwick 1886) both agree that the abolition of infanticide was perhaps the greatest ethical achievement of early Christianity.

Issue Cannot Be Settled by Absolute Standards

Callahan, in *Abortion: Law, Choice and Morality*, has reviewed all the biological, social, legal, and moral issues that bear on decisions to terminate life in its early stages and argues convincingly that the issue cannot be settled by appeals to absolute rights or standards. Of particular importance for our purposes, perhaps, is his discussion of the principle of the "sanctity of life," since opposition to liberalizing the abortion laws is so largely based on the fear of weakening respect for the dignity of life in general. It is particularly reassuring, therefore, that Callahan finds no objective evidence to support this contention. Indeed, in several countries agitation for the liberalization of abortion laws has proceeded simultaneously with efforts to strengthen respect for life in other areas—the abolition of capital punishment, for example. Indeed, Callahan's major thesis is that modern moral decisions can seldom rest on a single, paramount principle; they must be made individually after a careful weighing of the facts and all the nuances in each particular case.

The same considerations that apply to abortion would appear to apply, in principle, to decisions at the other end of the life span. In practice, however, it has proven difficult to approach the latter decisions with quite the same degree of detachment as those involving the life and death of an unborn embryo. It is not easy to overlook the fact that the dying patient possesses at least the remnants of a personality that developed over many decades and that involved a complicated set of interrelationships with other human beings. In the case of the embryo, such relationships are only potential, and it is easier to ignore the future than to overlook the past. It can be argued, however, that it should be easier to terminate a life whose potentialities have all been realized than to interrupt a pregnancy the future of which remains to be unfolded.

Once it is recognized that the process of dying under modern conditions is at least partially controlled by the decisions made by individual human beings, it becomes necessary to think rather more fully and carefully about what human beings should be involved and what kinds of considerations should be taken into account in making the decisions.

Traditionally it has been the physician who has made the decisions, and he has made them almost exclusively on his own view of what is best for the patient. Only under conditions of special stress, where available medical resources have been clearly inadequate to meet current needs, has the physician taken the welfare of third parties or "society" into account in deciding whether to give or withhold therapy. Until recently, such conditions were only encountered on the battlefield or in times of civilian catastrophe such as great fires, floods, or shipwrecks. Increasingly, however, the availability of new forms of therapy that depend on inherently scarce resources demands that decisions be made about distribution. In other words, the physician who is considering putting a patient on an artificial kidney may sometimes be forced to consider the needs of other potential users of the same device. The situation is even more difficult when the therapeutic device is an organ from another human being. In some communities, the burden of such decisions is shifted from a single physician to a group or committee that may contain nonmedical members.

These dramatic instances are often thought of as being special cases without much relationship to ordinary life and death. On the other hand, one may look upon them as simply more brilliantly colored examples of what is generally true but is not always so easy to discern. Any dying patient whose life is unduly prolonged imposes serious costs on those immediately around him, and, in many cases, on a larger, less clearly defined "society." It seems probable that, as these complex interrelationships are increasingly recognized, society will develop procedures for sharing the necessary decisions more widely, following the examples of the committee structure now being developed to deal with the dramatic cases.

It is not only probable but highly desirable that society should proceed with the greatest caution and deliberation in proposing procedures that in any serious way threaten the traditional sanctity of the individual life. As a consequence, society will certainly move very slowly in developing formal arrangements for taking into account the interests of others in life-and-death decisions. It may not be improper, however, to suggest one step that could be taken right now. Such a step might ease the way for many dying patients without impairing the sanctity or dignity of the individual life: instead, it should be enhanced. I refer here to the possibility of changing social attitudes and laws that now restrain the individual from taking an intelligent interest in his own death.

The Judeo-Christian tradition has made suicide a sin of much the same character as murder. The decline of orthodox theology has tended to reduce the sinfulness of the act, but the feeling still persists that there must be something wrong with somebody who wants to end his own life. As a result, suicide, when it is not recognized as a sin, is regarded as a symptom of serious mental illness. In this kind of atmosphere, it is almost impossible for a patient to work out with his doctor a rational and esthetically satisfactory plan for conducting the terminating phase of his life. Only rarely can a great individualist like George Eastman or Percy Bridgman (Holton 1962) transcend the prevailing mores to show us a rational way out of current prejudice. Far from injuring the natural rights of the individual, such a move can be regarded as simply a restoration of a right once greatly valued by our Roman ancestors, who contributed so much to the "natural law" view of human rights. Seneca, perhaps the most articulate advocate of the Roman view that death should remain under the individual's control, put the matter this way (Lecky 1870): "To death alone it is due that life is not a punishment, that erect beneath the frowns of fortune, I can preserve my mind unshaken and master of myself."

References

Beecher, Henry K. et al. "A Definition of Irreversible Coma." *Journal of the American Medical Association* 205 (August 1968): 337–40.

Callahan, Daniel. *Abortion: Law, Choice and Morality.* New York: Macmillan, 1970.

Holton, Gerald. "Percy Williams Bridgman." *Bulletin of Atomic Scientists* 18 (February 1962): 22–23. .

Jonas, Hans. "Philosophical Reflections on Experimenting with Human Subjects." In *Experimentation with Human Subjects,* edited by Paul A. Freund. New York: George Braziller, 1970.

Lecky, W. E. H. *History of European Morals from Augustus to Charlemagne.* New York: Appleton, 1870.

Ramsey, Paul. "On Updating Death." In *Updating Life and Death,* edited by Donald R. Cutler. Boston: Beacon Press, 1969.

Sidgwick, Henry. *Outlines of the History of Ethics.* London: Macmillan, 1886.

Whitehead, Alfred N. *Science and the Modern World.* New York: Macmillan, 1967.

6

Death as an Event:
A Commentary on Robert Morison

LEON R. KASS

AS I understand R. S. Morison's argument, it consists of these parts, although presented in different order. First: He notes that we face serious practical problems as a result of our unswerving adherence to the principle, "always prolong life." Second: Although *some* of these problems could be solved by updating the "definition of death," such revisions are scientifically and philosophically unsound. Third: The reason for this is that life and death are part of a continuum; it will prove impossible, in practice, to identify any border between them because theory tells us that no such border exists. Thus: We need to abandon both the idea of death as a concrete event and the search for its definition; instead, we must face the fact that our practical problems can only be solved by difficult judgments, based upon a complex cost-benefit analysis, concerning the value of the lives that might or might not be prolonged.

I am in agreement with Morison only on the first point. I think he leads us into philosophical, scientific, moral, and political error. Let me try to show how.

Reprinted from *Science* 173 (August 20, 1971): 698–702, with the permission of the author and publisher. Copyright © 1971 by the American Association for the Advancement of Science. Some footnotes omitted.

Some Basic Distinctions

The difficulties begin in Morison's beginning, in his failure to distinguish clearly among aging, dying, and dead. His statement that "dying is seen as a long-drawn-out process that begins when life itself begins" would be remarkable, if true, since it would render dying synonymous with living. One consequence would be that murder could be considered merely a farsighted form of euthanasia, a gift to the dying of an early exit from their miseries. But we need not ponder these riddles, because what Morison has done is to confuse dying with aging. Aging (or senescence) apparently does begin early in life (though probably not at conception), but there is no clear evidence that it is ever the cause of death. As Sir Peter Medawar (1957) has pointed out:

> Senescence, then, may be defined as that change of the bodily faculties and sensibilities and energies which accompanies aging, and which renders the individual progressively more likely to die from accidental causes of random incidence. Strictly speaking, the word "accidental" is redundant, for all deaths are in some degree accidental. No death is wholly "natural"; no one dies *merely* of the burden of the years.

As distinguished from aging, dying would be the process leading from the incidence of the "accidental" cause of death to and beyond some border, however ill-defined, after which the organism (or its body) may be said to be dead.

Morison observes, correctly, that death and life are abstractions, not things. But to hold that "livingness" or "life" is the property shared by living things, and thus to abstract this property *in thought*, does not necessarily lead one to hold that "life" or "livingness" is a thing in itself with an existence apart from the objects said to "possess" it. For reification and personification of life and death, I present no argument. For the adequacy of the abstractions themselves, we must look to the objects described.

What about these objects: living, nonliving, and dead things? A person who belives that living things and nonliving things do not differ in kind would readily dismiss "death" as a meaningless concept. It is hard to be sure that this is not Morison's view. When he says, "These objects *we elect to call* 'living things' [emphasis added]," is he merely being overly formal in his presentation, or is he deliberately intimating that the destinction between living and nonliving is simply a convention of human speech and not inherent in the nature of things? My suspicions are increased by his suggestion that "substitutes can be devised for each of the major components [of a man], and the necessary integration can be provided by a computer." A living organism comprising mechanical parts with computerized "integration"? Morison should be asked to clarify this point: Does he hold that there is or is not a *natural* distinction between living and nonliving things? Are his arguments about the fallacy of misplaced concreteness of "death" and "life" merely secondary and derivative from his belief that living and nonliving or dead objects do not differ in kind?

If there is a natural distinction between living and nonliving things, what is the proper way of stating the nature of that difference? What is the real difference between something alive and that "same" something dead? To this crucial question, I shall return later. For the present, it is sufficient to point out that the real source of our confusion about death is probably our confusion about living things. The death of an organism is not understandable because its "aliveness" is not understood except in terms of nonliving matter and motion.

One further important distinction must be observed. We must keep separate two distinct and crucial questions facing the physician: (1) When, if ever, is a person's life no longer worth prolonging? and (2) when is a person in fact dead? The first question translates, in practice, to: When is it permissible or desirable for a physician to withhold or withdraw treatment so that a patient (still alive) may be allowed to die? The second question translates, in practice, to: When does the physician pronounce the (ex)patient fit for burial? Morison is concerned only with the first question. He commendably condemns attempts to evade this moral issue by definitional wizardry. But regardless of how one settles the question of whether and what kind of life should be prolonged, one will still need criteria for recognizing the end. The determination of death may not be a very interesting question, but it is an extremely important one. At stake are matters of homicide and inheritance, of burial and religious observance, and many others.

In considering the definition and determination of death, we note that there is a difference between the meaning of an abstract concept such as death (or mass or gravity or time) and the operations used to determine or measure it. There are two "definitions" that should not be confused. There is the conceptual "definition" or meaning and the operational "definition" or meaning. I think it would be desirable to use "definition of death" only with respect to the first, and to speak of "criteria for determining that a death has occurred" for the second. Thus, the various proposals for updating the definition of death, their own language to the contrary, are not offering a new definition of death but merely refining the procedure stating that a man has died. Although there is much that could be said about these proposals, my focus here is on Morison's challenge to the concept of death as an event, and to the possibility of determining it.

The Concept of Death

There is no need to abandon the tranditional understanding of the concept of death: Death is the transition from the state of being alive to the state of being dead. Rather than emphasize the opposition between death and life, an opposition that invites Morison to see the evils wrought by personification, we should concentrate, for our purposes, on the opposition between death and birth (or conception). Both are transitions, however fraught with ambiguities. Notice that the notion of transition leaves open the question of whether the change is abrupt or gradual and whether it is continuous or discontinuous. But these questions about *when* and *how* cannot be adequately discussed without some substantive understanding of *what* it is that dies.

What dies is the organism as a whole. It is this death, the death of the individual human being, that is important for physicians and for the community, not the "death" of organs or cells, which are mere parts.

> The ultimate, most serious effect of injury is death. Necrosis is death but with this limitation; it is death of cells or tissue *within a living organism*. Thus we differentiate between *somatic death*, which is death of the whole, and *necrosis*, which is death of the part.
>
> From a tissue viewpoint, even when the whole individual dies, he dies part by part and at different times. For instance, nerve cells die within a few minutes after circulation stops, whereas cartilage cells may remain alive for several days. Because of this variation in cellular susceptibility to injury, it is virtually impossible to say just when all the component parts of the body have died. Death of composite whole, the organism as an *integrated* functional unit, is a different matter. Within three or four minutes after the heart stops beating, hypoxia ordinarily leads to irreversible changes of certain vital tissues, particularly those of the central nervous system, and this causes the *individual* to die. (Hopps 1959)

The same point may perhaps be made clearer by means of an anecdote. A recent discussion on the subject of death touched on the postmortem perpetuation of cell lines in tissue culture. Someone commented, "For all I know, I myself might wind up in one of those tissue-culture flasks." The speaker was asked to reconsider whether he really meant "I myself" or merely some of his cells.

Is Death a Discrete Event?

A proof that death is not a discrete event—that life and death are part of a continuum—would thus require evidence that the organism as a whole died progressively and continuously. This evidence Morison does not provide. Instead he calls attention to the continuity of the different ages of man and to growth and decay, but he does not show that any of these changes are analogous to the transition of death. The continuity between childhood and adolescence says nothing about whether the transition between life and death is continuous. He also mentions the "postmortem" viability of cells and organs. He says that "various parts of the body can go on living for months after its central organization has disintegrated." It should be clear by now that the viability of *parts* has no necessary bearing on the question of the whole. His claim that the beginning of life is not a discrete event ("the living human being starts inconspicuously, unconsciously, and at an unknown time, with the conjugation of two haploid cells"), even granting the relevance of the analogy with death, is really only a claim that we do not see and hence cannot note the time of the event. Morison himself more than once identifies the beginning as the discrete event in which egg and sperm unite to form the zygote, with its unique chromosomal pattern.

Only in a few places does Morison even approach the question of the death of the organism as a whole. But his treatment only serves to discredit the question. ["The nervous system is, of course, more closely coupled to personality than are the heart and lungs (a fact that is utilized in developing the new definitions of death), but there is clearly something arbitrary in tying the sanctity of life to our ability to detect the electrical potential charges that managed to traverse the impedance of the skull."] Lacking a concept of the organism as a whole, and confusing the concept of death with the criteria for determining it, Morison errs by trying to identify the whole with one of its parts and by seeking a single "infallible physiological index" to human personhood. One might as well try to identify a watch with either its mainspring or its hands; the watch is neither of these, yet it is "dead" without either. Why is the concept of the organism as a whole so difficult to grasp? Is it because we have lost or discarded, in our reductionist biology, all notions of organism, of whole?

Morison also attempts to discredit the "last gasp" as indicative of death as a discrete event: "Observers of such a climactic agony have found it easy to believe that a special event of some consequence has taken place, that indeed Death has come and Life has gone away." But if we forget about reification, personification, spirits fleeing, Death coming, Life leaving—is this not a visible sign of the death of the organism as a whole? This is surely a reasonable belief, and one which, if it now seems unreasonable, seems so only because of our tinkering.

Morison credits "the constant tinkering of man with his own machinery" for making it "obvious that death is not really a very easily identifiable event. . . ." To be sure, our tinkering has, in some cases, made it difficult to decide when the moment of death occurs, but does it really reveal that no such moment exists? Tinkering can often obscure rather than clarify reality, and I think this is one such instance. I agree that we are now in doubt about some borderline cases. But is the confusion ours or nature's? This is a crucial question. If the indeterminacy lies in nature, as Morison believes, then all criteria for determining death are arbitrary and all moments of death a fiction. If, however, the indeterminacy lies in *our* confusion and ignorance, then we must simply do the best we can in approximating the time of transition.

We are likely to remain ignorant of the true source of the indeterminacy. If so, then there is absolutely no good reason for insisting that it is nature's, and at least two good reasons for blaming ourselves. (1) It is foolish to abandon or discredit nature as a standard in matters of fundamental human importance: birth, death, health, sickness, origin. In the absence of this standard, we are left to our tastes and our prejudices about the most important human matters; we can never have knowledge, but, at best, only social policy developed out of a welter of opinion. (2) We might thereby be permitted to see how we are responsible for confusing ourselves about crucial matters, how technological intervention (with all its blessings) can destroy the visible manifestations and signs of natural phenomena, the recognition of which is indispensable to human community. Death was once recognizable by any ordinary observer who could see (or feel or hear). Today, in some difficult cases, we require further technological manipulation (from testing of reflexes to the electroencephalogram) to make manifest latent signs of a phenomenon, the visible signs of which an earlier intervention has obscured.

In the light of these remarks, I would argue that we should not take our bearings from the small number of unusual cases in which there is doubt. In most cases, there is no doubt. There is no real need to blur the distinction between a man alive and a man dead or to undermine the concept of death as an event. Rather, we should ask, in the light of our traditional concepts (though not necessarily with traditional criteria), whether the persons in the twilight zone are alive or not, and find criteria on the far side of the twilight zone in order to remove any suspicion that a man may be pronounced dead while he is yet alive.

Determining Whether a Man Has Died

In my opinion, the question, "Is he dead?" can still be treated as a question of fact, albeit one with great moral and social consequences. I hold it to be a medical-scientific question in itself, not only in that physicians answer it for us. Morison treats it largely as a social-moral question. This is because, as I indicated above, he does not distinguish the question of when a man is dead from the question of when his life is not worth prolonging. Thus, there is a conjoined issue: Is the determination of death a matter of the true, or a matter of the useful or good?

The answer to this difficult question turns, in part, on whether or not medicine and science are in fact capable of determining death. Therefore, the question of the true versus the good (or useful) will be influenced by what is in fact true and knowable about death as a medical "fact." The question of the true versus the good (or useful) will also be influenced by the truth about what is good or useful, and by what people think to be good and useful. But we can and should also ask, "What is the truth?" about which one of these concerns—scientific truth or social good—is uppermost in the minds of people who write and speak about the determination of death.

To turn to Morison's paper in the light of the last question, it seems clear that his major concern is with utility. He abandons what he calls "esoteric philosophical concerns," his own characterization of his scientific discussion about death, to turn to "practical matters of great moment." Despite his vigorous scientific criticisms of the proposals for "redefining" death, he thinks they have "great practical merit," and thus he does not really oppose them as he would any other wrong idea. Am I unfair in thinking that his philosophical and scientific criticism of the concept of death is really animated by a desire to solve certain practical problems? Would the sweeping away of the whole concept of death for the unstated purpose of forcing a cost-benefit analysis of the value of prolonging lives be any less disingenuous than a redefinition of death for the sake of obtaining organs?

Morison properly criticizes those who would seek to define a man out of existence for the purpose of getting at his organs or of saving on scarce resources. He points out that the redefiners take unfair advantage of the commonly shared belief that a body, once declared dead, can be buried or otherwise used. His stand here is certainly courageous. But does he not show an excess of courage, indeed rashness, when he would decree death itself out of existence for the sake of similar social goods? Just how rash will be seen when his specific principles of social good are examined.

The Ethics of Prolonging Life

We are all in Morison's debt for inviting us to consider the suffering that often results from slavish and limitless attempts to prolong life. But there is no need to abandon traditional ethics to deal with this problem. The Judeo-Christian tradition, which teaches us the duty of preserving life, does not itself hold life to be the absolute value. The medical tradition, until very recently, shared this view. Indeed, medicine's purpose was originally *health*, not simply the unlimited prolongation of life or the conquest of disease and death. Both traditions looked upon death as a natural part of life, not as an unmitigated evil or as a sign of the physician's failure. We sorely need to recover this more accepting attitude toward death and, with it, a greater concern for the human needs of the dying patient. We need to keep company with the dying and to help them cope with terminal illness (Kübler-Ross 1969). We must learn to desist from those useless technological interventions and institutional practices that deny to the dying what we most owe them—a good end. These purposes could be accomplished in large measure by restoring to medical practice the ethic of allowing a person to die (Ramsey 1970).

But the ethic of allowing a person to die is based solely on a consideration of the welfare of the dying patient himself, rather than on a consideration of benefits that accrue to others. This is a crucial point. It is one thing to take one's bearings from the patient and his interests and attitudes, to protect his dignity and his right to a good death against the onslaught of machinery and institutionalized loneliness; it is quite a different thing to take one's bearings from the interests of, or costs and benefits to, relatives or society. The first is in keeping with the physician's duty to act as the loyal agent of his patient; the second is a perversion of that duty, because it renders the physician, in this decisive test of his loyalty, merely an agent of society, and ultimately, her executioner. The first upholds and preserves the respect for human life and personal dignity; the second sacrifices these on the evershifting altar of public opinion.

To be sure, the physician always operates within the boundaries set by the community—by its allocation of resources, by its laws, by its values. Each physician, as well as the profession as a whole, should perhaps work to improve these boundaries and especially to see that adequate resources are made available to better the public health. But in his relations with individual patients, the physician must serve the interest of the patient. Medicine cannot retain trustworthiness or trust if it does otherwise.

On this crucial matter, Morison seems to want to have it both ways. On the one hand, he upholds the interest of the deteriorating individual himself. Morison wants him to exercise a greater control over his own death, "to work out with his doctor a rational and esthetically satisfactory plan for conducting the terminating phase of his life." On the other hand, there are hints that Morison would like to see other interests served as well. For example, he says: "It appears that parts of the dying body may acquire values greater than the whole." Greater to whom? Certainly not to the patient. We are asked to consider that "any dying patient whose life is unduly prolonged imposes serious costs on those immediately around him, and, in many cases, on a larger, less clearly defined 'society.' " But cannot the same be said for any patient whose life is prolonged? Or is Morison suggesting that the "unduliness" of "undue" prolongation is to be defined in terms of social costs? In a strictly patient-centered ethic of allowing a person to die, these costs to others would not enter—except perhaps as they might influence the patient's own judgment about prolonging his own life.

In perhaps the most revealing passage, in which he merges both the interests of patient and society, Morison notes:

> . . . the life of the dying patient becomes steadily less complicated and rich, and, as a result, less worth living or preserving. The pain and suffering involved in maintaining what is left are inexorably mounting, while the benefits enjoyed by the patient himself, or that he can in any way confer on those around him, are just as inexorably declining. As the costs mount higher and higher and the benefits become smaller and smaller, one may well begin to wonder what the point of it all is. These are the unhappy facts of the matter, and we have to face them sooner or later.

What are the implications of this analysis of costs and benefits? What should we do when we face these "unhappy facts"? The implication is clear: We must take, as the new "moment," the point at which the rising cost and declining benefit curves intersect, the time when the costs of keeping someone alive outweigh the value of his life. I suggest that it is impossible, both in principle and in practice, to locate such a moment, dangerous to try, and dangerously misleading to suggest otherwise. One simply cannot write an equation for the value of a person's life, let alone for comparing two or more lives. Life is incommensurable with the cost of maintaining it, despite Morison's suggestion that each be entered as one term in an equation.

Morison's own analogy—abortion—provides the best clue to the likely consequences of a strict adoption of his suggestions. I know he would find these consequences as abhorrent as I. No matter what one can say in favor of abortion, one can't say that it is done for the benefit of the fetus. His interests are sacrificed to those of his mother or of society at large. The analogous approach to the problem of the dying, the chronically ill, the elderly, the vegetating, the hopelessly psychotic, the weak, the infirm, the retarded—and all others whose lives might be deemed "no longer worth preserving"—points not toward suicide, but toward murder. Our age has witnessed the result of one such social effort to dispense with "useless lives."

To be fair, in the end, Morison explicitly suggests only that we make acceptable the practices of suicide and assisted suicide, or euthanasia. But in offering this patient-centered suggestion for reform, he challenges the ethics of medical practice, which has always distinguished between allowing to die and deliberately killing. Morison questions the validity of this distinction: "The intent appears to be the same in the two cases, and it is the intent that would seem to be significant." But the intent is not the same, although the outcome may be. In the one case, the intent is to desist from engaging in useless "treatments" precisely because they are no longer treatments, and to engage instead in the positive acts of giving comfort to and keeping company with the dying patient. In the other case, the intent is indeed to directly hasten the patient's death. The agent of the death in the first case is the patient's disease; in the second case, his physician. The distinction seems to me to be valuable and worth preserving.

Nevertheless, it may be true that the notion of death with dignity encompasses, under such unusual conditions as protracted, untreatable pain, the right to have one's death directly hastened. It may be an extreme act of love on the part of a spouse or a friend to administer a death-dealing drug to a loved one in such agony. In time, such acts of mercy killing may be legalized. But when and if this happens, we should insist upon at least this qualification: The hastening of the end should never be undertaken for anyone's benefit but the dying patient's. Indeed, we should insist that he spontaneously demand such assistance while of sound mind, or, if he were incapable of communication at the terminal stage, that he have made previous and very explicit arrangements for such contingencies. But we might also wish to insist upon a second qualification—that the physician not participate in the hastening. Such a qualification would uphold a cardinal principle of medical ethics: Doctors must not kill.

Summary

1. We have no need to abandon either the concept of death as an event or the efforts to set forth reasonable criteria for determining that a man has indeed died.

2. We need to recover both an attitude that is more accepting of death and a greater concern for the human needs of the dying patient. But we should not contaminate these concerns with the interests of relatives, potential transplant recipients, or "society." To do so would be both wrong and dangerous.

3. We should pause to note some of the heavy costs of technological progress in medicine: the dehumanization of the end of life, both for those

who die and for those who live on; and the befogging of the minds of intelligent and moral men with respect to the most important human matters.

References

Hopps, H. C. *Principles of Pathology*. New York: Appleton-Century-Crofts, 1959.
Kübler-Ross, Elisabeth. *On Death and Dying*. New York: Macmillan, 1969.
Medawar, P. B. *The Uniqueness of the Individual*. New York: Basic Books, 1957.
Ramsey, Paul. *The Patient as Person*. New Haven: Yale University Press, 1970.

7

A Definition of Irreversible Coma

Ad Hoc Committee of the
Harvard Medical School
to Examine the Definition of Brain Death

OUR primary purpose is to define irreversible coma as a new criterion for death. There are two reasons why there is need for a definition: (1) Improvements in resuscitative and supportive measures have led to increased efforts to save those who are desperately injured. Sometimes these efforts have only partial success so that the result is an individual whose heart continues to beat but whose brain is irreversibly damaged. The burden is great on patients who suffer permanent loss of intellect, on their families, on the hospitals, and on those in need of hospital beds already occupied by these comatose patients. (2) Obsolete criteria for the definition of death can lead to controversy in obtaining organs for transplantation.

Irreversible coma has many causes, but *we are concerned here only with those comatose individuals who have no discernible central nervous system activity.* If the characteristics can be defined in satisfactory terms, translatable into action—and we believe this is possible—then several problems will either disappear or will become more readily soluble.

More than medical problems are present. There are moral, ethical, re-

Reprinted from the *Journal of the American Medical Association* 205 (August 5, 1968): 85–88, with the permission of the authors and the publisher. Copyright © 1968 by the American Medical Association.

ligious, and legal issues. Adequate definition here will prepare the way for better insight into all of these matters as well as for better law than is currently applicable.

Characteristics of Irreversible Coma

An organ, brain or other, that no longer functions and has no possibility of functioning again is for all practical purposes dead. Our first problem is to determine the characteristics of a *permanently* nonfunctioning brain.

A patient in this state appears to be in deep coma. The condition can be satisfactorily diagnosed by points 1, 2, and 3 to follow. The electroencephalogram (point 4) provides confirmatory data, and when available it should be utilized. In situations where for one reason or another electroencephalographic monitoring is not available, the absence of cerebral function has to be determined by purely clinical signs, to be described, or by absence of circulation as judged by standstill of blood in the retinal vessels, or by absence of cardiac activity.

1. *Unreceptivity and unresponsitivity*—There is a total unawareness to externally applied stimuli and inner need and complete unresponsiveness—our definition of irreversible coma. Even the most intensely painful stimuli evoke no vocal or other response, not even a groan, withdrawal of a limb, or quickening of respiration.

2. *No movements or breathing*—Observations covering a period of at least one hour by physicians is adequate to satisfy the criteria of no spontaneous muscular movements or spontaneous respiration or response to stimuli such as pain, touch, sound, or light. After the patient is on a mechanical respirator, the total absence of spontaneous breathing may be established by turning off the respirator for three minutes and observing whether there is any effort on the part of the subject to breathe spontaneously. (The respirator may be turned off for this time provided that at the start of the trial period the patient's carbon dioxide tension is within the normal range, and provided also that the patient had been breathing room air for at least 10 minutes prior to the trial.)

3. *No reflexes*—Irreversible coma with abolition of central nervous system activity is evidenced in part by the absence of elicitable reflexes. The pupil will be fixed and dilated and will not respond to a direct source of bright light. Since the establishment of a fixed, dilated pupil is clearcut in clinical

practice, there should be no uncertainty as to its presence. Ocular movement (to head turning and to irrigation of the ears with ice water) and blinking are absent. There is no evidence of postural activity (decerebrate or other). Swallowing, yawning, vocalization are in abeyance. Corneal and pharyngeal reflexes are absent.

As a rule the stretch of tendon reflexes cannot be elicited; i.e., tapping the tendons of the biceps, triceps, and pronator muscles, quadriceps and gastrocnemius muscles with the reflex hammer elicits no contraction of the respective muscles. Plantar or noxious stimulation gives no response.

4. *Flat electroencephalogram*—Of great confirmatory value is the flat or isoelectric EEG. We must assume that the electrodes have been properly applied, that the apparatus is functioning normally, and that the personnel in charge is competent. We consider it prudent to have one channel of the apparatus used for an electrocardiogram. This channel will monitor the ECG so that, if it appears in the electroencephalographic leads because of high resistance, it can be readily identified. It also establishes the presence of the active heart in the absence of the EEG. We recommend that another channel be used for a noncephalic lead. This will pick up space-borne or vibration-borne artifacts and identify them. The simplest form of such a monitoring noncephalic electrode has two leads over the dorsum of the hand, preferably the right hand, so the ECG will be minimal or absent. Since one of the requirements of this state is that there be no muscle activity, these two dorsal hand electrodes will not be bothered by muscle artifact. The apparatus should be run at standard gains $10\mu v/$ mm, $50\mu v/5$ mm. Also it should be isoelectric at double this standard gain which is $5\mu v/mm$ or $25\mu v/5$ mm. At least ten full minutes of recording are desirable, but twice that would be better.

It is also suggested that the gains at some point be opened to their full amplitude for a brief period (5 to 100 seconds) to see what is going on. Usually in an intensive care unit artifacts will dominate the picture, but these are readily identifiable. There shall be no electroencephalographic response to noise or to pinch.

All of the above tests shall be repeated at least 24 hours later with no change.

The validity of such data as indications of irreversible cerebral damage depends on the exclusion of two conditions: hypothermia (temperature below 90°F [32.2°C]) or central nervous system depressants, such as barbiturates.

Other Procedures

The patient's condition can be determined only by a physician. When the patient is hopelessly damaged as defined above, the family and all colleagues who have participated in major decisions concerning the patient, and all nurses involved, should be so informed. Death is to be declared and *then* the respirator turned off. The decision to do this and the responsibility for it are to be taken by the physician-in-charge, in consultation with one or more physicians who have been directly involved in the case. It is unsound and undesirable to force the family to make the decision.

Legal Commentary

The legal system of the United States is greatly in need of the kind of analysis and recommendations for medical procedures in cases of irreversible brain damage as described. At present, the law of the United States, in all 50 states and in the federal courts, treats the question of human death as a question of fact to be decided in every case. When any doubt exists, the courts seek medical expert testimony concerning the time of death of the particular individual involved. However, the law makes the assumption that the medical criteria for determining death are settled and not in doubt among physicians. Furthermore, the law assumes that the traditional method among physicians for determination of death is to ascertain the absence of all vital signs. To this extent, *Black's Law Dictionary* (4th ed., 1951) defines death as "the cessation of life; the ceasing to exist; *defined by physicians* as a total stoppage of the circulation of the blood, and a cessation of the animal and vital functions consequent thereupon, such as respiration, pulsation, etc." (emphasis added). In the few modern court decisions involving a definition of death, the courts have used the concept of the total cessation of all vital signs. Two cases are worthy of examination. Both involved the issue of which one of two persons died first.

In *Thomas* v. *Anderson*, (96 Cal App 2d 371, 211 P 2d 478) a California District Court of Appeal in 1950 said, "In the instant case the question as to which of the two men died first was a question of fact for the determination of the trial court. . . ."

The appellate court cited and quoted in full the definition of death from *Black's Law Dictionary* and concluded, ". . . death occurs precisely when life ceases and does not occur until the heart stops beating and respiration ends. Death is not a continuous event and is an event that takes place at a precise time."

The other case is *Smith* v. *Smith* (229 Ark, 579, 317 SW 2d 275) decided in 1958 by the Supreme Court of Arkansas. In this case the two people were husband and wife involved in an auto accident. The husband was found dead at the scene of the accident. The wife was taken to the hospital unconscious. It is alleged that she "remained in coma due to brain injury" and died at the hospital 17 days later. The petitioner in court tried to argue that the two people died simultaneously. The judge writing the opinion said the petition contained a "quite unusual and unique allegation." It was quoted as follows:

> That the said Hugh Smith and his wife, Lucy Coleman Smith, were in an automobile accident on the 19th day of April, 1957, said accident being instantly fatal to each of them at the same time, although the doctors maintained a vain hope of survival and made every effort to revive and resuscitate said Lucy Coleman Smith until May 6th, 1957, when it was finally determined by the attending physicians that their hope of resuscitation and possible restoration of human life to the said Lucy Coleman Smith was entirely vain, and
> That as a matter of modern medical science, your petitioner alleges and states, and will offer the Court competent proof that the said Hugh Smith, deceased, and said Lucy Coleman Smith, deceased, lost their power to will at the same instant, and that their demise as earthly human beings occurred at the same time in said automobile accident, neither of them ever regaining any consciousness whatsoever.

The court dismissed the petition as a *matter of law*. The court quoted *Black's* definition of death and concluded: "Admittedly, this condition did not exist, and as a matter of fact, it would be too much of a strain of credulity for us to believe any evidence offered to the effect that Mrs. Smith was dead, scientifically or otherwise, unless the conditions set out in the definition existed." Later in the opinion the court said, "Likewise, we take judicial notice that one breathing, though unconscious, is not dead."

"Judicial notice" of this definition of death means that the court did not consider that definition open to serious controversy; it considered the question as settled in responsible scientific and medical circles. The judge thus makes proof of uncontroverted facts unnecessary so as to prevent prolonging the trial with unnecessary proof and also to prevent fraud being committed upon the court by quasi "scientists" being called into court to controvert settled scientific principles at a price. Here, the Arkansas Supreme Court considered the definition of death to be a settled, scientific, biological fact. It refused to consider the plaintiff's offer of evidence that "modern medical science" might say otherwise. In simplified form, the above is the state of the law in the United States concerning the definition of death.

In this report, however, we suggest that responsible medical opinion is ready to adopt new criteria for pronouncing death to have occurred in an individual sustaining irreversible coma as a result of permanent brain damage. If this position is adopted by the medical community, it can form the basis for change in the current legal concept of death. No statutory change in the law should be necessary since the law treats this question essentially as one of fact to be determined by physicians. The only circumstance in which it would be necessary that legislation be offered in the various states to define "death" by law would be in the event that great controversy were engendered surrounding the subject and physicians were unable to agree on the new medical criteria.

It is recommended as a part of these procedures that judgment of the existence of these criteria is solely a medical issue. It is suggested that the physician in charge of the patient consult with one or more other physicians directly involved in the case before the patient is declared dead on the basis of these criteria. In this way, the responsibility is shared over a wider range of medical opinion, thus providing an important degree of protection against later questions which might be raised about the particular case. It is further suggested that the decision to declare the person dead, and then to turn off the respirator, be made by physicians not involved in any later effort to transplant organs or tissue from the deceased individual. This is advisable in order to avoid any appearance of self-interest by the physicians involved.

It should be emphasized that we recommend the patient be declared dead before any effort is made to take him off a respirator, if he is then on a respirator. This declaration should not be delayed until he has been taken off the respirator and all artificially stimulated signs have ceased. The reason for this recommendation is that in our judgment it will provide a greater degree of legal protection to those involved. Otherwise, the physicians would be turning off the respirator on a person who is, under the present strict, technical application of law, still alive.

Comment

Irreversible coma can have various causes: cardiac arrest; asphyxia with respiratory arrest; massive brain damage; intracranial lesions, neoplastic or vascular. It can be produced by other encephalopathic states such as the metabolic derangements associated, for example, with uremia. Respiratory failure and impaired circulation underlie all of these conditions. They result in hypoxia and ischemia of the brain.

From ancient times down to the recent past it was clear that, when the respiration and heart stopped, the brain would die in a few minutes; so the obvious criterion of no heartbeat as synonymous with death was sufficiently accurate. In those times the heart was considered to be the central organ of the body; it is not surprising that its failure marked the onset of death. This is no longer valid when modern resuscitative and supportive measures are used. These improved activities can now restore "life" as judged by the ancient standards of persistent respiration and continuing heartbeat. This can be the case even when there is not the remotest possibility of an individual recovering consciousness following massive brain damage. In other situations "life" can be maintained only by means of artificial respiration and electrical stimulation of the heartbeat, or in temporarily bypassing the heart, or, in conjunction with these things, reducing with cold the body's oxygen requirement.

In an address, "The Prolongation of Life" (1957), Pope Pius XII raised many questions; some conclusions stand out: (1) In a deeply unconscious individual vital functions may be maintained over a prolonged period only by extraordinary means. Verification of the moment of death can be determined, if at all, only by a physician. Some have suggested that the moment of death is the moment when irreparable and overwhelming brain damage occurs. Pius XII acknowledged that it is not "within the competence of the Church" to determine this. (2) It is incumbent on the physician to take all reasonable, ordinary means of restoring the spontaneous vital functions and conciousness, and to employ such extraordinary means as are available to him to this end. It is not obligatory, however, to continue to use extraordinary means indefinitely in hopeless cases. "But normally one is held to use only ordinary means—according to circumstances of persons, places, times, and cultures—that is to say, means that do not involve any grave burden for oneself or another." It is the church's view that a time comes when resuscitative efforts should stop and death be unopposed.

Summary

The neurological impairment to which the terms "brain-death syndrome" and "irreversible coma" have become attached indicates diffuse disease. Function is abolished at cerebral, brainstem, and often spinal levels. This should be evident in all cases from clinical examination alone. Cerebral, cortical, and thalamic involvement are indicated by a complete absence of receptivity of all forms of sensory stimulation and a lack of response to stimuli and to inner need. The term "coma" is used to designate this state of unreceptivity and unresponsivity. But there is always coincident paralysis of brainstem and basal ganglionic mechanisms as manifested by an abolition of all postural reflexes, including induced decerebrate postures; a complete paralysis of respiration; widely dilated, fixed pupils; paralysis of ocular movements; swallowing; phonation; face and tongue muscles. Involvement of spinal cord, which is less constant, is reflected usually in loss of tendon reflex and all flexor withdrawal or nocifensive reflexes. Of the brainstem-spinal mechanisms which are conserved for a time, the vasomotor reflexes are the most persistent, and they are responsible in part for the paradoxical state of retained cardiovascular function, which is to some extent independent of nervous control, in the face of widespread disorder of cerebrum, brainstem, and spinal cord.

Neurological assessment gains in reliability if the aforementioned neurological signs persist over a period of time, with the additional safeguards that there is no accompanying hypothermia or evidence of drug intoxication. If either of the latter two conditions exist, interpretation of the neurological state should await the return of body temperature to normal level and elimination of the intoxicating agent. Under any other circumstances, repeated examinations over a period of 24 hours or longer should be required in order to obtain evidence of the irreversibility of the condition.

8

Refinements in Criteria for the Determination of Death: An Appraisal

TASK FORCE ON DEATH AND DYING OF THE INSTITUTE OF SOCIETY, ETHICS, AND THE LIFE SCIENCES

THE growing powers of medicine to combat disease and to prolong life have brought longer, healthier lives to many people. They have also brought new and difficult problems, including some which are not only medical but also fundamentally moral and political. An important example is the problem of determining whether and when a person has died—a determination that is sometimes made difficult as a direct result of new technological powers to sustain the signs of life in the severly ill and injured.

Death was (and in the vast majority of cases still is) a phenomenon known to the ordinary observer through visible and palpable manifestations, such as the cessation of respiration and heartbeat. However, in a small but growing number of cases, technological intervention has rendered insufficient these traditional signs as signs of continuing life. The heartbeat can be stimulated electrically; the heart itself may soon be replaceable by a mechanical pump. Respiration can be sustained entirely artificially with a mechanical respira-

Reprinted from the *Journal of the American Medical Association* 229 (July 3, 1972): 48–53, with the permission of the authors and publisher. Copyright © 1972 by the American Medical Association.

tor. If the patient requiring these artificial supports of vital functions is also comatose (as is often the case), there is likely to be confusion about his status and about his proper disposition.

Such confusion and uncertainty can have far-reaching and distressing consequences. Many social institutions, arrangements, and practices depend upon a clear notion of whether a person is still alive or not. At stake are matters pertaining to homicide, burial, family relations, inheritance, and indeed, all the legal and moral rights possessed by and the duties owed to a living human being. Also at stake is the role of the physician as the agent of the community empowered to determine, pronounce, and certify death. Thus, the establishment of criteria and procedures to help the physician answer the question "Is the patient dead?" would seem to be both necessary and desirable, and in the interests of everyone—patients, physicians, families, and the community.

In an effort to clear up the confusion and to provide the necessary guidelines, various individuals and groups have set forth proposals offering specific procedures, criteria, and tests to help the physician determine whether his patient has died. These proposals have been widely discussed, both by physicians and the public. While they have gained acceptance in some quarters, they have stimulated considerable controversy and criticism, and have given rise to some public disquiet. In an effort to clarify this state of affairs, an interdisciplinary task force of the Institute of Society, Ethics, and the Life Sciences has undertaken an appraisal of the proposed new criteria for determining death and of the sources of public disquiet. This article reports the results of our deliberations.

Some Basic Questions and Distinctions

An exploration of the meaning and definition of death unavoidably entails an exploration of some profound and enduring questions. To ask "What is death?" is to ask simultaneously "What makes living things alive?" To understand death as the transition between something alive and that "same" something dead presupposes that one understands the difference between "alive" and "dead," that one understands what it is that dies. Some people point out that it is possible to speak of life and death on many levels: the life and death of civilizations, families, individuals, organs, cells. Both clinical medicine and the community (and hence, also our task force) are concerned primarily with the life and death of individual human beings. The boundary between living and dead that we are seeking is the boundary that marks the death of a human organism.

Yet, even with this clarification, difficulties persist. First, the terms "human" and "organism" are ambiguous. Their meaning has been and remains the subject of intense controversy among and within many disciplines. Second, in addition to the ambiguity of each of the terms taken separately, it may make a considerable difference which of the two terms—"human" or "organism"—is given priority. Emphasis on the former might mean that the concepts of life and death would be most linked to the higher human functions, and hence, to the functioning of the central nervous system (CNS), and ultimately, of the cerebral cortex. Emphasis on the latter might mean that the concepts of life and death would be most linked to mere vegetative existence, and hence, to the functioning of the circulatory system and the heart. Finally, the concept of a "boundary" itself invites questions. How "wide" is the line between living and dead? Is there any line at all, or are "living" and "dead" parts of a continuum? Is death a process or an event? The various answers to these last questions very much depend upon the various understandings of the more fundamental ideas of "living," "dead," "human," and "organism."

We have considered some of these philosophical questions about the concept of death. . . . Not surprisingly, we have been unable to resolve many of the fundamental issues. We are convinced that some controversy concerning proper procedures for determining death is likely to persist so long as there is controversy concerning the proper concept of death. However, the present and persisting practical problems facing physicians, families, and the community need to be and can be addressed at a more practical level—by means of refinements in the criteria for determining whether death has already occurred. Hopefully, criteria can be developed that will be acceptable to persons holding various concepts of death. The rest of this report concerns itself with efforts to provide such refined criteria.

Some Criteria for Good Criteria of Death

When approaching the problem of setting down or evaluating criteria and procedures for determining death, it is worthwhile to keep in mind some formal characteristics that a set of criteria or procedures should share. We suggest that at least the following characteristics be considered.

1. The criteria should be clear and distinct, and the operational tests that are performed to see if the criteria are met should be expected to yield vivid and unambiguous results. Tests for presence or absence are to be preferred to tests for gradations of function.

2. The tests themselves should be simple, both easily and conveniently performed and interpreted by an ordinary physician (or nurse), and should depend as little as possible on the use of elaborate equipment and machinery. The determination of death should not require special consultation with specialized practitioners.

3. The procedure should include an evaluation of the permanence and irreversibility of the absence of functions and a determination of the absence of other conditions that may be mistaken for death (e.g., hypothermia, drug intoxication.)

4. The determination of death should not rely exclusively on a single criterion or on the assessment of a single function. The more comprehensive the criteria, the less likely will be the occurrence of alleged or actual errors in the final determination.

5. The criteria should not undermine but should be compatible with the continued use of the traditional criteria (cessation of spontaneous heartbeat and respiration) in the vast majority of cases where artificial maintenance of vital functions has not been in use. The revised criteria should be seen as providing an alternative means for recognizing the *same* phenomenon of death.

6. The alternative criteria, when they are used, should determine the physician's actions in the same way as the traditional criteria; that is, all individuals who fulfill either set of criteria should be declared dead by the physician as soon as he discerns that they have been fulfilled.

7. The criteria and procedures should be easily communicable, both to relatives and other laymen as well as to physicians. They should be acceptable by the medical profession as a basis for uniform practice, so that a man determined to be dead in one clinic, hospital, or jurisdiction would not be held to be alive in a different clinic, hospital, or jurisdiction, and so that all individuals who equally meet the same criteria would be treated equally, that is, declared dead. The criteria and procedures should be acceptable as

appropriate by the general public, so as to provide the operational basis for handling the numerous social matters which depend upon whether a person is dead or alive, and so as to preserve the public trust in the ability of the medical profession to determine that death has occurred.

8. The reasonableness and adequacy of the criteria and procedures should be vindicated by experience in their use and by autopsy findings.

Appraising a Specific Proposal

The most prominent proposal of new criteria and procedures for determining, in the difficult cases, that death has occurred has been offered in a Report of the Ad Hoc Committee of the Harvard Medical School to Examine the Definition of Brain Death (1968). The following criteria were presented, and described in some detail: (1) unreceptivity and unresponsivity to externally applied stimuli and inner need; (2) no spontaneous muscular movements or spontaneous respiration; (3) no elicitable brain reflexes; and (4) flat electroencephalogram. . . . In addition, the report suggests that the above findings again be verified on a repeat testing at least 24 hours later, and that the existence of hypothermia and CNS depressants be excluded. It is also recommended that, if the criteria are fulfilled, the patient be declared dead before any effort is made to disconnect a respirator. . . .

The criteria of the Harvard Committee Report meet the formal characteristics of "good" criteria, as outlined in this communication. The criteria are clear and distinct, the tests are easily performed and interpreted by an ordinary physician, and the results of the tests generally unambiguous. Some question has been raised about the ease of obtaining an adequate electroencephalographic assessment, but the report does not consider the electroencephalographic examination mandatory. It holds that the EEG provides only confirmatory data for what is, in fact, a clinical diagnosis. Recognizing that electroencephalographic monitoring may be unavailable, the report states, "when available it should be utilized."

On the score of comprehensiveness, the tests go beyond an assessment of higher brain function to include a measure of various lower brainstem (vegetative) functions, and go beyond an assessment just of brain activity by including the vital function of spontaneous respiration. It is true that the circulatory system is not explicitly evaluated. However, because of the close link between circulation and respiration, a heartbeat in a patient on a mechanical respirator (i.e., in a patient who has permanently lost his spontaneous capacity to breathe) should not be regarded as a sign of continued life. The continued beating of the heart in such cases may be regarded as an "artifact," as sustained only by continued artificial respiration.

The new criteria are meant to be necessary for only that small percentage of cases where there is irreversible coma with permanent brain damage, and where the traditional signs of death are obscured because of the intervention of resuscitation machinery. The proposal is meant to complement, not to replace, the traditional criteria of determining death. Where the latter can be clearly established, they are still determinative.

The Harvard Committee Report does not explicitly require that the physician declare the patient dead when the criteria are fulfilled; because it was a novel and exploratory proposal, it was more concerned to permit, rather than to oblige him to do so. However, once the criteria are accepted as valid by the medical profession and the community, nothing in the report would oppose making the declaration of death mandatory on fulfillment of the criteria. Thus, the alternative criteria and the traditional criteria could be—and should be—used identically in determining the physician's actions.

Experience to date in the use of these criteria and procedures for determining death suggests them to be reasonable and appropriate. Support for their validity has come from postmortem studies of 128 individuals who fulfilled the Harvard criteria. On autopsy, the brains of all 128 subjects were found to be obviously destroyed (E. Richardson, unpublished results). The electroencephalographic criterion has received an independent evaluation. The largest single study (Silverman et al. 1970), done with 2,642 comatose patients with isoelectric (i.e., flat) EEGs of 24-hours' duration, revealed that not one patient recovered (excepting three who had received anesthetic doses of CNS depressants, and who were, therefore, outside the class of patients covered by the report). Although further evidence is desirable and is now being accumulated (in studies by the American EEG Society and by the National Institute of Neurological Diseases and Stroke, among others), the criteria seem well suited to the detection of whether the patient has indeed died.

We are not prepared to comment on the precise technical aspects of each of the criteria and procedures. Medical groups, and especially neurologists and neurosurgeons, may have some corrections and refinements to offer. Nevertheless, we can see no medical, logical, or moral objection to the criteria as set forth in the Harvard Committee Report. The criteria and procedures seem to provide the needed guidelines for the physician. If adopted, they will greatly diminish the present perplexity about the status of some "patients," and will thus put an end to needless, useless, time-consuming, time-consuming, and upsetting ministrations on the part of physicians and relatives.

Causes of Concern

Despite the obvious utility and advantages of the proposed criteria and procedures, the Report of the Ad Hoc Committee of the Harvard Medical School has met with opposition, both within and outside the medical profession. Some public disquiet is to be expected when matters of life and death are at stake. In fact, little concern has been generated by the criteria themselves. Rather, the concern which has been expressed is largely due to the ways in which some people have spoken about the new criteria, and especially about the reasons why they are needed. Four causes of concern have been identified: (1) problems with concepts and language; (2) reasons behind the new criteria and the relationship of organ transplantation; (3) problems concerning the role of the physician and the procedures for establishing the new criteria; and (4) fears concerning possible further updatings of the criteria.

Problems with Concepts and Language

Some of the difficulties go back to the unresolved ambiguities surrounding the concept of death. The proliferation and indiscriminate use of terms such as clinical death, physiological death, biological death, spiritual death, mind death, brain death, cerebral death, neocortical death, body death, heart death, irreversible coma, irreversible loss of consciousness, and virtual death only add to the confusion. The multiplicity of these terms and the difficulties encountered in defining them and in relating them to one another and to the idea of death of a person testify to the need for greater clarity in our understanding of the concept of death. Pending the advent of such clarity, it should be remembered that what is needed are criteria and procedures for determining that a man has died. The various abstract terms listed above do not contribute to the devising of such criteria. They are, perhaps, best avoided. Even more to be avoided is the notion that the new criteria constitute a new or an alternative *definition* of death, rather than a refined and alternative means for detecting the same "old" phenomenon of death.

A second confusion concerns the relation of the "medical" and "legal" definitions of death. Some commentators have drawn a sharp distinction between these two definitions, and have even gone so far as to say that a given individual died medically on one day and legally on another. This is loose, misleading, and probably incorrect usage. It is true that the law offers its own various "definitions" of "death" to serve its own various purposes—for example, in deciding about inheritance or survivorship. But these so-called "definitions" of "death" are in fact only definitions of "who shall inherit." With regard to the actual biological phenomenon of death, the law generally treats the matter as a medical question of fact, to be determined according to criteria established by physicians. No statutory change in the law will be necessary once the medical profession itself adopts the new criteria—provided, of course, that the public does not object.

A third confusion concerns the use of the term "arbitrary" to describe the new criteria. It is the arbitrary (in the sense of "capricious," "without justification") conduct of physicians that the public fears in regard to the definition of death. To be sure, the criteria are manmade, the result of human decision and arbitrament, but they are in no sense capricious. The selection of 24 hours as the waiting period between examinations is, it is true, arbitrary in the sense that it could just as well have been 20 hours or 30 hours. But the selection of 24 hours was considered reasonable, i.e., sufficient to check for any reversibility in the signs of death. The criteria themselves, far from being arbitrary, have been selected as best suited to reveal the phenomenon of death.

A fourth confusion is especially serious, since it goes to the very heart of what is being done and why. Some have spoken of the criteria enunciated by the Harvard Committee Report as criteria for stopping the use of extraordinary means to keep a patient alive. (Actually, the report itself invokes the statement of Pope Pius XII to the effect that there is no obligation on the part of the physician to employ extraordinary means to prolong life.) This language serves to confuse the question of the determination of death with a second important question facing the physician, namely, "When is it desirable or permissible to withdraw or withhold treatment so that a patient (unquestionably still alive) may be allowed to die?" The only question being considered in this communication, and by the Ad Hoc Committee, is

"When does the physician pronounce the (ex)patient dead?" The two questions need to be kept apart.

Reasons behind the New Criteria:
The Relation of Transplantation

Following the first heart transplantation, there appeared in the medical literature and in the popular press a series of articles calling for clarification of the criteria for determining death. Some called for an "updating" of the criteria to facilitate the work of the transplant surgeons and the taking of organs. Others asked for the establishment of agreed-upon guidelines to protect the integrity of the donor against possible premature organ removal or to protect the physician against possible charges of malpractice, or even of homicide. The frequent mention of organ transplantation in connection with proposals offering new criteria of death has created an uneasiness on the part of many people—including some physicians (Rutstein 1969; Toole 1971) and also a few members of this task force (Jonas 1969; Ramsey 1970)—that the need for organs for transplant has influenced, or might sometime in the future influence, the criteria and procedures actually proposed for determining that death has occurred.

While we cannot deny the fact that the growth of the practice of transplantation with cadaveric organs provided a powerful stimulus to reassess the criteria for determining death, the members of this task force are in full agreement that the need for organs is not and should not be a reason for changing these criteria, and especially for selecting any given criterion or procedure. Choice of the criteria for pronouncing a man dead ought to be completely independent of whether or not he is a potential donor of organs. The procedures, criteria, and the actual judgment in determining the death of one human being must not be contaminated with the needs of others, no matter how legitimate those needs may be. The medical profession cannot retain trust if it does otherwise, or if the public suspects (even wrongly) that it does otherwise.

There are ample reasons, both necessary and sufficient, and independent of the needs of potential transplant recipients, of the patient's family and of society, for clarifying and refining the criteria and procedures for pronouncing a man dead. It is the opinion of the task force that the widespread adoption and use of the Harvard Committee's (or similar) clearly defined criteria will, in fact, allay public fears of possibly arbitrary or mischievous practices on the part of some physicians. We also believe that if the criteria for determining death are set wholly independently of the need for organs, there need be no reticence or embarrassment in making use of any organs which may actually become more readily available if the criteria are clarified (provided, of course, that other requirements of ethical medical practice are met).

Problems Concerning the Role of the Physician and the Procedures for Establishing the New Criteria

Even if it has been agreed that there is a need for a revision of the traditional definition or criteria of death, there remain questions of who is to make the revision, and how (i.e., according to what procedure) that revision is to be made. There are at least five levels where decisions are made with respect to the death of a human being: (1) establishing a concept of death; (2) selecting general criteria and procedures for determining that a patient has died; (3) determining in the particular case that the patient meets the criteria; (4) pronouncing him dead; and (5) certifying the death on a certificate of record. Until recently, because there was tacit agreement on the concept of death, our society was content to leave the last four matters solely in the hands of physicians. At the present time, opinion is divided on the proper role and authority of the physician, especially with respect to the first two decisions. Some have questioned the status and authority of the various groups who have proposed new criteria. Some have questioned whether the decision to move to a "brain-centered" concept of life and death is a decision to be left to the medical profession, whereas others have questioned whether any other profession or group may be any more qualified. Some have called for the establishment of a definition of death by legal statute.

The state of Kansas has recently enacted a statute which establishes two alternative concepts of death (it refers to them as "definitions of death"): permanent absence of spontaneous respiratory and cardiac function, and permanent absence of spontaneous brain activity. The specific criteria are left to "ordinary standards of medical practice." Both the desirability of this law and its specific language have recently been attacked (Kennedy 1971) and defended (Curran 1971; Mills 1971). The controversy over the Kansas statute has illuminated some of the advantages and disadvantages of legislation in this area. We are sympathetic to the value of having any changes in the concept of death, or even major changes in criteria for determining death, ratified by the community, as a sign of public acceptance and for the legal protection of physicians. On the other hand, we are concerned about the possibility of confused, imprecisely drafted, or overly rigid statutes. Moreover, we do not believe that legislation is absolutely necessary in order to permit physicians to use the new criteria, once these receive the endorsement and support of the medical profession. Clearly, these matters of decision making and the role of law need further and widespread discussion. The acceptability of any new concept or criteria of death will depend at least as much on the acceptability of the procedure by which they are adopted as on their actual content. The precedents now established are likely to be very important, given the likelihood that the increase of organ transplantation or the rising costs of caring for the terminally ill will produce renewed pressures to alter again concepts and criteria of death.

Fears Concerning Possible Further Updatings of the Criteria

The fear of being pronounced dead prematurely is an understandable human fear, and, in some earlier ages, a justifiable fear based upon actual premature burials. A similar fear may be behind the concern that current revisions in criteria for determining death will serve as precedents for future updatings, with the result that persons who would be considered alive by today's criteria will be declared dead by tomorrow's criteria. In protest against this prospect, one commentary (Rot and VanTill 1971) has put the matter succinctly and well: "A living body turns into a corpse by biological reasons only—not by declarations, or the signing of certificates."

Recent proposals to place exclusive reliance on electroencephalography for the determination of death may be said to represent a current example of efforts to further update the criteria. In accord with other commentators (Toole), we view this prospect with some concern. Leaving aside technical questions having to do with the reliability of the electroencephalographic evaluations, we wish to comment on some of the assumptions underlying the proposed shift away from the recommendation that the EEG be used as a *confirmatory* adjunct to the clinical determination of death, and not as a definitive criterion.

Most such proposals appear to rest on three assumptions: (1) that the existence of human life, no less than its essence, is defined in terms of activities normally associated with higher brain function; (2) that such activities are exclusively centered in the anatomical locus known as the neocortex; and (3) that the EEG provides a full and complete measure of neocortical function. From these assumptions, the following conclusion is drawn: In the absence of a functioning neocortex, as determined by an isoelectric EEG, human life has ceased.

These assumptions appear to be sufficiently questionable to rule out exclusive reliance on the EEG for determinations of death: the first on purely philosophical grounds, and the second and third on the strength of preliminary experimental findings. For example, the second assumption that activities like instrumental learning and cognition reside entirely in the neocortex has now been called into question by a recent report (Oakley 1971) describing evidence for instrumental learning in neodecorticate rabbits.

The overall conclusion that an isoelectric EEG signifies the end of human life must be questioned in the light of a recent article (Brierly et al. 1971) reporting that patients with isoelectric EEGs (and subsequently verified anatomical death of their neocortices) continued to breathe spontaneously for up to six months. The authors of this study express uncertainty as to whether or not such decorticate patients should be declared dead. While they agree that the Harvard criteria pointed clearly to a diagnosis of "alive," they imply that they have some difficulty with this conclusion. While an isoelectric EEG may be grounds for interrupting all forms of treatment and allowing these patients to die, it cannot itself be the basis for declaring dead someone who is still spontaneously breathing and who still has intact cerebral reflexes. It is inconceivable that society or the medical profession would allow the preparation of such persons for burial. To prevent such confusion and the possible dangerous practices that might result from a shift to exclusive reliance on the EEG, we urge that the clinical and more comprehensive criteria of the Harvard Report be adopted. We are supported in this conclusion by the report (Silverman et al. 1969) that a majority of neurologists have rejected the proposition that EEG determinations are sufficient as the sole basis for a determination of death.

References

Brierley, J. B.; D. I. Graham; J. H. Adams; and J. A. Simpson. "Neocortical Death after Cardiac Arrest." *Lancet* 2 (September 1971): 560–65.

Curran, William J. "Legal and Medical Death: Kansas Takes the First Step." *New England Journal of Medicine* 284 (1971): 260–61.

Jonas, Hans. "Philosophical Reflections on Experimenting with Human Subjects." *Daedalus* 98 (Spring 1969); 219–47.

Kennedy, Ian McColl. "The Kansas Statute on Death—An Appraisal." *New England Journal of Medicine* 285 (October 1971): 946–50.

Mills, Don Harper. "The Kansas Death Statute—Bold and Innovative." *New England Journal of Medicine* 285 (October 1971); 968–69.

Oakley, David A. "Instrumental Learning in Neodecorticate Rabbits." *Nature: New Biology* 233 (October 1971): 185–87.

Ramsey, Paul. *The Patient as Person*. New Haven: Yale University Press, 1970.

Rot, Anne, and H. A. H. vanTill. "Neocortical Death after Cardiac Arrest." *Lancet* 2 (November 1971): 1099–1100.

Rutstein, David D. "The Ethical Design of Human Experiments." *Daedalus* 98 (Spring 1969): 523–41.

Silverman, Daniel; Richard L. Masland; Michael G. Saunders; and Robert S. Schwab. "EEG and Cerebral Death: the Neurologist's View." *Electroencephalography and Clinical Neurophysiology* 27 (November 1969): 549.

—— "Irreversible Coma Associated with Electrocerebral Silence." *Neurology* 20 (June 1970); 525–33.

Toole, James F. "The Neurologist and the Concept of Brain Death." *Perspectives in Biology and Medicine* 14 (Summer 1971); 599–607.

9

A Statutory Definition of the Standards for Determining Human Death: An Appraisal and a Proposal

ALEXANDER MORGAN CAPRON AND LEON R. KASS

IN RECENT years, there has been much discussion of the need to refine and update the criteria for determining that a human being has died. In light of medicine's increasing ability to maintain certain signs of life artificially and to make good use of organs from newly dead bodies, new criteria of death have been proposed by medical authorities. Several states have enacted or are considering legislation to establish a statutory "definition of death," at the prompting of some members of the medical profession who apparently feel that existing, judicially framed standards might expose physicians, particularly transplant surgeons, to civil or criminal liability. Although the leading statute in this area (Kansas 1970) appears to create more problems than it resolves, some legislation may be needed for the protection of the public as well as the medical profession, and, in any event, many more states will probably be enacting such statutes in the near future.

Reprinted from the *University of Pennsylvania Law Review* 121 (November 1972): 87–118, with the permission of the publisher. Copyright © 1972 by the University of Pennsylvania. Some footnotes omitted.

I. Background

Courts and physicians can no longer assume that determining whether and when a person has died is always a relatively simple matter. The development and use of sophisticated machinery to maintain artificially both respiration and circulation has introduced difficulties in making this determination in some instances. In such cases, the use of a cardiac pacemaker or a mechanical respirator renders doubtful the significance of the traditional "vital signs" of pulse, heartbeat, and respiratory movements as indicators of continuing life. Similarly, the ability of an organ recipient to go on living after his own heart has been removed and replaced by another's has further undermined the status of the beating heart as one of the most reliable—if not *the* most reliable—signs that a person is still alive. In addition, the need of transplant surgeons to obtain organs in good condition from cadavers has stimulated the search for tests that would permit the death of the organism as a whole to be declared before the constituent organs have suffered extensive deterioration. Consequently, new criteria for judging a person dead have been proposed and are gaining acceptance among physicians. The most prominent are those formulated in 1968 by the Harvard Medical School's Ad Hoc Committee to Examine the Definition of Brain Death, chaired by Dr. Henry K. Beecher.

The Harvard Committee described in considerable detail three criteria of "irreversible coma": (1) "unreceptivity and unresponsivity" to "externally applied stimuli and inner need"; (2) absence of spontaneous muscular movements or spontaneous respiration; and (3) no elicitable reflexes. In addition, a flat (isoelectric) electroencephalogram was held to be "of great confirmatory value" for the clinical diagnosis. Although generally referred to as criteria for "cerebral death" or "brain death," these criteria assess not only higher brain functions but brainstem and spinal cord activity and spontaneous respiration as well. The accumulating scientific evidence (Silverman et al. 1970) indicates that patients who meet the Harvard criteria will not recover and on autopsy will be found to have brains which are obviously destroyed, and supports the conclusion that these criteria may be useful for determining that death has occurred. The Harvard Committee's views were apparently well received in the medical community. Not all physicians have been enthusiastic, however. Professor David Rutstein (1969) of the Harvard Medical School, for example, expressed concern over "this major ethical change [which] has occurred right before our eyes . . . with little public discussion of its significance."

Not surprisingly, disquiet over the change in medical attitude and practice arose in lay as well as medical circles. The prospect of physicians agreeing amongst themselves to change the rules by which life is measured in order to salvage a larger number of transplantable organs met with something short of universal approval. Especially with increasing disenchantment over heart transplantation (the procedure in which the traditional criteria for determining death posed the most difficulties), some doubt arose whether it was wise to adopt measures which encouraged a medical "advance" that seemed to have gotten ahead of its own basic technology. Furthermore, many people—doctors included—found themselves with nagging if often unarticulated doubts about how to proceed in the situation, far more common than transplantation, in which a long-comatose patient shows every prospect of "living" indefinitely with artificial means of support. As a result of this growing public and professional concern, elected officials, with the encouragement of the medical community, have urged public discussion and action to dispel the apprehension created by the new medical knowledge and to clarify and reformulate the law. Some commentators (Kennedy 1971), however, have argued that public bodies and laymen in general have no role to play in this process of change. Issue is therefore joined on at least two points: (1) ought the public to be involved in "defining" death? and (2) if so, how ought it to be involved—specifically, should governmental action, in the form of legislation, be taken?

II. Public Involvement or Professional Prerogative?

In considering the possible need for and the desirability of public involvement, the central question appears to be to what extent, if at all, the "defining" of death is a medical matter, properly left to physicians because it lies within their particular sphere of competence. The belief that the matter of "defining death" is wholly medical is frequently expressed, and not only by physicians. Indeed, when a question concerning the moment at which a person died has arisen in litigation, common-law courts have generally regarded this as "a question of fact" for determination at trial on the basis (partially but not exclusively) of expert medical testimony. Yet the standards which are applied in arriving at a conclusion, although based on medical knowledge, are established by the courts "as a matter of law."

Thus while it is true that the application of particular criteria or tests to determine the death of an individual may call for the expertise of a physician, there are other aspects of formulating a "definition" of death that are not particularly within medical competence. To be sure, in practice, so long as the standards being employed are stable and congruent with community opinion about the phenomena of death, most people are content to leave the matter in medical hands. But the underlying extramedical aspects of the "definition" become visible, as they have recently, when medicine departs (or appears to depart) from the common or traditional understanding of the concept of death. The formulation of a concept of death is neither simply a technical matter nor one susceptible of empirical verification. The idea of death is at least partly a philosophical question, related to such ideas as "organism," "human," and "living." Physicians *qua* physicians are not expert on these philosophical questions, nor are they expert on the question of which physiological functions decisively identify a "living, human organism." They, like other scientists, can suggest which "vital signs" have what significance for which human functions. They may, for example, show that a person in an irreversible coma exhibits "total unawareness to externally applied stimuli and inner need and complete unresponsiveness" (Harvard report), and they may predict that when tests for this condition yield the same results over a 24-hour period there is only a very minute chance that the coma will ever be "reversed" (Silverman et al.). Yet the judgment that "total unawareness . . . and complete unresponsiveness" are the salient characteristics of death, or that a certain level of risk of error is acceptable, requires more than technical expertise and goes beyond medical authority, properly understood.

The proposed departure from the traditional standards for determining death not only calls attention to the extramedical issues involved, but is itself a source of public confusion and concern. The confusion can perhaps be traced to the fact that the traditional signs of life (the beating heart and the expanding chest) are manifestly accessible to the senses of the layman, whereas some of the new criteria require sophisticated intervention to elicit latent signs of life such as brain reflexes. Furthermore, the new criteria may disturb the layman by suggesting that these visible and palpable traditional signs, still useful in most cases, may be deceiving him in cases where supportive machinery is being used. The anxiety may also be attributable to the apparent intention behind the "new definition," which is, at least in part, to facilitate other developments such as the transplantation of cadaver organs. Such confusion and anxiety about the standards for determining death can have far-reaching and distressing consequences for the patient's family, for the physician, for other patients, and for the community at large. If the uncertainties surrounding the question of determining death are to be laid to rest, a clear and acceptable standard is needed. And if the formulation and adoption of this standard are not to be abdicated to the medical fraternity under an expanded view of its competence and authority, then the public and its representatives ought to be involved. Even if the medical profession takes the lead—as indeed it has—in promoting new criteria of death, members of the public should at least have the opportunity to review, and either to affirm or reject the standards by which they are to be pronounced dead.

III. What Manner of Public Involvement?

There are a number of potential means for involving the public in this process of formulation and review, none of them perfect. The least ambitious or comprehensive is simply to encourage discussion of the issues by the lay press, civic groups, and the community at large. This public consideration might be directed or supported through the efforts of national organizations such as the American Medical Association, the National Institutes of Health, or the National Academy of Sciences. A resolution calling for the establishment of an ad hoc body to evaluate public attitudes toward the changes wrought by biomedical advances has been sponsored by Senator Mondale since 1967 and was adopted by the Senate in December 1971.[1] Mondale's proposed National Advisory Commission on Health Science and Society, under the direction of a board of 15 members of the general public and professionals from "medicine, law, theology, biological science, physical science, social science, philosophy, humanities, health administration, government, and public affairs," would conduct "seminars and public hearings" as part of its two-year study. As important as it is to ventilate the issues,

[1] S.J. Res. 75, 92d Cong., 1st sess. 1971, in 117 Cong. Rec. S20, 089-93 (daily ed. Dec. 2, 1971).

studies and public discussions alone may not be adequate to the task. They cannot by themselves dispel the ambiguities which will continue to trouble decision makers and the public in determining whether an artificially maintained, comatose "patient" is still alive.

A second alternative, reliance upon the judicial system, goes beyond ascertaining popular attitudes and could provide an authoritative opinion that might offer some guidance for decision makers. Reliance on judge-made law would, however, neither actively involve the public in the decision-making process nor lead to a prompt, clear, and general "definition." The courts, of course, cannot speak in the abstract prospectively, but must await litigation, which can involve considerable delay and expense, to the detriment of both the parties and society. A need to rely on the courts reflects an uncertainty in the law which is unfortunate in an area where private decision makers (physicians) must act quickly and irrevocably. An ambiguous legal standard endangers the rights—and in some cases the lives—of the participants. In such circumstances, a person's choice of one course over another may depend more on his willingness to test his views in court than on the relative merits of the courses of action.

Once called upon to "redefine" death—for example, in a suit brought by a patient's relatives or, perhaps, by a revived "corpse" against the physician declaring death—the judiciary may be as well qualified to perform the task as any governmental body. If the issue could be resolved solely by a process of reasoning and of taking "judicial notice" of widely known and uncontroverted facts, a court could handle it without difficulty. If, on the other hand, technical expertise is required problems may arise. Courts operate within a limited compass—the facts and contentions of a particular case—and with limited expertise; they have neither the staff nor the authority to investigate or to conduct hearings in order to explore such issues as public opinion or the scientific merits of competing "definitions." Consequently, a judge's decision may be merely a rubberstamping of the opinions expressed by the medical experts who appear before him. Indeed, those who believe that the "definition of death" should be left in the hands of physicians favor the judicial route over the legislative on the assumption that, in the event of a lawsuit, the courts will approve "the consensus view of the medical profession" (Kennedy 1971) in favor of the new standards. Leaving the task of articulating a new set of standards to the courts may prove unsatisfactory, however, if one believes, as suggested previously, that the formulation of such standards, as opposed to their application in particular cases, goes beyond the authority of the medical profession.

Uncertainties in the law are, to be sure, inevitable at times and are often tolerated if they do not involve matters of general applicability or great moment. Yet the question of whether and when a person is dead plainly seems the sort of issue that cannot escape the need for legal clarity on these grounds. Therefore, it is not surprising that although they would be pleased simply to have the courts endorse their views, members of the medical profession are doubtful that the judicial mode of lawmaking offers them adequate protection in this area. There is currently no way to be certain that a doctor would not be liable, criminally or civilly, if he ceased treatment of a person found to be dead according to the Harvard Committee's criteria but not according to the "complete cessation of all vital functions" test presently employed by the courts. Although such "definitions" were adopted in cases involving inheritors' rights and survivorship rather than a doctor's liability for exercising his judgment about when a person has died, physicians have with good reason felt that this affords them little assurance that the courts would not rely upon those cases as precedent. On the contrary, it is reasonable to expect that the courts would seek precedent in these circumstances. Adherence to past decisions is valued because it increases the likelihood that an individual will be treated fairly and impartially; it also removes the need to relitigate every issue in every case. Most importantly, courts are not inclined to depart from existing rules because to do so may upset the societal assumption that one may take actions, and rely upon the actions of others, without fear that the ground rules will be changed retroactively.

Considerations of precedent as well as other problems with relying on the judicial formulation of a new definition were made apparent in *Tucker* v. *Lower*,[2] the first case to present the question of the "definition of death" in the context of organ transplantation. Above all, this case demonstrates the uncertainty that is inherent in the process of litigation, which was touch and go for the medical profession as well as the defendents. *Tucker* involved a $100,000 damage action against Drs. David Hume and Richard Lower and other defendant doctors on the Medical College of Virginia transplant team, brought by William E. Tucker, whose brother's heart was removed on May 25, 1968, in the world's seven-

[2] No. 2831 (Richmond, Va., L. & Eq. Ct., May 23, 1972).

teenth human heart transplant. The plaintiff claimed that the heart was taken without approval of the next of kin and that the operation was commenced before his brother had died. On the latter point, William Tucker offered evidence that his brother was admitted to the hospital with severe head injuries sustained in a fall and that after a neurological operation he was placed on a respirator. At the time he was taken to the operating room to have his organs removed "he maintained vital signs of life, that is, . . . normal body temperature, normal pulse, normal blood pressure and normal rate of respiration." Based on the neurologist's finding that the brother was dead from a neurological standpoint, the respirator was turned off and he was pronounced dead. The defendants moved to strike the plaintiff's evidence and for summary judgment in their favor, but the trial judge denied the motions.

The function of This Court is to determine the state of the law on this or any other subject according to legal precedent and principle. The courts which have had occasion to rule upon the nature of death and its timing have all decided that death occurs at a precise time, and that it is defined as the cessation of life; the ceasing to exist; a total stoppage of the circulation of the blood, and a cessation of the animal and vital functions consequent thereto such as respiration and pulsation.

The court adhered to "the legal concept of death" and rejected "the invitation offered by the defendants to employ a medical concept of neurological death in establishing a rule of law." The court ruled that the jury would be allowed to assess damages if it concluded "that the decedent's life was terminated at a time earlier than it would ordinarily have ended had all reasonable medical efforts been continued to prolong his life."

When he sent the case to the jurors, however, the judge permitted them to consider all possible causes of death, including injury to the brain as well as cessation of breathing or heartbeat, and a verdict was returned for the defendants. Unfortunately, the discrepancy between the initial ruling and the subsequent instructions to the jury did little to resolve the legal uncertainty. The plaintiff has announced that he plans to appeal to the Supreme Court of Virginia, and the creation of a clear and binding rule will depend on the action of that court.

In declining the defendants' suggestion that he adopt a standard based on neurological signs, the judge stated that application for "such a radical change" in the law should be made "not to the courts but to the legislature wherein the basic concepts of our society relating to the preservation and extension of life could be examined, and, if necessary, reevaluated." A statutory "definition" of death would have notable advantages as an alternative to a judicial promulgation. Basically, the legislative process permits the public to play a more active role in decision making and allows a wider range of information to enter into the framing of criteria for determining death. Moreover, by providing prospective guidance, statutory standards could dispel public and professional doubt, and could provide needed reassurance for physicians and patients' families, thereby reducing both the fear and the likelihood of litigation for malpractice (or even for homicide).

The legislative alternative also has a number of drawbacks, however. Foremost among these is the danger that a statute "defining" death may be badly drafted. It may be either too general or too specific, or it may be so poorly worded that it will leave physicians or laymen unsure of its intent. There is also the danger that the statutory language might seem to preclude future refinements that expanding medical knowledge would introduce into the tests and procedures for determining death. The problem of bad draftsmanship is compounded by the fact that a statute once enacted may be difficult to revise or repeal, leaving to the slow and uncertain process of litigation the clarification of its intent and meaning. By contrast, although judges usually espouse the doctrine of stare decisis, flexibility over time is a hallmark of the common law. An additional practical problem is the possibility that the statutes enacted may reflect primarily the interests of powerful lobbying groups—for example, state medical societies or transplant surgeons. This possibility—similar to the danger of judicial "rubberstamping" of medical experts' opinions—may be avoided by legislatures' holding open and well-publicized hearings at which sociologists, lawyers, theologians, and representatives of various viewpoints are also called upon to testify.

Professor Ian Kennedy (1971) has suggested the further danger that a statutory "definition," rather than protecting the public, may leave it vulnerable to physicians who through "liberal interpretation and clever argument" might take actions "just within the letter if not the spirit of the law." Kennedy would rely instead on the medical profession's generalized "consensus view" of the proper "definition of death." It is, however, far from clear why physicians who would violate a statute are unlikely to depart from such an informal "consensus," which may or may not eventually be sanctioned by the courts. Legislation will not remove the need for reasoned interpretation—first by physicians and perhaps then by judges—but it can restrict the compass within which they make their choices to one which has been found acceptable by the public.

Finally, the legislative route may reduce the likelihood that conflicting "definitions" of death will be employed in different jurisdictions in this country. Theoretically, uniformity is also possible in judicial opinions, but it occurs infrequently. If the formulation and reception of the Uniform Anatomical Gift Act provide any precedent, the Commissioners on Uniform State Laws appear to be well situated to provide leadership in achieving an intelligent response to changes in medical procedure.

In sum, then, official action, as opposed to mere discussion of the issues, is needed if the conflict between current medical practice and present law is to be eliminated. A reformulation of the standards for determining death should thus be undertaken by either courts or legislatures. There are strengths and weaknesses in both law-creating mechanisms, but on balance we believe that if legislators approach the issues with a critical and inquiring attitude, a statutory "definition" of death may be the best way to resolve the conflicting needs for definiteness and flexibility, for public involvement and scientific accuracy. Moreover, since pressures for a legislative response to the problem appear to be mounting, careful examination of the proper scope and content of such a statute seems to be called for.

IV. What Can and Should Be Legislated?

Arguments both for and against the desirability of legislation "defining" deaths often fail to distinguish among the several different subjects that might be touched on by such legislation. As a result, a mistaken impression may exist that a single statutory model is, and must be, the object of debate. An appreciation of the multiple meanings of a "definition of death" may help to refine the deliberations.

Death, in the sense the term is of interest here, can be defined purely formally as the transition, however abrupt or gradual, between the state of being alive and the state of being dead. There are at least four levels of "definitions" that would give substance to this formal notion; in principle, each could be the subject of legislation: (1) the basic concept or idea; (2) general physiological standards; (3) operational criteria, and (4) specific tests or procedures.

The *basic concept* of death is fundamentally a philosophical matter. Examples of possible "definitions" of death at this level include "permanent cessation of the integrated functioning of the organism as a whole" "departure of the animating or vital principle," or "irreversible loss of personhood." These abstract definitions offer little concrete help in the practical task of determining whether a person has died, but they may very well influence how one goes about devising standards and criteria.

In setting for the *general physiological standard(s)* for recognizing death, the definition moves to a level which is more medioco-technical, but not wholly so. Philosophical issues persist in the choice to define death in terms of organ systems, physiological functions, or recognizable human activities, capacities, and conditions. Examples of possible general standards include "irreversible cessation of spontaneous respiratory and/or circulatory functions," "irreversible loss of spontaneous brain functions," "irreversible loss of the ability to respond or communicate," or some combination of these.

Operational criteria further define what is meant by the general physiological standards. The absence of cardiac contraction and lack of movement of the blood are examples of traditional criteria for "cessation of spontaneous circulatory functions," whereas deep coma, the absence of reflexes, and the lack of spontaneous muscular movements and spontaneous respiration are among criteria proposed for "cessation of spontaneous brain functions" by the Harvard Committee.

Fourth, there are the *specific tests and procedures* to see if the criteria are fulfilled. Pulse, heartbeat, blood pressure, electrocardiogram, and examination of blood flow in the retinal vessels are among the specific tests of cardiac contraction and movement of the blood. Reaction to painful stimuli, appearance of the pupils and their responsiveness to light, and observation of movement and breathing over a specified time period are among specific tests of the "brain function" criteria enumerated above.

There appears to be general agreement that legislation should not seek to "define death" at either the most general or the most specific levels (the first and fourth). In the case of the former, differences of opinion would seem hard to resolve, and agreement, if it were possible, would provide little guidance for practice. In the case of the latter, the specific tests and procedures must be kept open to changes in medical knowledge and technology. Thus, arguments concerning the advisability and desirability of a statutory definition of death are usually confined to the two levels we have called "standards" and "criteria," yet often without any apparent awareness of the distinction between them. The need for flexibility in the face of medical advance would appear to be a persuasive argument for not legislating any specific operational criteria. Moreover, these are almost exclusively technical matters, best left to the judgment of physicians. Thus, the kind of "definition" suitable for legislation would be a definition of the general physiological standard or standards. Such a definition, while not immutable, could be expected to be useful for a long period of time and would therefore not require frequent amendment.

There are other matters that could be comprehended in legislation "defining" death. The statute could specify who (and how many) shall make the determination. In the absence of a compelling reason to change past practices, this may continue to be set at "a physician" (Uniform Anatomical Gift Act), usually the doctor attending a dying patient or the one who happens to be at the scene of an accident. Moreover, the law ought probably to specify the "time of death." The statute may seek to fix the precise time when death may be said to have occurred, or it may merely seek to define a time that is clearly after "the precise moment," that is, a time when it is possible to say "the patient is dead," rather than "the patient has just now died." If the medical procedures used in determining that death has occurred call for verification of the findings after a fixed period of time (for example, the Harvard Committee's recommendation that the tests be repeated after 24 hours), the statute could in principle assign the "moment of death" to either the time when the criteria were first met or the time of verification. The former has been the practice with the traditional criteria for determining death.

Finally, legislation could speak to what follows upon the determination. The statute could be permissive or prescriptive in determining various possible subsequent events, including especially the pronouncement and recording of the death, and the use of the body for burial or other purposes. It is our view that these matters are best handled outside of a statute which has as its purpose to "define death."

V. Principles Governing the Formulation of a Statute

In addition to carefully selecting the proper degree of specificity for legislation, there are a number of other principles we believe should guide the drafting of a statute "defining" death. First, the phenomenon of interest to physicians, legislators, and laymen alike is human death. Therefore, the statute should concern the death of a human being, not the death of his cells, tissues, or organs, and not the "death" or cessation of his role as a fully functioning member of his family or community. This point merits considerable emphasis. There may be a proper place for a statutory standard for deciding when to turn off a respirator which is ventilating a patient still clearly alive, or, for that matter, to cease giving any other form of therapy. But it is crucial to distinguish this question of "when to allow to die?" from the question with which we are here concerned, namely, "when to declare dead?" Since very different issues and purposes are involved in these questions, confusing the one with the other clouds the analysis of both. The problem of determining when a person is dead is difficult enough without its being tied to the problem of whether physicians, or anyone else, may hasten the death of a terminally ill patient, with or without his consent or that of his relatives, in order to minimize his suffering or to conserve scarce medical resources. Although the same set of social and medical conditions may give rise to both problems, they must be kept separate if they are to be clearly understood.

Distinguishing the question "is he dead?" from the question "should he be allowed to die?" also assists in preserving the continuity with tradition, a second important principle. By restricting itself to the "is he dead?" issue, a revised "definition" permits practices to move incrementally, not by replacing traditional cardiopulmonary standards for the determination of death but rather by supplementing them. These standards are, after all, still adequate in the majority of cases, and are the ones that both physicians and the public are in the habit of employing and relying on. The supplementary standards are needed primarily for those cases in which artificial means of support of comatose patients render the traditional standards unreliable.

Third, this incremental approach is useful for the additional and perhaps most central reason that any new means for judging death should be seen as just that and nothing more—a change in method dictated by advances in medical practice, but not an alteration of the meaning of "life" and "death." By indicating that the various standards for measuring death relate to a single phenomenon, legislation can serve to reduce a primary source of public uneasiness on this subject. Once it has been established that certain consequences—for example, burial, autopsy, transfer of property to the heirs, and so forth—follow from a determination of death, definite problems would arise if there were a number of "definitions" according to which some people could be said to be "more dead" than others.

There are, of course, many instances in which the law has established differing definitions of a term, each framed to serve a particular purpose. One wonders, however, whether it does not appear somewhat foolish for the law to offer a number of arbitrary definitions of a natural phenomenon such as death. Nevertheless, legislators might seek to identify a series of points during the process of dying, each of which might be labeled "death" for certain purposes. Yet so far as we know, no arguments have been presented for special-purpose standards except in the area of organ transplantation. Such a separate "definition of death," aimed at increasing the supply of viable organs, would permit physicians to declare a patient dead before his condition met the generally applicable standards for determining death if his organs are of potential use in transplantation. The adoption of a special standard risks abuse and confusion, however. The status of a prospective organ donor is an arbitrary one to which a person can be assigned by relatives or physicians and is unrelated to anything about the extent to which his body's functioning has deteriorated. A special "definition" of death for transplantation purposes would thus need to be surrounded by a set of procedural safeguards that would govern not only the method by which a person is to be declared dead but also those by which he is to be classified as an organ donor. Even more troublesome is the confusion over the meaning of death that would probably be engendered by multiple "definitions." Consequently, it would be highly desirable if a statute on death could avoid the problems with a special "definition." Should the statute happen to facilitate organ transplantation, either by making more organs available or by making prospective donors and transplant surgeons more secure in knowing what the law would permit, so much the better.

If, however, more organs are needed for transplantation than can be legally obtained, the question whether the benefits conferred by transplantation justify the risks associated with a broader "definition" of death should be addressed directly rather than by attempting to subsume it under the question "what is death?" Such a direct confrontation with the issue could lead to a discussion about the standards and procedures under which organs might be taken from persons near death, or even those still quite alive, at their own option or that of relatives, physicians, or representatives of the state. The major advantage of keeping the issues separate is not, of course, that this will facilitate transplantation, but that it will remove a present source of concern: it is unsettling to contemplate that as you lie slowly dying physicians are free to use a more "lenient" standard to declare you dead if they want to remove your organs for transplantation into other patients.

Fourth, the standards for determining death ought not only to relate to a single phenomenon but should also be applied uniformly to all persons. A person's wealth or his "social utility" as an organ donor should not affect the way in which the moment of his death is determined.

Finally, while there is a need for uniformity of application at any one time, the fact that changes in medical technology brought about the present need for "redefinition" argues that the new formulation should be flexible. As suggested in the previous section, such flexibility is most easily accomplished if the new "definition" confines itself to the general standards by which death is to be determined and leaves to the continuing exercise of judgment by physicians the establishment and application of appropriate criteria and specific tests for determining that the standards have been met.

VI. The Kansas Statute

The first attempt at a legislative resolution of the problems discussed here was made in 1970 when the State of Kansas adopted "An Act relating to and defining death." [3] The Kansas statute has received a good deal of attention; similar legislation was enacted in the spring of 1972 in Maryland and is presently under consideration in a number of other jurisdictions. [4] The Kansas legislation, which was drafted in response to developments in organ transplantation and medical support of dying patients, provides "alternative definitions of death," set forth in two paragraphs. Under the first, a person is considered "medically and legally dead" if a physician determines "there is the absence of spontaneous respiratory and cardiac function and . . . attempts at resuscitation are considered hopeless." In the second "definition," death turns on the absence of spontaneous brain function if during "reasonable attempts" either to "maintain or restore spontaneous circulatory or respiratory function," it appears that "further attempts at resuscitation or supportive maintenance will not succeed." The purpose of the latter "definition" is made clear by the final sentence of the second paragraph:

[3] Law of Mar. 17, 1970, ch. 378, Kan. Laws 994.
[4] Maryland Sessions Laws ch. 693 (1972).

"Death is to be pronounced before artificial means of supporting respiratory and circulatory function are terminated and *before any vital organ is removed for the purpose of transplantation*" [emphasis added].

The primary fault with this legislation is that it appears to be based on, or at least gives voice to, the misconception that there are two separate phenomena of death. This dichotomy is particularly unfortunate because it seems to have been inspired by a desire to establish a special definition for organ transplantation, a definition which physicians would not, however, have to apply, in the draftsman's words, "to prove the irrelevant deaths of most persons" (Taylor 1971). Although there is nothing in the Act itself to indicate that physicians will be less concerned with safeguarding the health of potential organ donors, the purposes for which the Act was passed are not hard to decipher, and they do little to inspire the average patient with confidence that his welfare (including his not being prematurely declared dead) is of as great concern to medicine and the State of Kansas as is the facilitation of organ transplantation. As Professor Kennedy (1971) cogently observes, "public disquiet [over transplantation] is in no way allayed by the existence in legislative form of what appear to be alternative definitions of death." One hopes that the form the statute takes does not reflect a conclusion on the part of the Kansas legislature that death occurs at two distinct points during the process of dying. Yet this inference can be derived from the Act, leaving open the prospect "that X at a certain stage in the process of dying can be pronounced dead, whereas Y, having arrived at the same point, is not said to be dead" (Kennedy).

The Kansas statute appears also to have attempted more than the "definition" of death, or rather, to have tried to resolve related questions by erroneously treating them as matters of "definition." One supporter of the statute (Mills 1971) praises it, we think mistakenly, for this reason: "Intentionally, the statute extends to these questions: When can a physician avoid attempting resuscitation? When can he terminate resuscitative efforts? When can he discontinue artificial maintenance?" To be sure, "when the patient is dead" is one obvious answer to these questions, but by no means the only one. As indicated above, we believe that the question "when is the patient dead?" needs to be distinguished and treated separately from the questions "when may the doctor turn off the respirator?" or "when may a patient—dying yet still alive—be allowed to die?"

VII. A Statutory Proposal

As an alternative to the Kansas statute we propose the following:

A person will be considered dead if in the announced opinion of a physician, based on ordinary standards of medical practice, he has experienced an irreversible cessation of spontaneous respiratory and circulatory functions. In the event that artificial means of support preclude a determination that these functions have ceased, a person will be considered dead if in the announced opinion of a physician, based on ordinary standards of medical practice, he has experienced an irreversible cessation of spontaneous brain functions. Death will have occurred at the time when the relevant functions ceased.

This proposed statute provides a "definition" of death confined to the level of *general physiological standards*, and it has been drafted in accord with the five principles set forth above in section V. First, the proposal speaks in terms of the *death* of a *person*. The determination that a person has died is to be based on an evaluation of certain vital bodily functions, the permanent absence of which indicates that he is no longer a living human being. By concentrating on the death of a human being as a whole, the statute rightly disregards the fact that some cells or organs may continue to "live" after this point, just as others may have ceased functioning long before the determination of death. This statute would leave for resolution by other means the question of when the absence or deterioration of certain capacities, such as the ability to communicate, or functions, such as the cerebral, indicates that a person may or should be allowed to die without further medical intervention.

Second, the proposed legislation is predicated upon the single phenomenon of death. Moreover, it applies uniformly to all persons, by specifying the circumstances under which each of the standards is to be used rather than leaving this to the unguided discretion of physicians. Unlike the Kansas law, the model statute does not leave to arbitrary decision a choice between two apparently equal yet different "alternative definitions of death." Rather, its second standard is applicable only when "artificial means of support preclude" use of the first. It does not establish a separate kind of death, called "brain death." In other words, the proposed law would provide two standards gauged by different functions, for measuring different manifestations of the same phenomenon. If cardiac and pulmonary functions have ceased, brain functions cannot continue; if there is no brain activity and respiration has to be maintained artificially, the same state (i.e., death) exists. Some people might prefer a single standard, one based either on cardiopulmonary or brain functions. This would have the advantage of removing the last trace of the "two deaths" image, which any reference to alternative standards may still leave. Respiratory and circulatory indicators, once the only touchstone, are no longer adequate in some situations. It would be possible, however, to adopt the alternative, namely that death is always to be established by assessing spontaneous brain functions. Reliance only on brain activity, however, would represent a sharp and unnecessary break with tradition. Departing from continuity with tradition is not only theoretically unfortunate in that it violates another principle of good legislation suggested previously, but also practically very difficult, since most physicians customarily employ cardiopulmonary tests for death and would be slow to change, especially when the old tests are easier to perform, more accessible and acceptable to the lay public, and perfectly adequate for determining death in most instances.

Finally, by adopting standards for death in terms of the cessation of certain vital bodily functions but not in terms of the specific criteria or tests by which these functions are to be measured, the statute does not prevent physicians from adapting their procedures to changes in medical technology.

A basic substantive issue remains: what are the merits of the proposed standards? For ordinary situations, the appropriateness of the traditional standard, "an irreversible cessation of spontaneous respiratory and circulatory functions," does not require elaboration. Indeed, examination by a physician may be more a formal than a real requirement in determining that most people have died. In addition to any obvious injuries, elementary signs of death such as absence of heartbeat and breathing, cold skin, fixed pupils, and so forth, are usually sufficient to indicate even to a layman that the accident victim, the elderly person who passes away quietly in the night, or the patient stricken with a sudden infarct has died. The difficulties arise when modern medicine intervenes to sustain a patient's respiration and circulation. As we noted in discussing the Harvard Committee's conclusions, the indicators of brain damage appear reliable, in that studies have shown that patients who fit the Harvard criteria have suffered such extensive damage that they do not recover. Of course, the task of the neurosurgeon or physician is simplified in the common case where an accident victim has suffered such gross, apparent injuries to the head that it is not necessary to apply the Harvard criteria in order to establish cessation of brain functioning.

The statutory standard, "irreversible cessation of spontaneous brain functions," is intended to encompass both higher brain activities and those of the brainstem. There must, of course, also be no spontaneous respiration; the second standard is applied only when breathing is being artificially maintained. The major emphasis placed on brain functioning, although generally consistent with the common view of what makes man distinctive as a living creature, brings to the fore a basic issue: What aspects of brain function should be decisive? The question has been reframed by some clinicians (Brierley et al. 1971) in light of their experience with patients who have undergone what they term "neocortical death" (that is, complete destruction of higher brain activity, demonstrated by a flat EEG). "Once neocortical death has been unequivocally established and the possibility of any recovery of consciousness and intellectual activity [is] thereby excluded, . . . although [the] patient breathes spontaneously, is he or she alive?" While patients with irreversible brain damage from cardiac arrest seldom survive more than a few days, cases have recently been reported of survival for up to two and one-quarter years. Nevertheless, though existence in this state falls far short of a full human life, the very fact of spontaneous respiration, as well as coordinated movements and reflex activities at the brainstem and spinal cord levels, would exclude these patients from the scope of the statutory standards. The condition of "neocortical death" may well be a proper justification for interrupting all forms of treatment and allowing these patients to die, but this moral and legal problem cannot and should not be settled by "defining" these people "dead."

The legislation suggested here departs from the Kansas statute in its basic approach to the problem of "defining" death: the proposed statute does not set about to establish a special category of "brain death" to be used by transplanters. Further, there are a number of particular points of difference between them. For example, the proposed statute does not speak of persons being "medically and legally dead," thus avoiding redundancy, and, more importantly, the mistaken implication that the "medical" and "legal" definitions could differ. Also, the proposed legislation does not include the provision that "death is to be pronounced before" the machine is turned off or any organs removed. Such a *modus operandi*, which was incorporated by

Kansas from the Harvard Committee's report, may be advisable for physicians on public relations grounds but it has no place in a statute "defining" death. The proposed statute already provides that "death will have occurred at the time when the relevant functions ceased." If supportive aids, or organs, are withdrawn after this time, such acts cannot be implicated as having caused death. The manner in which, or exact time at which, the physician should articulate his finding is a matter best left to the exigencies of the situation, to local medical customs or hospital rules, or to statutes on the procedures for certifying death or on transplantation if the latter is the procedure which raises the geatest concern of medical impropriety. The real safeguard against doctors killing patients is not to be found in a statute "defining" death. Rather, it inheres in physicians' ethical and religious beliefs, which are also embodied in the fundamental professional ethic of *primum non nocere* and are reinforced by homicide and "wrongful death" laws and the rules governing medical negligence applicable in license-revocation proceedings or in private actions for damages.

The proposed statute shares with the Kansas legislation two features of which Professor Kennedy is critical. First, it does not require that two physicians participate in determining death, as recommended by most groups which set forth suggestions about transplantation. The reasons for the absence of such a provision should be obvious. Since the statute deals with death in general and not with death in relation to transplantation, there is no reason for it to establish a general rule which is required only in that unusual situation. If particular dangers lurk in the transplantation setting, they should be dealt with in legislation on that subject, such as the Uniform Anatomical Gift Act. If all current means of determining "irreversible cessation of spontaneous brain functions" are inherently so questionable that they should be double-checked by a second (or third, fourth, etc.) physician to be trustworthy, or if a certain means of measuring brain function requires as a technical matter the cooperation of two, or twenty, physicians, then the participation of the requisite number of experts would be part of the "ordinary standards of medical practice" that circumscribe the proper, nonnegligent use of such procedures. It would be unfortunate, however, to introduce such a requirement into legislation which sets forth the general standards for determining who is dead, especially when it is done in such a way as to differentiate between one standard and another.

Kennedy's second objection, that a death statute ought to provide "for the separation and insulation of the physician (or physicians) attending the patient donor and certifying death, from the recipient of any organ that may be salvaged from the cadaver," is likewise unnecessary. As was noted previously, language that relates only to transplantation has no place in a statute on the determination of death.

VIII. Conclusion

Changes in medical knowledge and procedures have created an apparent need for a clear and acceptable revision of the standards for determining that a person has died. Some commentators have argued that the formulation of such standards should be left to physicians. The reasons for rejecting this argument seem compelling: the "definition of death" is not merely a matter for technical expertise, the uncertainty of the present law is unhealthy for society and physicians alike, there is a great potential for mischief and harm through the possibility of conflict between the standards applied by some physicians and those assumed to be applicable by the community at large and its legal system, and patients and their relatives are made uneasy by physicians apparently being free to shift around the meaning of death without any societal guidance. Accordingly, we conclude the public has a legitimate role to play in the formulation and adoption of such standards. This article has proposed a model statute which bases a determination of death primarily on the traditional standard of final respiratory and circulatory cessation; where the artificial maintenance of these functions precludes the use of such a standard, the statute authorizes that death be determined on the basis of irreversible cessation of spontaneous brain functions. We believe the legislation proposed would dispel public confusion and concern and protect physicians and patients, while avoiding the creation of "two types of death," for which the statute on this subject first adopted in Kansas has been justly criticized. The proposal is offered not as the ultimate solution to the problem, but as a catalyst for what we hope will be a robust and well-informed public debate over a new "definition." Finally, the proposed statute leaves for future resolution the even more difficult problems concerning the conditions and procedures under which a decision may be reached to cease treating a terminal patient who does not meet the standards set forth in the statutory "definition of death."

References

Brierley, J. B.; D. I. Graham; J. H. Adams; and J. A. Simpson. "Neocortical Death after Cardiac Arrest." *Lancet* 2 (September 1971): 560–65.

Kennedy, Ian McColl. "The Kansas Statute on Death—An Appraisal." *New England Journal of Medicine* 285 (October 1971): 946–50.

Mills, Don Harper. "The Kansas Death Statute—Bold and Innovative." *New England Journal of Medicine* 285 (October 1971): 968–69.

Rutstein, David D. "The Ethical Design of Human Experiments." *Daedalus* 98 (Spring 1969): 523–41.

Silverman, Daniel; Richard L. Masland; Michael G. Saunders; and Robert S. Schwab. "Irreversible Coma Associated with Electrocerebral Silence." *Neurology* 20 (June 1970): 525–33.

Taylor, Loren F. "A Statutory Definition of Death in Kansas." *Journal of the American Medical Association* 215 (January 11, 1971): 296.

10

Tucker v. Lower

WILLIAM E. TUCKER, Administrator of
the Estate of BRUCE O. TUCKER, deceased,
                                    Plaintiff,
                        vs.

DR. RICHARD R. LOWER
DR. DAVID M. HUME
DR. DAVID H. SEWELL
DR. H. M. LEE
AND DR. ABDULLAH FATTEH,   MEMORANDUM
                        Defendants.
                                            OPINION

THE FACTS thus far are, in the main, uncontradicted. The decedent, Bruce O. Tucker, age 54, was brought unconscious to the emergency room of the Medical College of Virginia Hospital by the personnel of a local ambulance company on Friday, May 24, 1968, and was registered therein at 6:05 P.M. He had suffered a fall at another location in the City and the evidence shows that he was not accompanied to the hospital by any relative or friend.

Upon examination, the decedent was found to have sustained severe head injuries, including a large right-sided lateral basilar skull fracture. He was admitted to the neurosurgical service of the hospital and upon further examination and tests, a diagnosis of subdural hematoma on the left and brain-stem contusion was made prior to the performance at 11:00 P.M. on May 24 of an operation described as a right temporoparietal craniotomy and right parietal bur hole. A tracheostomy was also performed at the same time.

Following this operation, which was completed about 2:05 A.M. on May 25, the decedent left the operating room in slightly better condition than preoperatively and was placed in the recovery room, where he was to remain until the afternoon of that day.

In the recovery room he was being fed intravenously and he was receiving medication each hour until 11:30 A.M., when he was placed on a respirator, which kept him "mechanically alive." At 11:45 A.M. the treating physician, Dr. Brawley, noted that "[his] prognosis for recovery is nil and death imminent." At 1:00 P.M. on that day, Dr. Hooshmand, a neurologist, was called upon to obtain an EEG to determine the state of the patient's brain activity. Between 1:00 P.M. and 2:00 P.M. he examined the decedent and made a single EEG recording which showed flat lines with occasional artifact. He found no clinical evidence of viability and no evidence of cortical activity. Based upon this examination, he was of the opinion that the patient was then dead from a neurological standpoint.

At this time, the neurologist also found that the decedent's heart was beating and that his body temperature, pulse, and blood pressure were all normal for a patient in his condition. In addition to theological death, the neurologist defined two other types of death. First, he defined clinical or neurological death as total cessation of function of the central nervous system or brain. He then defined biological death as the death of an organ or a part of the body or a cell. He described death as a continuing thing since tissue and organs live after the brain dies, but he stated that in his opinion the individual dies when the brain dies. In his opinion, the decedent's brain was dead prior to the time he ran the EEG. The patient showed no evidence of being able to breathe spontaneously at all. The respirator was doing all the breathing, he said.

Dr. Hooshmand was of the opinion that it was "very likely" the decedent's condition was "irreversible" at the time the patient was admitted to the hospital on May 24.

At 2:45 P.M., the decedent was taken back into the operating room in preparation for the removal of his heart and both kidneys, this being the operation participated in by the defendants Lower, Hume, Sewell, and Lee.

Sometime before 2:45 P.M., Dr. Campbell was requested to give anesthesia in the form of oxygen to the decedent during the operation. The patient was receiving oxygen to continue viability of certain organs. Dr. Sewell had told Campbell after 12:00 noon on that day that his services would be needed because "we have a prospective donor for a heart transplant."

From the time (2:45 P.M.) that the patient was taken from the recovery room to the operating room, until 4:30 P.M., he maintained vital signs of life, that is, he maintained, for the most part, normal body temperature, normal pulse, normal blood pressure and normal rate of respiration. During the same period, he was receiving dextrose and saline to furnish nourishment to the organs.

At 3:30½ the respirator was cut off by Dr. Bralley and at 3:35½ the patient was pronounced dead by Dr. Bralley. At 4:25 the incision was made to remove the heart and it was taken out at 4:32 P.M. by Dr. Sewell, who was assisted by Dr. Hume. The heart was then placed in the body of the recipient, Joseph Klett, by his treating physician, Dr. Lower, who had made the incision in Klett at 3:33 P.M. . . .

Since the decedent was unconscious from the time he arrived at the hospital, no information as to the whereabouts of his relatives had been obtained from him nor was any consent for any surgical procedure given by him. . . .

Having viewed the evidence in the light most favorable to the plaintiff, as the court is bound to do at this stage of the proceeding, it is apparent to the court that the plaintiff has established a *prima facie* case for recovery under the Virginia Death by Wrongful Act Statutes.

The plaintiff has not, however, made out any case of medical malpractice in the customary and strict sense of that term. The duty of the physician or surgeon to exercise reasonable and ordinary care and diligence in the exertion of his skill and application of his knowledge as to the treatment of the case intrusted to him is usually based upon the contractual relationship between the patient and his physician. As the defendants point out, none of them had the relationship to Bruce O. Tucker of a treating physician. Therefore, unless there is some other basis for liability of these defendants, the plaintiff has not made out a case and his action must fail. . . .

The first important consideration, then, raised by the facts of this case and the argument of the defendants in support of their motions relates to the meaning of the word "death" as used in the [Virginia Death by Wrongful

Act] statute. Under the law, does death occur at a particular moment in time or is it continuing? This determination must necessarily include a decision by the court upon the question of whether death must be defined by the law or whether the definition must be controlled entirely by, or in part by, medical opinion.

The function of This Court is to determine the state of the law on this or any other subject according to legal precedent and principle. The courts which have had occasion to rule upon the nature of death and its timing have all decided that death occurs at a precise time, and that it is defined as the cessation of life; the ceasing to exist; a total stoppage of the circulation of the blood, and a cessation of the animal and vital functions consequent thereto such as respiration and pulsation (*Black's Law Dictionary,* 4th ed.). . . .

This court adopts the legal concept of death and rejects the invitation offered by the defendants to employ a medical concept of neurological death in establishing a rule of law. . . .

A. Christian Compton
May 23, 1972

THREE
Allowing to Die

infants

11

Moral and Ethical Dilemmas in the Special-Care Nursery

RAYMOND S. DUFF AND A. G. M. CAMPBELL

BETWEEN 1940 and 1970 there was a 58 percent decrease in the infant death rate in the United States (Wegman 1971). This reduction was related in part to the application of new knowledge to the care of infants. Neonatal mortality rates in hospitals having infant intensive-care units have been about one-half those reported in hospitals without such units (Swyer 1970). There is now evidence (Rawlings et al. 1971) that in many conditions of early infancy the long-term morbidity may also be reduced. Survivors of these units may be healthy, and their parents grateful, but some infants continue to suffer from such conditions as chronic cardiopulmonary disease, short-bowel-syndrome or various manifestations of brain damage; others are severely handicapped by a myriad of congenital malformations that in previous times would have resulted in early death. Recently, both lay and professional persons have expressed increasing concern about the quality of life for these severely impaired survivors and their families. Many pediatricians and others are distressed with the long-term results of pressing on and on to save life at all costs and in all circumstances. Eliot Slater (1971) stated, "If this is one of the consequences of the sanctity-of-life ethic, perhaps our formulation of the principle should be revised."

Reprinted from *The New England Journal of Medicine* 289 (October 25, 1973): 890–94, with the permission of the publisher. Copyright © 1973 by the Massachusetts Medical Society.

The experiences described in this communication document some of the grave moral and ethical dilemmas now faced by physicians and families. They indicate some of the problems in a large special-care nursery where medical technology has prolonged life and where "informed" parents influence the management decisions concerning their infants.

Background and Methods

The special-care nursery of the Yale-New Haven Hospital not only serves an obstetric service for over 4,000 live births annually but also acts as the principal referral center in Connecticut for infants with major problems of the newborn period. From January 1, 1970, through June 30, 1972, 1,615 infants born at the hospital were admitted, and 556 others were transferred for specialized care from community hospitals. During this interval, the average daily census was 26, with a range of 14 to 37.

For some years the unit has had a liberal policy for parental visiting, with the staff placing particular emphasis on helping parents adjust to and participate in the care of their infants with special problems. By encouraging visiting, attempting to create a relaxed atmosphere within the unit, exploring carefully the special needs of the infants, and familiarizing parents with various aspects of care, it was hoped to remove much of the apprehension—indeed, fear—with which parents at first view an intensive-care nursery. At any time, parents may see and handle their babies. They commonly observe or participate in most routine aspects of care and are often present when some infant is critically ill or moribund. They may attend, as they choose, the death of their own infant. Since an average of two to three deaths occur each week and many infants are critically ill for long periods, it is obvious that the concentrated, intimate social interactions between personnel, infants, and parents in an emotionally charged atmosphere often make the work of the staff very difficult and demanding. However, such participation and recognition of parents' rights to information about their infant appear to be the chief foundations of "informed consent" for treatment.

Each staff member must know how to cope with many questions and problems brought up by parents, and if he or she cannot help, they must have access to those who can. These requirements can be met only when staff members work closely with each other in all the varied circumstances from simple to complex, from triumph to tragedy. Formal and informal meetings take place regularly to discuss the technical and family aspects of care. As a given problem may require, some or all of several persons (including families, nurses, social workers, physicians, chaplains, and others) may convene to exchange information and reach decisions. Thus, staff and parents function more or less as a small community in which a concerted attempt is made to ensure that each member may participate in and know about the major decisions that concern him or her. However, the physician takes appropriate initiative in final decision making, so that the family will not have to bear that heavy burden alone.

For several years, the responsibilities of attending pediatrician have been assumed chiefly by ourselves, who, as a result, have become acquainted intimately with the problems of the infants, the staff, and the parents. Our almost constant availability to staff, private pediatricians, and parents has resulted in the raising of more and more ethical questions about various aspects of intensive care for critically ill and congenitally deformed infants. The penetrating questions and challenges, particularly of knowledgeable parents (such as physicians, nurses, or lawyers), brought increasing doubts about the wisdom of many of the decisions that seemed to parents to be predicated chiefly on technical considerations. Some thought their child had a right to die since he could not live well or effectively. Others thought that society should pay the costs of care that may be so destructive to the family economy. Often, too, the parents' or siblings' rights to relief from the seemingly pointless, crushing burdens were important considerations. It seemed right to yield to parent wishes in several cases as physicians have done for generations. As a result, some treatments were withheld or stopped with the knowledge that earlier death and relief from suffering would result. Such options were explored with the less knowledgeable parents to ensure that their consent for treatment of their defective children was truly informed. As Eisenberg (1972) pointed out regarding the application of technology, "At long last, we are beginning to ask, not *can* it be done, but *should* it be done?" In lengthy, frank discussions, the anguish of the parents was shared, and attempts were made to support fully the reasoned choices, whether for active treatment and rehabilitation or for an early death.

To determine the extent to which death resulted from withdrawing or withholding treatment, we examined the hospital records of all children who died from January 1, 1970, through June 30, 1972.

Results

In total, there were 299 deaths. Each was classified in one of two categories. Deaths in category 1 resulted from pathologic conditions in spite of the treatment given; 256 (86 percent) were in this category. Of these, 66 percent were the result of respiratory problems or complications associated with extreme prematurity (birth weight under 1,000 g). Congenital heart disease and other anomalies accounted for an additional 22 percent (Table 11.1).

Deaths in category 2 were associated with severe impairment, usually from congenital disorders: 43 (14 percent) were in this group (Table 11.2). These deaths or their timing was associated with discontinuance or withdrawal of treatment. The mean duration of life in category 2 (Table 11.3) was greater than that in category 1. This was the result of a mean life of 55 days for eight infants who became chronic cardiopulmonary cripples but for whom prolonged and intensive efforts were made in the hope of eventual recovery. They were infants who were dependent on oxygen, digoxin, and diuretics, and most of them had been treated for the idiopathic respiratory-distress syndrome with high oxygen concentrations and positive-pressure ventilation.

Some examples of management choices in category 2 illustrate the problems. An infant with Down's syndrome and intestinal atresia, like the much-publicized one at Johns Hopkins Hospital [see Gustafson article], was not treated because his parents thought that surgery was wrong for their baby and themselves. He died seven days after birth. Another child had chronic pulmonary disease after positive-pressure ventilation with high oxygen concentrations for treatment of severe idiopathic respiratory-distress syndrome. By five months of age, he still required 40 percent oxygen to survive, and even then, he was chronically dyspneic and cyanotic. He also suffered from

Table 11.1 Problems Causing Death in Category 1

Problem	No. of Deaths	Percentage
Respiratory	108	42.2
Extreme prematurity	60	23.4
Heart disease	42	16.4
Multiple anomalies	14	5.5
Other	32	12.5
Totals	256	100.0

Table 11.2 Problems Associated with Death in Category 2

Problem	No. of Deaths	Percentage
Multiple anomalies	15	34.9
Trisomy	8	18.6
Cardiopulmonary	8	18.6
Meningomyelocele	7	16.3
Other central nervous system defects	3	7.0
Short-bowel syndrome	2	4.6
Totals	43	100.0

cor pulmonale, which was difficult to control with digoxin and diuretics. The nurses, parents, and physicians considered it cruel to continue, and yet difficult to stop. All were attached to this child, whose life they had tried so hard to make worthwhile. The family had endured high expenses (the hospital bill exceeding $15,000), and the strains of the illness were believed to be threatening the marriage bonds and to be causing sibling behavioral disturbances. Oxygen supplementation was stopped, and the child died in about three hours. The family settled down and 18 months later had another baby, who was healthy.

A third child had meningomyelocele, hydrocephalus, and major anomalies of every organ in the pelvis. When the parents understood the limits of medical care and rehabilitation, they believed no treatment should be given. She died at five days of age.

We have maintained contact with most families of children in category 2. Thus far, these families appear to have experienced a normal mourning for their losses. Although some have exhibited doubts that the choices were correct, all appear to be as effective in their lives as they were before this experience. Some claim that their profoundly moving experience has provided a

Table 11.3 Selected Comparisons of 256 Cases in Category 1 and 43 in Category 2

Attribute	Category 1	Category 2
Mean length of life	4.8 days	7.5 days
Standard deviation	8.8	34.3
Range	1–69	1–150
Portion living for < 2 days	50.0%	12.0%

deeper meaning in life, and from this they believe they have become more effective people.

Members of all religious faiths and atheists were participants as parents and as staff in these experiences. There appeared to be no relation between participation and a person's religion. Repeated participation in these troubling events did not appear to reduce the worry of the staff about the awesome nature of the decisions.

Discussion

That decisions are made not to treat severely defective infants may be no surprise to those familiar with special-care facilities. All laymen and professionals familiar with our nursery appeared to set some limits upon their application of treatment to extend life or to investigate a pathologic process. For example, an experienced nurse said about one child, "We lost him several weeks ago. Isn't it time to quit?" In another case, a house officer said to a physician investigating an aspect of a child's disease, "For this child, don't you think it's time to turn off your curiosity so you can turn on your kindness?" Like many others, these children eventually acquired the "right to die."

Arguments among staff members and families for and against such decisions were based on varied notions of the rights and interests of defective infants, their families, professionals, and society. They were also related to varying ideas about prognosis. Regarding the infants, some contended that individuals should have a right to die in some circumstances such as anencephaly, hydranencephaly, and some severely deforming and incapacitating conditions. Such very defective individuals were considered to have little or no hope of achieving meaningful "humanhood" (Fletcher 1972). For example, they have little or no capacity to love or be loved. They are often cared for in facilities that have been characterized as "hardly more than dying bins" (Freeman et al. 1970), an assessment with which, in our experience, knowledgeable parents (those who visited chronic-care facilities for placement of their children) agreed. With institutionalized well children, social participation may be essentially nonexistent, and maternal deprivation severe; this is known to have an adverse, usually disastrous, effect upon the child. The situation for the defective child is probably worse, for he is restricted socially both by his need for care and by his defects. To escape "wrongful life" (Engelhardt 1973), a fate rated as worse than death, seemed right. In this regard, Lasagna (1968) notes, "We may, as a society, scorn the civilizations that slaughtered their infants, but our present treatment of the retarded is in some ways more cruel."

Others considered allowing a child to die wrong for several reasons. The person most involved, the infant, had no voice in the decision. Prognosis was not always exact, and a few children with extensive care might live for months, and occasionally years. Some might survive and function satisfactorily. To a few persons, withholding treatment and accepting death was condemned as criminal.

Families had strong but mixed feelings about management decisions. Living with the handicapped is clearly a family affair, and families of deformed infants thought there were limits to what they could bear or should be expected to bear. Most of them wanted maximal efforts to sustain life and to rehabilitate the handicapped; in such cases, they were supported fully. However, some families, especially those having children with severe defects, feared that they and their other children would become socially enslaved, economically deprived, and permanently stigmatized, all perhaps for a lost cause. Such a state of "chronic sorrow" until death has been described by Olshansky (1962). In some cases, families considered the death of the child right both for the child and for the family. They asked if that choice could be theirs or their doctors.

As Feifel (1969) has reported, physicians on the whole are reluctant to deal with the issues. Some, particularly specialists based in the medical center, gave specific reasons for this disinclination. There was a feeling that to "give up" was disloyal to the cause of the profession. Since major research, teaching, and patient-care efforts were being made, professionals expected to discover, transmit, and apply knowledge and skills; patients and families were supposed to cooperate fully even if they were not always grateful. Some physicians recognized that the wishes of families went against their own, but they were resolute. They commonly agreed that if they were the parents of very defective children, withholding treatment would be most desirable for them. However, they argued that aggressive management was indicated for others. Some believed that allowing death as a management option was euthanasia and must be stopped for fear of setting a "poor ethical example" or for fear of personal prosecution or damage to their clinical departments or to the medical center as a whole. Alexander's report (1949) on Nazi Germany was cited in some cases as providing justification for pressing the effort to combat disease. Some persons were concerned about the loss through death of "teaching material." They feared the training of professionals for the care of defective children in the future and the advancing of the state of the art would be compromised. Some parents who became aware of this concern thought their children should not become experimental subjects.

Practicing pediatricians, general practitioners, and obstetricians were often familiar with these families and were usually sympathetic with their views. However, since they were more distant from the special-care nursery than the specialists of the medical center, their influence was often minimal. As a result, families received little support from them, and tension in community-medical relations was a recurring problem.

Infants with severe types of meningomyelocele precipitated the most controversial decisions. Several decades ago, those who survived this condition beyond a few weeks usually became hydrocephalic and retarded, in addition to being crippled and deformed. Without modern treatment, they died earlier. Some may have been killed or at least not resuscitated at birth. From the early 1960s, the tendency has been to treat vigorously all infants with meningomyelocele. As advanced by Zachary (1968) and Shurtleff (1968), aggressive management of these children became the rule in our unit as in many others. Infants were usually referred quickly. Parents routinely signed permits for operation though rarely had they seen their children's defects or had the nature of various management plans and their respective prognoses clearly explained to them. Some physicians believed that parents were too upset to understand the nature of the problems and the options for care. Since they believed informed consent had no meaning in these circumstances, they either ignored the parents or simply told them that the child needed an operation on the back as the first step in correcting several defects. As a result, parents often felt completely left out while the activities of care proceeded at a brisk pace.

Some physicians experienced in the care of these children and familiar with the impact of such conditions upon families had early reservations about this plan of care (Matson 1968). More recently, they were influenced by the pessimistic appraisal of vigorous management schemes in some cases (Lorber 1971). Meningomyelocele, when treated vigorously, is associated with higher survival rates, but the achievement of satisfactory rehabilitation is at best difficult and usually impossible for almost all who are severely affected. Knowing this, some physicians and some families decide against treatment of the most severely affected. Knowing this, some physicians and some families decide against treatment of the most severely affected. If treatment is not carried out, the child's condition will usually deteriorate from further brain damage, urinary-tract infections, and orthopedic difficulties, and death can be expected much earlier. Two-thirds may be dead by three months, and over 90 percent by one year of age. However, the quality of life during that time is poor, and the strains on families are great, but not necessarily greater than with treatment (Hide et al. 1972). Thus, both treatment and nontreatment constitute unsatisfactory dilemmas for everyone, especially for the child and his family. When maximum treatment was viewed as unacceptable by families and physicians in our unit, there was a growing tendency to seek early death as a management option, to avoid that cruel choice of gradual, often slow, but progressive deterioration of the child who was required under these circumstances in effect to kill himself. Parents and the staff then asked if his dying needed to be prolonged. If not, what were the most appropriate medical responses?

Is it possible that some physicians and some families may join in a conspiracy to deny the right of a defective child to live or to die? Either could occur. Prolongation of the dying process by resident physicians having a vested interest in their careers has been described by Sudnow (1967). On the other hand, from the fatigue of working long and hard some physicians may give up too soon, assuming that their cause is lost. Families, similarly, may have mixed motives. They may demand death to obtain relief from the high costs and the tensions inherent in suffering, but their sense of guilt in this thought may produce the opposite demand, perhaps in violation of the sick person's rights. Thus, the challenge of deciding what course to take can be most tormenting for the family and the physician. Unquestionably, not facing the issue would appear to be the easier course, at least temporarily; no doubt many patients, families, and physicians decline to join in an effort to solve the problems. They can readily assume that what is being done is right and sufficient and ask no questions. But pretending there is no decision to be made is an arbitrary and potentially devastating decision of default. Since families and patients must live with the problems one way or another in any case, the physician's failure to face the issues may constitute a victimizing abandonment of patients and their families in times of greatest need. As Lasagna pointed out, "There is no place for the physician to hide."

Can families in the shock resulting from the birth of a defective child understand what faces them? Can they give truly "informed consent" for treatment or withholding treatment? Some of our colleagues answer no to both questions. In our opinion, if families regardless of background are heard sympathetically and at length and are given information and answers to their questions in words they understand, the problems of their children as well as the expected benefits and limits of any proposed care can be understood clearly in practically all instances. Parents *are* able to understand the implications of such things as chronic dyspnea, oxygen dependency, incontinence, paralysis, contractures, sexual handicaps, and mental retardation.

Another problem concerns who decides for a child. It may be acceptable for a person to reject treatment and bring about his own death. But it is quite a different situation when others are doing this for him. We do not know how often families and their physicians will make just decisions for severely handicapped children. Clearly, this issue is central in evaluation of the process of decision making that we have described. But we also ask, if these parties cannot make such decisions justly, who can?

We recognize great variability and often much uncertainty in prognoses and in family capacities to deal with defective newborn infants. We also acknowledge that there are limits of support that society can or will give to assist handicapped persons and their families. Severely deforming conditions that are associated with little or no hope of a functional existence pose painful dilemmas for the laymen and professionals who must decide how to cope with severe handicaps. We believe the burdens of decision making must be borne by families and their professional advisers because they are most familiar with the respective situations. Since families primarily must live with and are most affected by the decisions, it therefore appears that society and the health professions should provide only general guidelines for decision making. Moreover, since variations between situations are so great, and the situations themselves so complex, it follows that much latitude in decision making should be expected and tolerated. Otherwise, the rules of society or the policies most convenient for medical technologists may become cruel masters of human beings instead of their servants. Regarding any "allocation of death" policy (Manning 1970) we readily acknowledge that the extreme excesses of Hegelian "rational utility" under dictatorships must be avoided (Alexander). Perhaps it is less recognized that the uncontrolled application of medical technology may be detrimental to individuals and families. In this regard, our views are similar to those of Waitzkin and Stoekle (1972). Physicians may hold excessive power over decision making by limiting or controlling the information made available to patients or families. It seems appropriate that the profession be held accountable for presenting fully all management options and their expected consequences. Also, the public should be aware that professionals often face conflicts of interest that may result in decisions against individual preferences.

What are the legal implications of actions like those described in this paper? Some persons may argue that the law has been broken, and others would contend otherwise. Perhaps more than anything else, the public and professional silence on a major social taboo and some common practices has been broken further. That seems appropriate, for out of the ensuing dialogue perhaps better choices for patients and families can be made. If working out these dilemmas in ways such as those we suggest is in violation of the law, we believe the law should be changed.

References

Alexander, Leo. "Medical Science under Dictatorship." *New England Journal of Medicine* 241 (July 14, 1949): 39–47.

Eisenberg, Leon. "The Human Nature of Human Nature." *Science* 176 (April 1972): 123–28.

Engelhardt, H. Tristram. "Euthanasia and Children: the Injury of Continued Existence." *Journal of Pediatrics* 83 (July 1973): 170–71.

Feifel, Herman. "Perception of Death." *Annals of the New York Academy of Science* 164 (December 1969): 669–77.

Fletcher, Joseph. "Indicators of Humanhood: a Tentative Profile of Man." *Hastings Center Report* 2 (November 1972): 1–4.

Freeman, Howard E.; Orville G. Brim, Jr.; and Greer Williams. "New Dimensions of Dying." In *The Dying Patient*, edited by Orville G. Brim, Howard Freeman, Sol Levine, and Norman A. Scotch. New York: Russell Sage Foundation, 1970.

Hide, D. W.; H. Perry Williams; and H. L. Ellis. "The Outlook for the Child with a Myelomeningocele for Whom Early Surgery Was Considered Inadvisable." *Developmental Medicine and Child Neurology* 14 (February 1972): 304–7.

Lasagna, Louis. *Life, Death and the Doctor*. New York: Knopf, 1968.

Lorber, J. "Results of Treatment of Myelomeningocele." *Developmental Medicine and Child Neurology* 13 (June 1971): 279–303.

Manning, Bayless. "Legal and Policy Issues in the Allocation of Death." In *The Dying Patient*, edited by Orville G. Brim, Jr., Howard Freeman, Sol Levine, and Norman A. Scotch. New York: Russell Sage Foundation, 1970.

Matson, Donald D. "Surgical Treatment of Myelomeningocele." *Pediatrics* 42 (August 1968): 225–27.

Olshansky, Simon. "Chronic Sorrow: a Response to Having a Mentally Defective Child." *Social Casework* 43 (April 1962): 190–93.

Rawlings, Grace; Ann Stewart; E. O. R. Reynolds; and L. B. Strang. "Changing Prognosis for Infants of Very Low Birth Weight." *Lancet* 1 (March 1971): 516–19.

Shurtleff, D. B. "Care of the Myelodysplastic Patient." In *Ambulatory Pediatrics*, edited by Morris Green and Robert Haggerty. Philadelphia: Saunders, 1968.

Slater, Eliot. "Health Service or Sickness Service?" *British Medical Journal* 4 (December 1971): 734–36.

Sudnow, David. *Passing On*. Englewood Cliffs, N.J.: Prentice-Hall, 1967.

Swyer, P. R. "The Regional Organization of Special Care for the Neonate." *Pediatric Clinics of North America* 17 (November 1970): 761–76.

Waitzkin, H., and J. D. Stoeckle. "The Communication of Information about Illness." *Advances in Psychosomatic Medicine* 8 (1972): 180–215.

Wegman, Myron E. "Annual Summary of Vital Statistics—1970." *Pediatrics* 48 (December 1971): 979–83.

Zachary, R. B. "Ethical and Social Aspects of Treatment of Spina Bifida." *Lancet* 2 (August 1968): 274–76.

12

Mongolism, Parental Desires, and the Right to Life

JAMES M. GUSTAFSON

The Problem

The Family Setting

Mother, 34 years old, hospital nurse.
Father, 35 years old, lawyer.
Two normal children in the family.

In late fall of 1963, Mr. and Mrs. —— gave birth to a premature baby boy. Soon after birth, the child was diagnosed as a "mongoloid" (Down's syndrome) with the added complication of an intestinal blockage (duodenal atresia). The latter could be corrected with an operation of quite nominal risk. Without the operation, the child could not be fed and would die.

At the time of birth Mrs. —— overheard the doctor express his belief that the child was a mongol. She immediately indicated she did not want the child. The next day, in consultation with a physician, she maintained this position, refusing to give permission for the corrective operation on the intestinal block. Her husband supported her in this position, saying that his

Reprinted from *Perspectives in Biology and Medicine* 16 (Summer 1973): pp. 529-57, with the permission of the author and the University of Chicago Press. Copyright 1973 by the University of Chicago.

wife knew more about these things (i.e., mongoloid children) than he. The reason the mother gave for her position—"It would be unfair to the other children of the household to raise them with a mongoloid."

The physician explained to the parents that the degree of mental retardation cannot be predicted at birth—running from very low mentality to borderline subnormal. As he said: "Mongolism, it should be stressed, is one of the milder forms of mental retardation. That is, mongols' IQs are generally in the 50–80 range, and sometimes a little higher. That is, they're almost always trainable. They can hold simple jobs. And they're famous for being happy children. They're perennially happy and usually a great joy." Without other complications, they can anticipate a long life.

Given the parents' decision, the hospital staff did not seek a court order to override the decision (see "Legal Setting" below). The child was put in a side room and, over an 11-day period, allowed to starve to death.

Following this episode, the parents undertook genetic counseling (chromosome studies) with regard to future possible pregnancies.

The Legal Setting

Since the possibility of a court order reversing the parents' decision naturally arose, the physician's opinion in this matter—and his decision not to seek such an order—is central. As he said: "In the situation in which the child has a known, serious mental abnormality, and would be a burden both to the parents financially and emotionally and perhaps to society, I think it's unlikely that the court would sustain an order to operate on the child against the parents' wishes." He went on to say: "I think one of the great difficulties, and I hope [this] will be part of the discussion relative to this child, is what happens in a family where a court order is used as the means of correcting a congenital abnormality. Does that child ever really become an accepted member of the family? And what are all of the feelings, particularly guilt and coercion feelings, that the parents must have following that type of extraordinary force that's brought to bear upon them for making them accept a child that they did not wish to have?"

Both doctors and nursing staff were firmly convinced that it was "clearly illegal" to hasten the child's death by the use of medication.

One of the doctors raised the further issue of consent, saying: "Who has the right to decide for a child anyway? . . . The whole way we handle life and death is the reflection of the long-standing belief in this country that children don't have any rights, that they're not citizens, that their parents can decide to kill them or to let them live, as they choose."

The Hospital Setting

When posed the question of whether the case would have been taken to court had the child had a normal IQ, with the parents refusing permission for the intestinal operation, the near unanimous opinion of the doctors: "Yes, we would have tried to override their decision." Asked why, the doctors replied: "When a retarded child presents us with the same problem, a different value system comes in; and not only does the staff acquiesce in the parent's decision to let the child die, but it's probable that the courts would also. That is, there is a different standard. . . . There is this tendency to value life on the basis of intelligence. . . . [It's] a part of the American ethic."

The treatment of the child during the period of its dying was also interesting. One doctor commented on "putting the child in a side room." When asked about medication to hasten the death, he replied: "No one would ever do that. No one would ever think about it, because they feel uncomfortable about it. . . . A lot of the way we handle these things has to do with our own anxieties about death and our own desires to be separated from the decisions that we're making."

The nursing staff who had to tend to the child showed some resentment at this. One nurse said she had great difficulty just in entering the room and watching the child degenerate—she could "hardly bear to touch him." Another nurse, however, said: "I didn't mind coming to work. Because like I would rock him. And I think that kind of helped me some—to be able to sit there and hold him. And he was just a tiny little thing. He was really a very small baby. And he was cute. He had a cute little face to him, and it was easy to love him, you know?" And when the baby died, how did she feel?—"I was glad that it was over. It was an end for him."

The Resolution

This complex of human experiences and decisions evokes profound human sensibilities and serious intellectual examination. One sees in and beyond it dimensions that could be explored by practitioners of various academic disciplines. Many of the standard questions about the ethics of medical care are pertinent, as are questions that have been long discussed by philosophers and theologians. One would have to write a full-length book to plow up, cultivate, and bring to fruition the implications of this experience.

I am convinced that, when we respond to a moral dilemma, the way in which we formulate the dilemma, the picture we draw of its salient features, is largely determinative of the choices we have. If the war in Vietnam is pictured as a struggle between the totalitarian forces of evil seeking to suppress all human values on the one side, and the forces of righteousness on the other, we have one sort of problem with limited choice. If, however, it is viewed as a struggle of oppressed people to throw off the shackles of colonialism and imperialism, we have another sort of problem. If it is pictured as more complex, the range of choices is wider, and the factors to be considered are more numerous. If the population problem is depicted as a race against imminent self-destruction of the human race, an ethics of survival seems to be legitimate and to deserve priority. If, however, the population problem is depicted more complexly, other values also determine policy, and our range of choices is broader.

One of the points under discussion in this medical case is how we should view it. What elements are in the accounts that the participants give to it? What elements were left out? What "values" did they seem to consider, and which did they seem to ignore? Perhaps if one made a different montage of the raw experience, one would have different choices and outcomes.

Whose picture is correct? It would not be difficult for one moral philosopher or theologian to present arguments that might undercut, if not demolish, the defenses made by the participants. Another moralist might make a strong defense of the decisions by assigning different degrees of importance to certain aspects of the case. The first might focus on the violation of individual rights, in this case the rights of the infant. The other might claim that the way of least possible suffering for the fewest persons over the longest range of time was the commendable outcome of the account as we have it. Both would be accounts drawn by external observers, not by active, participating agents. There is a tradition that says that ethical reflection by an ideal external observer can bring morally right answers. I have an observer's perspective, though not that of an "ideal observer." But I believe that it is both charitable and intellectually important to try to view the events as the major participants viewed them. The events remain closer to the confusions of the raw experience that way; the passions, feelings, and emotions have some echo of vitality remaining. The parents were not without feeling, the nurses not without anguish. The experiences could become a case in which x represents the rights of the infant to life, y represents the consequences of continued life as a mongoloid person, and z represents the consequences of his continued life for the family and the state. But such abstraction has a way of oversimplifying experience. One would "weigh" x against y and z. I cannot reproduce the drama even of the materials I have read, the interviews with doctors and nurses, and certainly even those are several long steps from the thoughts and feelings of the parents and the staff at that time. I shall, however, attempt to state the salient features of the dilemma for its participants; features that are each value laden and in part determinative of their decisions. In the process of doing that for the participants, I will indicate what reasons might justify their decisions. Following that I will draw a different picture of the experience, highlighting different values and principles, and show how this would lead to a different decision. Finally, I shall give the reasons why I, an observer, believe they, the participants, did the wrong thing. Their responsible and involved participation, one must remember, is very different from my detached reflection on documents and interviews almost a decade later.

The Mother's Decision

Our information about the mother's decision is secondhand. We cannot be certain that we have an accurate account of her reasons for not authorizing the surgery that could have saved the mongoloid infant's life. It is not my role to speculate whether her given reasons are her "real motives"; that would involve an assessment of her "unconscious." When she heard the child was probably a mongol, she "expressed some negative feeling" about it, and "did not want a retarded child." Because she was a nurse she understood what mongolism indicated. One reason beyond her feelings and wants is given: to raise a mongoloid child in the family would not be "fair" to the other children. That her decision was anguished we know from several sources.

For ethical reflection, three terms I have quoted are important: "negative feeling," "wants" or "desires," and "fair." We need to inquire about the status of each as a justification for her decision.

What moral weight can a negative feeling bear? On two quite different grounds, weight could be given to her feelings in an effort to sympathetically understand her decision. First, at the point of making a decision, there is always an element of the rightness or wrongness of the choice that defies full rational justification. When we see injustice being done, we have strong negative feelings; we do not need a sophisticated moral argument to tell us that the act is unjust. We "feel" that it is wrong. It might be said that the mother's "negative feeling" was evoked by an intuition that it would be wrong to save the infant's life, and that feeling is a reliable guide to conduct.

Second, her negative response to the diagnosis of mongolism suggests that she would not be capable of giving the child the affection and the care that it would require. The logic involved is an extrapolation from that moment to potential consequences for her continued relationship to the child in the future. The argument is familiar; it is common in the literature that supports abortion on request—"no unwanted child ought to be born." Why? Because unwanted children suffer from hostility and lack of affection from their mothers, and this is bad for them.

The second term is "wants" or "desires." The negative feelings are assumed to be an indication of her desires. We might infer that at some point she said, "I do not want a retarded child." The status of "wanting" is different, we might note, if it expresses a wish before the child is born, or if it expresses a desire that leads to the death of the infant after it is born. No normal pregnant woman would wish a retarded child. In this drama, however, it translates into: "I would rather not have the infant kept alive." Or, "I will not accept parental responsibilities for a retarded child." What is the status of a desire or a want as an ethical justification for an action? To discuss that fully would lead to an account of a vast literature. The crucial issue in this case is whether the existence of the infant lays a moral claim that supersedes the mother's desires.

If a solicitor of funds for the relief of refugees in Bengal requested a donation from her and she responded, "I do not want to give money for that cause," some persons would think her to be morally insensitive, but none could argue that the refugees in Bengal had a moral claim on her money which she was obligated to acknowledge. The existence of the infant lays a weightier claim on her than does a request for a donation. We would not say that the child's right to surgery, and thus to life, is wholly relative to, and therefore exclusively dependent upon, the mother's desires or wants.

Another illustration is closer to her situation than the request for a donation. A man asks a woman to marry him. Because she is asked, she is under no obligation to answer affirmatively. He might press claims upon her—they have expressed love for each other; or they have dated for a long time; he has developed his affection for her on the assumption that her responsiveness would lead to marriage. But none of these claims would be sufficient to overrule her desire not to marry him. Why? Two sorts of reasons might be given. One would refer to potential consequences: a marriage in which one partner does not desire the relationship leads to anxiety and suffering. To avoid needless suffering is obviously desirable. So in this case, it might be said that the mother's desire is to avoid needless suffering and anxiety: the undesirable consequences can be avoided by permitting the child to die.

The second sort of reason why a woman has no obligation to marry her suitor refers to her rights as an individual. A request for marriage does not constitute a moral obligation, since there is no prima facie claim by the suitor. The woman has a right to say no. Indeed, if the suitor sought to coerce her into marriage, everyone would assert that she has a right to refuse him. In our case, however, there are some differences. The infant is incapable of expressing a request or demand. Also, the relationship is different; the suitor is not dependent upon his girlfriend in the same way that the infant is dependent upon his mother. Dependence functions in two different senses; the necessary conditions for the birth of the child were his conception and *in utero* nourishment—thus, in a sense the parents "caused" the child to come into being. And, apart from instituting adoption procedures, the parents are the only ones who can provide the necessary conditions for sustaining the child's life. The infant is dependent on them in the sense that he must rely upon their performance of certain acts in order to continue to exist. The ethical question to the mother is, Does the infant's physical life lay an unconditioned moral claim on the mother? She answered, implicitly, in the negative.

What backing might the negative answer be given? The most persuasive justification would come from an argument that there are no unconditioned moral claims upon one when those presumed claims go against one's desires and wants. The claims of another are relative to my desires, my wants. Neither the solicitor for Bengal relief nor the suitor has an unconditioned claim to make; in both cases a desire is sufficient grounds for denying such a claim. In our case, it would have to be argued that the two senses of dependence that the infant has on the mother are not sufficient conditions for a claim on her that would morally require the needed surgery. Since there are no unconditioned claims, and since the conditions in this drama are not sufficient to warrant a claim, the mother is justified in denying permission for the surgery.

We note here that in our culture there are two trends in the development of morality that run counter to each other: one is the trend that desires of the ego are the grounds for moral and legal claims. If a mother does not desire the fetus in her uterus, she has a right to an abortion. The other increasingly limits individual desires and wants. An employer might want to hire only white persons of German ancestry, but he has no right to do so.

The word "fair" appeals to quite different warrants. It would not be "fair" to the other children in the family to raise a mongoloid with them. In moral philosophy, fairness is either the same as justice or closely akin to it. Two traditional definitions of justice might show how fairness could be used in this case. One is "to each his due." The other children would not get what is due them because of the inordinate requirements of time, energy, and financial resources that would be required if the mongoloid child lived. Or, if they received what was due to them, there would not be sufficient time, energy, and other resources to attend to the particular needs of the mongoloid; his condition would require more than is due him. The other traditional definition is "equals shall be treated equally." In principle, all children in the family belong to a class of equals and should be treated equally. Whether the mongoloid belongs to that class of equals is in doubt. If he does, to treat him equally with the others would be unfair to him because of his particular needs. To treat him unequally would be unfair to the others.

Perhaps "fairness" did not imply "justice." Perhaps the mother was thinking about such consequences for the other children as the extra demands that would be made upon their patience, the time they would have to give the care of the child, the emotional problems they might have in coping with a retarded sibling, and the sense of shame they might have. These consequences also could be deemed to be unjust from her point of view. Since they had no accountability for the existence of the mongoloid, it was not fair to them that extra burdens be placed upon them.

To ask what was due the mongoloid infant raises harder issues. For the mother, he was not due surgical procedure that would sustain his life. He was "unequal" to her normal children, but the fact of his inequality does not necessarily imply that he has no right to live. This leads to a matter at the root of the mother's response which has to be dealt with separately.

She (and as we shall see, the doctors also) assumed that a factual distinction (between normal and mongoloid) makes the moral difference. Factual distinctions do make moral differences. A farmer who has no qualms about killing a runt pig would have moral scruples about killing a deformed infant. If the child had not been mongoloid and had an intestinal blockage, there would have been no question about permitting surgery to be done. The value of the infant is judged to be relative to a quality of its life that is predictable on the basis of the factual evidences of mongolism. Value is relative to quality: that is the justification. Given the absence of a certain quality, the value is not sufficient to maintain life; given absence of a quality, there is no right to physical life. (Questions about terminating life among very sick adults are parallel to this instance.)

What are the qualities, or what is *the* quality that is deficient in this infant? It is not the capacity for happiness, an end that Aristotle and others thought to be sufficient in itself. The mother and the doctors knew that mongoloids can be happy. It is not the capacity for pleasure, the end that the hedonistic utilitarians thought all men seek, for mongoloids can find pleasure in life. The clue is given when a physician says that the absence of the capacity for normal intelligence was crucial. He suggested that we live in a society in which intelligence is highly valued. Perhaps it is valued as a quality in itself, or as an end in itself by some, but probably there is a further point, namely that intelligence is necessary for productive contribution to one's own well-being and to the well-being of others. Not only will a mongoloid make a minimal contribution to his own well-being and to that of others, but also others must contribute excessively to his care. The right of an infant, the value of his life, is relative to his intelligence; that is the most crucial factor in enabling or limiting his contribution to his own welfare and that of others. One has to defend such a point in terms of the sorts of contributions that would be praiseworthy and the sorts of costs that would be detrimental. The contribution of a sense of satisfaction to those who might enjoy caring for the mongoloid would not be sufficient. Indeed, a full defense would require a quantification of qualities, all based on predictions at the point of birth, that would count both for and against the child's life in a cost-benefit analysis.

The judgment that value is relative to qualities is not implausible. In our society we have traditionally valued the achiever more than the nonachievers. Some hospitals have sought to judge the qualities of the contributions of patients to society in determining who has access to scarce medical resources. A mongoloid is not valued as highly as a fine musician, an effective politician, a successful businessman, a civil rights leader whose actions have brought greater justice to the society, or a physician. To be sure, in other societies and at other times other qualities have been valued, but we judge by the qualities valued in our society and our time. Persons are rewarded according to their contributions to society. A defense of the mother's decision would have to be made on these grounds, with one further crucial step. That is, when the one necessary condition for productivity is deficient (with a high degree of certitude) at birth, there is no moral obligation to maintain that life. That the same reasoning would have been sufficient to justify overtly taking the infant's life seems not to have been the case. But that point emerges later in our discussion.

The reliance upon feelings, desires, fairness, and judgments of qualities of life makes sense to American middle-class white families, and anguished decisions can very well be settled in these terms. The choice made by the mother was not that of an unfeeling problem-solving machine, nor that of a rationalistic philosopher operating from these assumptions. It was a painful, conscientious decision, made apparently on these bases. One can ask, of course, whether her physicians should not have suggested other ways of perceiving and drawing the contours of the circumstances, other values and ends that she might consider. But that points to a subsequent topic.

The Father's Decision

The decision of the father is only a footnote to that of the mother. He consented to the choice of not operating on the infant, though he did seek precise information about mongolism and its consequences for the child. He was "willing to go along with the mother's wishes," he "understood her feelings, agreed with them," and was not in a position to make "the same intelligent decision that his wife was making."

Again we see that scientific evidence based on professional knowledge is determinative of a moral decision. The physician was forthright in indicating what the consequences would be of the course of action they were taking. The consequences of raising a mongoloid child were presumably judged to be more problematic than the death of the child.

The Decision of the Physicians

A number of points of reference in the contributions of the physicians to the case study enable us to formulate a constellation of values that determined their actions. After I have depicted that constellation, I shall analyze some of the points of reference to see how they can be defended.

The constellation can be stated summarily. The physicians felt no moral or legal obligation to save the life of a mongoloid infant by an ordinary surgical procedure when the parents did not desire that it should live. Thus, the infant was left to die. What would have been a serious but routine procedure was omitted in this instance on two conditions, both of which were judged to be necessary, but neither of which was sufficient in itself: the mongolism and the parents' desires. If the parents had desired the mongoloid infant to be saved, the surgery would have been done. If the infant had not been mongoloid and the parents had refused permission for surgery to remove a bowel obstruction, the physicians would at least have argued against them and probably taken legal measures to override them. Thus, the value-laden points of reference appear to be the desires of the parents, the mongolism of the infant, the law, and choices about ordinary and extraordinary medical procedures.

One of the two most crucial points was the obligation the physicians felt to acquiesce to the desires of the parents. The choice of the parents not to operate was made on what the physicians judged to be adequate information: it was an act of informed consent on the part of the parents. There is no evidence that the physicians raised questions of a moral sort with the parents that they subsequently raised among themselves. For example, one physician later commented on the absence of rights for children in our society and in our legal system and on the role that the value of intelligence seems to have in judging worthiness of persons. These were matters, however, that the physicians did not feel obligated to raise with the distressed parents. The physicians acted on the principle that they are only to do procedures that the patient (or crucially in this case, the parents of the patient) wanted. There was no overriding right to life on the part of a mongoloid infant that led them to argue against the parents' desires or to seek a court order requiring the surgical procedure. They recognized the moral autonomy of the parents, and thus did not interfere; they accepted as a functioning principle that the parents have the right to decide whether an infant shall live.

Elaboration of the significance of parental autonomy is necessary in order to see the grounds on which it can be defended. First, the physicians apparently recognized that the conscientious parents were the moral supreme court. There are grounds for affirming the recognition of the moral autonomy of the principal persons in complex decisions. In this case, the principals were the parents: the infant did not have the capacities to express any desires or preferences he might have. The physicians said, implicitly, that the medical profession does not have a right to impose certain of its traditional values on persons if these are not conscientiously held by those persons.

There are similarities, but also differences, between this instance and that of a terminal patient. If the terminally ill patient expresses a desire not to have his life prolonged, physicians recognize his autonomy over his own body and thus feel under no obligation to sustain his life. Our case, however, would be more similar to one in which the terminally ill patient's family decided that no further procedures ought to be used to sustain life. No doubt there are many cases in which the patient is unable to express a preference due to his physical conditions, and in the light of persuasive medical and familial reasons the physician agrees not to sustain life. A difference between our case and that, however, has to be noted in order to isolate what seems to be the crucial point. In the case of the mongoloid infant, a decision is made at the beginning of his life and not at the end; the effect is to cut off a life which, given proper care, could be sustained for many years, rather than not sustaining a life which has no such prospects.

Several defenses might be made of their recognition of the parents' presumed rights in this case. The first is that parents have authority over their children until they reach an age of discretion, and in some respects until they reach legal maturity. Children do not have recognized rights over against parents in many respects. The crucial difference here, of course, is the claimed parental right in this case to determine that an infant shall not live. What grounds might there be for this? Those who claim the moral right to an abortion are claiming the right to determine whether a child shall live, and this claim is widely recognized both morally and legally. In this case we have an extension of that right to the point of birth. If there are sufficient grounds to indicate that the newborn child is significantly abnormal, the parents have the same right as they have when a severe genetic abnormality is detected prenatally on the basis of amniocentesis. Indeed, the physicians could argue that if a mother has a right to an abortion, she also has a right to determine whether a newborn infant shall continue to live.

One is simply extending the time span and the circumstances under which this autonomy is recognized.

A second sort of defense might be made: that of the limits of professional competence and authority. The physicians could argue that in moral matters they have neither competence nor authority. Perhaps they would wish to distinguish between competence and authority. They have a competence to make a moral decision on the basis of their own moral and other values, but they have no authority to impose this upon their patients. Morals, they might argue, are subjective matters, and if anyone has competence in that area, it is philosophers, clergymen, and others who teach what is right and wrong. If the parents had no internalized values that militated against their decision, it is not in the province of the physicians to tell them what they ought to do. Indeed, in a morally pluralistic society, no one group or person has a right to impose his views on another. In this stronger argument for moral autonomy no physician would have any authority to impose his own moral values on any patient. A social role differentiation is noted: the medical profession has authority only in medical matters—not in moral matters. Indeed, they have an obligation to indicate what the medical alternatives are in order to have a decision made by informed consent, but insofar as moral values or principles are involved in decisions, these are not within their professional sphere.

An outsider might ask what is meant by authority. He might suggest that surely it is not the responsibility (or at least not his primary responsibility) or the role of the physician to make moral decisions, and certainly not to enforce his decisions on others. Would he be violating his role if he did something less determinative than that, namely, in his counseling indicate to them what some of the moral considerations might be in choosing between medical alternatives? In our case the answer seems to be yes. If the principals desire moral counseling, they have the freedom to seek it from whomsoever they will. In his professional role he acknowledges that the recognition of the moral autonomy of the principals also assumes their moral self-sufficiency, that is, their capacities to make sound moral decisions without interference on his part, or the part of any other persons except insofar as the principals themselves seek such counsel. Indeed, in this case a good deal is made of the knowledgeability of the mother particularly, and this assumes that she is morally, as well as medically, knowledgeable. Or, if she is not, it is still not the physician's business to be her moral counselor.

The physicians also assumed in this case that the moral autonomy of the parents took precedence over the positive law. At least they felt no obligation to take recourse to the courts to save the life of this infant. On that issue we will reflect more when we discuss the legal point of reference.

Another sort of defense might be made. In the order of society, decisions should be left to the most intimate and smallest social unit involved. That is the right of such a unit, since the interposition of outside authority would be an infringement of its freedom. Also, since the family has to live with the consequences of the decision, it is the right of the parents to determine which potential consequences they find most desirable. The state, or the medical profession, has no right to interfere with the freedom of choice of the family. Again, in a formal way, the argument is familiar; the state has no right to interfere with the determination of what a woman wishes to do with her body, and thus antiabortion laws are infringements of her freedom. The determination of whether an infant shall be kept alive is simply an extension of the sphere of autonomy properly belonging to the smallest social unit involved.

In all the arguments for moral autonomy, the medical fact that the infant is alive and can be kept alive does not make a crucial difference. The defense of the decision would have to be made in this way: if one grants moral autonomy to mothers to determine whether they will bring a fetus to birth, it is logical to assume that one will grant the same autonomy after birth, at least in instances where the infant is abnormal.

We have noted in our constellation of factors that the desire of the parents was a necessary but not a sufficient condition for the decisions of the physicians. If the infant had not been mongoloid, the physicians would not have so readily acquiesced to the parents' desires. Thus, we need to turn to the second necessary condition.

The second crucial point is that the infant was a mongoloid. The physicians would not have acceded to the parents' request as readily if the child had been normal; the parents would have authorized the surgical procedure if the child had been normal. Not every sort of abnormality would have led to the same decision on the part of the physicians. Their appeal was to the consequences of the abnormality of mongolism: the child would be a burden financially and emotionally to the parents. Since every child, regardless of his capacities for intelligent action, is a financial burden, and at least at times an emotional burden, it is clear that the physicians believed that the quantity or degree of burden in this case would exceed any benefits that might be forthcoming if the child were permitted to live. One can infer that a principle was operative, namely, that mongoloid infants have no inherent right to life; their right to life is conditional upon the willingness of their parents to accept them and care for them.

Previously we developed some of the reasons why a mongoloid infant was judged undesirable. Some of the same appeals to consequences entered into the decisions of the physicians. If we are to seek to develop reasons why the decisions might be judged to be morally correct, we must examine another point, namely, the operating definition of "abnormal" or "defective." There was no dissent to the medical judgment that the infant was mongoloid, though precise judgments about the seriousness of the child's defect were not possible at birth.

Our intention is to find as precisely as possible what principles or values might be invoked to claim that the "defectiveness" was sufficient to warrant not sustaining the life of this infant. As a procedure, we will begin with the most general appeals that might have been made to defend the physician's decision in this case. The most general principle would be that any infant who has any empirically verifiable degree of defect at birth has no right to life. No one would apply such a principle. Less general would be that all infants who are carriers of a genetic defect that would have potentially bad consequences for future generations have no right to life. A hemophiliac carrier would be a case in point. This principle would not be applicable, even if it were invoked with approval, in this case.

Are the physicians prepared to claim that all genetically "abnormal" infants have no claim to life? I find no evidence that they would. Are they prepared to say that where the genetic abnormality affects the capacity for "happiness" the infant has no right to live? Such an appeal was not made in this case. It appears that "normal" in this case has reference to a capacity for a certain degree of intelligence.

A presumably detectable physical norm now functions as a norm in a moral sense, or as an ideal. The ideal cannot be specified in precise terms, but there is a vague judgment about the outer limits beyond which an infant is judged to be excessively far from the norm or ideal to deserve sustenance. Again, we come to the crucial role of an obvious sign of the lack of capacity for intelligence of a certain measurable sort in judging a defect to be intolerable. A further justification of this is made by an appeal to accepted social values, at least among middle- and upper-class persons in our society. Our society values intelligence; that value becomes the ideal norm from which abnormality or deficiencies are measured. Since the infant is judged not to be able to develop into an intelligent human being (and do all that "normal" intelligence enables a human being to do), his life is of insufficient value to override the desires of the parents not to have a retarded child.

Without specification of the limits to the sorts of cases to which it could be applied, the physicians would probably not wish to defend the notion that the values of a society determine the right to life. To do so would require that there be clear knowledge of who is valued in our society (we also value aggressive people, loving people, physically strong people, etc.), and in turn a procedure by which capacities for such qualities could be determined in infancy so that precise judgments could be made about what lives should be sustained. Some members of our society do not value black people; blackness would obviously be an insufficient basis for letting an infant die. Thus, in defense of their decision the physicians would have to appeal to "values generally held in our society." This creates a different problem of quantification: what percentage of dissent would count to deny a "general" holding of a value? They would also have to designate the limits to changes in socially held values beyond which they would not consent. If the parents belonged to a subculture that valued blue eyes more than it valued intelligence, and if they expressed a desire not to have a child because it had hazel eyes, the problem of the intestinal blockage would not have been a sufficient condition to refrain from the surgical procedure.

In sum, the ideal norm of the human that makes a difference in judging whether an infant has the right to life in this case is "the capacity for normal intelligence." For the good of the infant, for the sake of avoiding difficulties for the parents, and for the good of society, a significant deviation from normal intelligence, coupled with the appropriate parental desire, is sufficient to permit the infant to die.

A third point of reference was the law. The civil law and the courts figure in the decisions at two points. First, the physicians felt no obligation to seek a court order to save the life of the infant if the parents did not want it. Several possible inferences might be drawn from this. First, one can infer that the infant had no legal right to life; his legal right is conditional upon parental desires. Second, as indicated in the interviews, the physicians believed that the court would not insist upon the surgical procedure to save the infant since it was a mongoloid. Parental desires would override legal rights in such a case. And third (an explicit statement by the physician), if the infant's life had been saved as the result of a court order, there were doubts that it would have been "accepted" by the parents. Here is an implicit appeal to potential consequences: it is not beneficial for a child to be raised by parents who do not "accept" him. The assumption is that they could not change their attitudes.

If the infant had a legal right to life, this case presents an interesting instance of conscientious objection to law. The conscientious objector to military service claims that the power of the state to raise armies for the defense of what it judges to be the national interest is one that he conscientiously refrains from sharing. The common good, or the national interest, is not jeopardized by the granting of a special status to the objector because there are enough persons who do not object to man the military services. In this case, however, the function of the law is to protect the rights of individuals to life, and the physician-objector is claiming that he is under no obligation to seek the support of the legal system to sustain life even when he knows that it could be sustained. The evidence he has in hand (the parental desire and the diagnosis of mongolism) presumably provides sufficient moral grounds for his not complying with the law. From the standpoint of ethics, an appeal could be made to conscientious objection. If, however, the appropriate law does not qualify its claims in such a way as to (a) permit its nonapplicability in this case or (b) provide for exemption on grounds of conscientious objection, the objector is presumably willing to accept the consequences for his conscientious decision. This would be morally appropriate. The physician believed that the court would not insist on saving the infant's life, and thus he foresaw no great jeopardy to himself in following conscience rather than the law.

The second point at which the law figures is in the determination of how the infant should die. The decision not to induce death was made in part in the face of the illegality of overt euthanasia (in part, only, since also the hospital staff would "feel uncomfortable" about hastening the death). Once the end or purpose of action (or inaction) was judged to be morally justified, and judged likely to be free from legal censure, the physicians still felt obliged to achieve that purpose within means that would not be subject to legal sanctions. One can only speculate whether the physicians believed that a court that would not order an infant's life to be saved would in turn censure them for overtly taking the life, or whether the uncomfortable feelings of the hospital staff were more crucial in their decision. Their course of decisions could be interpreted as at one point not involving obligation to take recourse to the courts and at the other scrupulously obeying the law. It should be noted, however, that there is consistency of action on their part; in neither instance did they intervene in what was the "natural" course of developments. The moral justification to fail to intervene in the second moment had to be different from that in the first. In the first it provides the reasons for not saving a life; in the second, for not taking a life. This leads to the last aspect of the decisions of the physicians that I noted, namely, that choices were made between ordinary and extraordinary means of action.

There is no evidence in the interviews that the language of ordinary and extraordinary means of action was part of the vocabulary of the medical staff. It is, however, an honored and useful distinction in Catholic moral theology as it applies to medical care. The principle is that a physician is under no obligation to use extraordinary means to sustain life. The difficulty in the application of the principle is the choice of what falls under ordinary and what under extraordinary means. Under one set of circumstances a procedure may be judged ordinary, and under another extraordinary. The surgery required to remove the bowel obstruction in the infant was on the whole an ordinary procedure; there were no experimental aspects to it, and there were no unusual risks to the infant's life in having it done. If the infant had had no other genetic defects, there would have been no question about using it. The physicians could make a case that when the other defect was mongolism, the procedure would be an extraordinary one. The context of the judgment about ordinary and extraordinary was a wider one than the degree of risk to the life of the patient from surgery. It included his other defect, the desires of the family, the potential costs to family and society, etc. No moralists, to my knowledge, would hold them culpable if the infant were so deformed that he would be labeled (nontechnically) a monstrosity. To heroically maintain the life of a monstrosity as long as one could would be most extraordinary. Thus, we return to whether the fact of mongolism and its consequences is a sufficient justification to judge the lifesaving procedure to be extraordinary in this instance. The physicians would argue that it is.

The infant was left to die with a minimum of care. No extraordinary means were used to maintain its life once the decision not to operate had been made. Was it extraordinary not to use even ordinary procedures to maintain the life of the infant once the decision not to operate had been made? The judgment clearly was in the negative. To do so would be to prolong a life that would not be saved in any case. At that point the infant was in a class of terminal patients, and the same justifications used for not prolonging the life of a terminal patient would apply here. Patients have a right to die, and physicians are under no moral obligation to sustain their lives when it is clear that they will not live for long. The crucial difference between a terminal cancer patient and this infant is that in the situation of the former, all procedures which might prolong life for a goodly length of time are likely to have been exhausted. In the case of the infant, the logic of obligations to terminal patients takes its course as a result of a decision not to act at all.

To induce death by some overt action is an extraordinary procedure. To justify overt action would require a justification of euthanasia. This case would be a good one from which to explore euthanasia from a moral point of view. Once a decision is made not to engage in a life-sustaining and life-saving procedure, has not the crucial corner been turned? If that is a reasonable and moral thing to do, on what grounds would one argue that it is wrong to hasten death? Most obviously it is still illegal to do it, and next most obviously people have sensitive feelings about taking life. Further, it goes against the grain of the fundamental vocation of the medical profession to maintain life. But, of course, the decision not to operate also goes against that grain. If the first decision was justifiable, why was it not justifiable to hasten the death of the infant? We can only assume at this point traditional arguments against euthanasia would have been made.

The Decisions of the Nurses

The nurses, as the interviews indicated, are most important for their expressions of feelings, moral sensibilities, and frustrations. They demonstrate the importance of deeply held moral convictions and of profound compassion in determining human responses to ambiguous circumstances. If they had not known that the infant could have survived, the depth of their frustrations and feelings would have not been so great. Feelings they would have had, but they would have been compassion for an infant bound to die. The actual range of decision for them was clearly circumscribed by the role definitions in the medical professions; it was their duty to carry out the orders of the physicians. Even if they conscientiously believed that the orders they were executing were immoral, they could not radically reverse the course of events; they could not perform the required surgery. It was their lot to be the immediate participants in a sad event but to be powerless to alter its course.

It would be instructive to explore the reasons why the nurses felt frustrated, were deeply affected by their duties in this case. Moral convictions have their impact upon the feelings of persons as well as upon their rational decisions. A profound sense of vocation to relieve suffering and to preserve life no doubt lies behind their responses, as does a conviction about the sanctity of human life. For our purposes, however, we shall leave them with the observation that they are the instruments of the orders of the physicians. They have no right of conscientious objection, at least not in this set of circumstances.

Before turning to another evaluative description of the case, it is important to reiterate what was said in the beginning. The decisions by the principals were conscientious ones. The parents anguished. The physicians were informed by a sense of compassion in their consent to the parents' wishes; they did not wish to be party to potential suffering that was avoidable. Indeed, in the way in which they formulated the dilemma, they did what was reasonable to do. They chose the way of least possible suffering to the fewest persons over a long range of time, with one exception, namely, not taking the infant's life. By describing the dilemma from a somewhat different set of values, or giving different weight to different factors, another course of action would have been reasonable and justified. The issue, it seems to me, is at the level of what is to be valued more highly, for one's very understanding of the problems he must solve are deeply affected by what one values most.

The Dilemma from a Different Moral Point of View

Wallace Stevens wrote in poetic form a subtle account of "Thirteen Ways of Looking at a Blackbird." Perhaps there are 13 ways of looking at this medical case. I shall attempt to look at it from only one more way. By describing the dilemma from a perspective that gives a different weight to some of the considerations that we have already exposed, one has a different picture, and different conclusions are called for. The moral integrity of any of the original participants is not challenged, not because of a radical relativism that says they have their points of view and I have mine, but out of respect for their conscientiousness. For several reasons, however, more consideration ought to have been given to two points. A difference in evaluative judgments would have made a difference of life or death for the infant, depending upon : (1) whether what one ought to do is determined by what one desires to do and (2) whether a mongoloid infant has a claim to life.

To restate the dilemma once again: If the parents had "desired" the mongoloid infant, the surgeons would have performed the operation that would have saved its life. If the infant had had a bowel obstruction that could be taken care of by an ordinary medical procedure, but had not been a mongoloid, the physicians would probably have insisted that the operation be performed.

Thus, one can recast the moral dilemma by giving a different weight to two things: the desires of the parents and the value or rights of a mongoloid infant. If the parents and the physicians believed strongly that there are things one ought to do even when one has no immediate positive feelings about doing them, no immediate strong desire to do them, the picture would have been different. If the parents and physicians believed that mongoloid children have intrinsic value, or have a right to life, or if they believed that mongolism is not sufficiently deviant from what is normatively human to merit death, the picture would have been different.

Thus, we can redraw the picture. To be sure, the parents are ambivalent about their feelings for a mongoloid infant, since it is normal to desire a normal infant rather than an abnormal infant. But (to avoid a discussion of abortion at this point) once an infant is born its independent existence provides independent value in itself, and those who brought it into being and those professionally responsible for its care have an obligation to sustain its life regardless of their negative or ambiguous feelings toward it. This probably would have been acknowledged by all concerned if the infant had not been mongoloid. For example, if the pregnancy had been accidental, and in this sense the child was not desired, and the infant had been normal, no one would have denied its right to exist once it was born, though some would while still in utero, and thus would have sought an abortion. If the mother refused to accept accountability for the infant, alternative means of caring for it would have been explored.

To be sure, a mongoloid infant is genetically defective, and raising and caring for it put burdens on the parents, the family, and the state beyond the burdens required to raise a normal infant. But a mongoloid infant is human, and thus has the intrinsic value of humanity and the rights of a human being. Further, given proper care, it can reach a point of significant fulfillment of its limited potentialities; it is capable of loving and responding to love; it is capable of realizing happiness; it can be trained to accept responsibility for itself within its capacities. Thus, the physicians and parents have an obligation to use all ordinary means to preserve its life. Indeed, the humanity of mentally defective children is recognized in our society by the fact that we do not permit their extermination and do have policies which provide, all too inadequately, for their care and nuture.

If our case had been interpreted in the light of moral beliefs that inform the previous two paragraphs, the only reasonable conclusion would be that the surgery ought to have been done.

The grounds for assigning the weights I have to these crucial points can be examined. First, with reference simply to common experience, we all have obligations to others that are not contingent upon our immediate desires. When the registrar of my university indicates that senior grades have to be in by May 21, I have an obligation to read the exams, term papers, and senior essays in time to report the grades, regardless of my negative feelings toward those tasks or my preference to be doing something else. I have an obligation to my students, and to the university through its registrar, which I accepted when I assumed the social role of an instructor. The students have a claim on me; they have a right to expect me to fulfill my obligations to them and to the university. I might be excused from the obligation if I suddenly became too ill to fulfill it; my incapacity to fulfill it would be a temporarily excusing condition. But negative feelings toward that job, or toward any students, or a preference for writing a paper of my own at that time, would not constitute excusing conditions. I must consider, in determining what I do, the relationships that I have with others and the claims they have on me by virtue of those relationships.

In contrast to this case, it might be said that I have a contractual obligation to the university into which I freely entered. The situation of the parents is not the same. They have no legal contractual relationship with the infant, and thus their desires are not bound by obligations. Closer to their circumstances, then, might be other family relationships. I would argue that the fact that we brought our children into being lays a moral obligation on my wife and me to sustain and care for them to the best of our ability. They did not choose to be; and their very being is dependent, both causally and in other ways, upon us. In the relationship of dependence, there is a claim of them over against us. To be sure, it is a claim that also has its rewards and that we desire to fulfill within a relationship of love. But until they have reached an age when they can accept full accountability (or fuller accountability) for themselves, they have claims upon us by virtue of our being their parents, even when meeting those claims is to us financially costly, emotionally distressing, and in other ways not immediately desirable. Their claims are independent of our desires to fulfill them. Particular claims they might make can justifiably be turned down, and others can be negotiated, but the claim against us for their physical sustenance constitutes a moral obligation that we have to meet. That obligation is not conditioned by their IQ scores, whether they have cleft palates or perfectly formed faces, whether they are obedient or irritatingly independent, whether they are irritatingly obedient and passive or laudably self-determining. It is not conditioned by any predictions that might be made about whether they will become the persons we might desire that they become. The infant in our case has the same sort of claim, and thus the parents have a moral obligation to use all ordinary means to save its life.

An objection might be made. Many of my fellow Christians would say that the obligation of the parents was to do that which is loving toward the infant. Not keeping the child alive was the loving thing to do with reference both to its interests and to the interests of the other members of the family. To respond to the objection, one needs first to establish the spongy character of the words "love" or "loving." They can absorb almost anything. Next one asks whether the loving character of an act is determined by feelings or by motives, or whether it is also judged by what is done. It is clear that I would argue for the latter. Indeed, the minimal conditions of a loving relationship included respect for the other, and certainly for the other's presumption of a right to live. I would, however, primarily make the case that the relationship of dependence grounds the claim, whether or not one feels loving toward the other.

The dependence relationship holds for the physicians as well as the parents in this case. The child's life depended utterly upon the capacity of the physicians to sustain it. The fact that an infant cannot articulate his claim is irrelevant. Physicians will struggle to save the life of a person who has attempted to commit suicide even when the patient might be in such a drugged condition that he cannot express his desire—a desire expressed already in his effort to take his life and overridden by the physician's action to save it. The claim of human life for preservation, even when such a person indicates a will not to live, presents a moral obligation to those who have the capacity to save it.

A different line of argument might be taken. If the decisions made were as reliant upon the desires of the parents as they appear to be, which is to say, if desire had a crucial role, what about the desire of the infant? The infant could not give informed consent to the nonintervention. One can hypothesize that every infant desires to live, and that even a defective child is likely to desire life rather than death when it reaches an age at which its desires can be articulated. Even if the right to live is contingent upon a desire, we can infer that the infant's desire would be for life. As a human being, he would have that desire, and thus it would constitute a claim on those on whom he is dependent to fulfill it.

I have tried to keep a persuasive case to indicate why the claim of the infant constitutes a moral obligation on the parents and the physicians to keep the child alive. The intrinsic value or rights of a human being are not qualified by any given person's intelligence or capacities for productivity, potential consequences of the sort that burden others. Rather, they are constituted by the very existence of the human being as one who is related to others and dependent upon others for his existence. The presumption is always in favor of sustaining life through ordinary means; the desires of persons that run counter to that presumption are not sufficient conditions for abrogating that right.

The power to determine whether the infant shall live or die is in the hands of others. Does the existence of such power carry with it the moral right to such determination? Long history of moral experience indicates not only that arguments have consistently been made against the judgment that the capacity to do something constitutes a right to do it, or put in more familiar terms, that might makes right. It also indicates that in historical situations where persons have claimed the right to determine who shall live because they have the power to do so, the consequences have hardly been beneficial to mankind. This, one acknowledges, is a "wedge" argument or a "camel's nose under the tent" argument. As such, its limits are clear. Given a culture in which humane values are regnant, it is not likely that the establishment of a principle that some persons under some circumstances claim the right to determine whether others shall live will be transformed into the principle that the right of a person to live is dependent upon his having the qualities approved by those who have the capacity to sustain or take his life. Yet while recognizing the sociological and historical limitations that exist in a humane society, one still must recognize the significance of the precedent. To cite an absurd example, what would happen if we lived in a society in which the existence of hazel eyes was considered a genetic defect by parents and physicians? The absurdity lies in the fact that no intelligent person would consider hazel eyes a genetic defect; the boundaries around the word defect are drawn by evidences better than eye color. But the precedent in principle remains; when one has established that the capacity to determine who shall live carries with it the right to determine who shall live, the line of discussion has shifted from a sharp presumption (of the right of all humans to live) to the softer, spongier determination of the qualities whose value will be determinative.

Often we cannot avoid using qualities and potential consequences in the determination of what might be justifiable exceptions to the presumption of the right to life on the part of any infant—indeed, any person. No moralist would insist that the physicians have an obligation to sustain the life of matter born from human parents that is judged to be a "monstrosity." Such divergence from the "normal" qualities presents no problem, and potential consequences for its continued existence surely enter into the decision. The physicians in our case believed that in the absence of a desire for the child on the part of the parents, mongolism was sufficiently removed from an ideal norm of the human that the infant had no overriding claim on them. We are in a sponge. Why would I draw the line on a different side of mongolism than the physicians did? While reasons can be given, one must recognize that there are intuitive elements, grounded in beliefs and profound feelings, that enter into particular judgments of this sort. I am not prepared to say that my respect for human life is "deeper," "profounder," or "stronger" than theirs. I am prepared to say that the way in which, and the reasons why, I respect life orient my judgment toward the other side of mongolism than theirs did.

First, the value that intelligence was given in this instance appears to me to be simplistic. Not all intelligent persons are socially commendable (choosing socially held values as the point of reference because one of the physicians did). Also, many persons of limited intelligence do things that are socially commendable, if only minimally providing the occasion for the expression of profound human affection and sympathy. There are many things we value about human life; that the assumption that one of them is the *sine qua non*, the necessary and sufficient condition for a life to be valued at all, oversimplifies human experience. If there is a *sine qua non*, it is physical life itself, for apart from it, all potentiality of providing benefits for oneself or for others is impossible. There are occasions on which other things are judged to be more valuable than physical life itself; we probably all would admire the person whose life is martyred for the sake of saving others. But the qualities or capacities we value exist in bundles, and not each as overriding in itself. The capacity for self-determination is valued, and on certain occasions we judge that it is worth dying, or taking life, for the sake of removing repressive limits imposed upon persons in that respect. But many free, self-determining persons are not very happy; indeed, often their anxiety increases with the enlargement of the range of things they must and can determine for themselves. Would we value a person exclusively because he is happy? Probably not, partly because his happiness has at least a mildly contagious effect on some other persons, and thus we value him because he makes others happy as well. To make one quality we value (short of physical life itself, and here there are exceptions) determinative over all other qualities is to impoverish the richness and variety of human life. When we must use the sponge of qualities to determine exceptions to the presumption of the right to physical life, we need to face their variety, their complexity, the abrasiveness of one against the other, in the determination of action. In this case the potentialities of a mongoloid for satisfaction in life, for fulfilling his limited capacities, for happiness, for providing the occasions of meaningful (sometimes distressing and sometimes joyful) experience for others are sufficient so that no exception to the right to life should be made. Put differently, the anguish, suffering, embarrassment, expenses of family and state (I support the need for revision of social policy and practice) are not sufficiently negative to warrant that a mongoloid's life not be sustained by ordinary procedures.

Second, and harder to make persuasive, is that my view of human existence leads to a different assessment of the significance of suffering than appears to be operative in this case. The best argument to be made in support of the course of decisions as they occurred is that in the judgment of the principals involved, they are able to avoid more suffering and other costs for more people over a longer range of time than could have been avoided if the infant's life had been saved. To suggest a different evaluation of suffering is not to suggest that suffering is an unmitigated good, or that the acceptance of suffering when it could be avoided is a strategy that ought to be adopted for the good life, individually and collectively. Surely it is prudent and morally justifiable to avoid suffering if possible under most normal circumstances of life. But two questions will help to designate where a difference of opinion between myself and the principals in our drama can be located. One is, At what cost to others is it justifiable to avoid suffering for ourselves? On the basis of my previous exposition, I would argue that in this instance the avoidance of potential suffering at the cost of that life was not warranted. The moral claims of others upon me often involve emotional and financial stress, but that stress is not sufficient to warrant my ignoring the claims. The moral and legal claim of the government to the right to raise armies in defense of the national interest involves inconvenience, suffering, and even death for many; yet the fact that meeting that claim will cause an individual suffering is not sufficient ground to give conscientious objection. Indeed, we normally honor those who assume suffering for the sake of benefits to others.

The second question is, Does the suffering in prospect appear to be bearable for those who have to suffer? We recognize that the term "bearable" is a slippery slope and that fixing an answer to this question involves judgments that are always hypothetical. If, however, each person has a moral right to avoid all bearable inconvenience of suffering that appears to run counter to his immediate or long-range self-interest, there are many things necessary for the good of other individuals and for the common good that would not get done. In our case, there appear to be no evidences that the parents with assistance from other institutions would necessarily find the raising of a mongoloid child to bring suffering that they could not tolerate. Perhaps there is justifying evidence to which I do not have access, such as the possibility that the mother would be subject to severe mental illness if she had to take care of the child. But from the information I received, no convincing case could be made that the demands of raising the child would present intolerable and unbearable suffering to the family. That it would create greater anguish, greater inconvenience, and greater demands than raising a normal child would is clear. But that meeting these demands would cause greater suffering to this family than it does to thousands of others who raise mongoloid children seems not to be the case.

Finally, my view, grounded ultimately in religious convictions as well as moral beliefs, is that to be human is to have a vocation, a calling, and the calling of each of us is "to be for others" at least as much as "to be for ourselves." The weight that one places on "being for others" makes a difference in one's fundamental orientation toward all of his relationships, particularly when they conflict with his immediate self-interest. In the Torah we have that great commandment, rendered in the New English Bible as "you shall love your neighbour as a man like yourself" (Lev. 19:18). It is reiterated in the records we have of the words of Jesus, "Love your neighbor as yourself" (Matt. 22:39, and several other places). Saint Paul makes the point even stronger at one point: "Each of you must regard, not his own interests, but the other man's" (1 Cor. 10:24, NEB). And finally, the minimalist saying accredited both to Rabbi Hillel and to Jesus in different forms, "Do unto others as you would have others do unto you."

The point of the biblical citations is not to take recourse to dogmatic religious authority, as if these sayings come unmediated from the ultimate power and orderer of life. The point is to indicate a central thrust in Judaism and Christianity, which has nourished and sustained a fundamental moral outlook, namely, that we are "to be for others" at least as much as we are "to be for ourselves." The fact that this outlook has not been adhered to consistently by those who professed it does not count against it. It remains a vocation, a calling, a moral ideal, if not a moral obligation. The statement of such an outlook does not resolve all the particular problems of medical histories such as this one, but it shapes a bias, gives a weight, toward the well-being of the other against inconvenience or cost to oneself. In this case, I believe that all the rational inferences to be drawn from it, and all the emotive power that this calling evokes, lead to the conclusion that the ordinary surgical procedure should have been done, and the mongoloid infant's life saved.

13

To Save or Let Die:
The Dilemma of Modern Medicine

Richard A. McCormick

ON February 24, the son of Mr. and Mrs. Robert H. T. Houle died following court-ordered emergency surgery at Maine Medical Center. The child
was born February 9, horribly deformed. His entire left side was malformed;
he had no left eye, was practically without a left ear, had a deformed left
hand; some of his vertebrae were not fused. Furthermore, he was afflicted
with a tracheal esophageal fistula and could not be fed by mouth. Air leaked
into his stomach instead of going to the lungs, and fluid from the stomach
pushed up into the lungs. As Dr. André Hellegers recently noted, "It takes
little imagination to think there were further internal deformities" (*Obstet-
rical and Gynecological News*, April 1974).

As the days passed, the condition of the child deteriorated. Pneumonia set
in. His reflexes became impaired and because of poor circulation, severe
brain damage was suspected. The tracheal esophageal fistula, the immediate
threat to his survival, can be corrected with relative ease by surgery. But in
view of the associated complications and deformities, the parents refused
their consent to surgery on "Baby Boy Houle." Several doctors in the Maine
Medical Center felt differently and took the case to court. Maine Superior

Reprinted from the *Journal of the American Medical Association*, 229 (July 8, 1974), 172–76,
and from *America*, 131 (July 13, 1974), 6–10, with the permission of the author and publishers. Copyright © 1974 by the American Medical Association and by *America* Press.

Court Judge David G. Roberts ordered the surgery to be performed. He ruled: "At the moment of live birth there does exist a human being entitled to the fullest protection of the law. The most basic right enjoyed by every human being is the right to life itself."

"Meaningful Life"

Instances like this happen frequently. In a recent issue of the *New England Journal of Medicine*, Drs. Raymond S. Duff and A. G. M. Campbell (1973) reported on 299 deaths in the special-care nursery of the Yale-New Haven Hospital between 1970 and 1972. Of these, 43 (14 percent) were associated with discontinuance of treatment for children with multiple anomalies, trisomy, cardiopulmonary crippling, meningomyelocele, and other central nervous system defects. After careful consideration of each of these 43 infants, parents and physicians in a group decision concluded that the prognosis for "meaningful life" was extremely poor or hopeless, and therefore rejected further treatment. The abstract of the Duff-Campbell report states: "The awesome finality of these decisions, combined with a potential for error in prognosis, made the choice agonizing for families and health professionals. Nevertheless, the issue has to be faced, for not to decide is an arbitrary and potentially devastating decision of default."

In commenting on this study in the Washington *Post* (Oct. 28, 1973), Dr. Lawrence K. Pickett, chief of staff at the Yale-New Haven Hospital, admitted that allowing hopelessly ill patients to die "is accepted medical practice." He continued: "This is nothing new. It's just being talked about now."

It has been talked about, it is safe to say, at least since the publicity associated with the famous "Johns Hopkins Case" some three years ago. In this instance, an infant was born with Down's syndrome and duodenal atresia. The blockage is reparable by relatively easy surgery. However, after consultation with spiritual advisers, the parents refused permission for this corrective surgery, and the child died by starvation in the hospital after 15 days. For to feed him by mouth in this condition would have killed him. Nearly everyone who has commented on this case has disagreed with the decision.

It must be obvious that these instances—and they are frequent—raise the most agonizing and delicate moral problems. The problem is best seen in the ambiguity of the term "hopelessly ill." This used to and still may refer to lives that cannot be saved, that are irretrievably in the dying process. It may also refer to lives that can be saved and sustained, but in a wretched, painful, or deformed condition. With regard to infants, the problem is, which infants, if any, should be allowed to die? On what grounds or according to what criteria, as determined by whom? Or again, is there a point at which a life that can be saved is not "meaningful life," as the medical community so often phrases the question? If our past experience is any hint of the future, it is safe to say that public discussion of such controversial issues will quickly collapse into slogans such as "There is no such thing as a life not worth saving" or "Who is the physician to play God?" We saw and continue to see this far too frequently in the abortion debate. We are experiencing it in the euthanasia discussion. For instance, "death with dignity" translates for many into a death that is fast, clean, painless. The trouble with slogans is that they do not aid in the discovery of truth; they co-opt this discovery and promulgate it rhetorically, often only thinly disguising a good number of questionable value judgments in the process. Slogans are not tools for analysis and enlightenment; they are weapons for ideological battle.

Thus far, the ethical discussion of these truly terrifying decisions has been less than fully satisfactory. Perhaps this is to be expected since the problems have only recently come to public attention. In a companion article to the Duff-Campbell report, Dr. Anthony Shaw (1973) of the Pediatric Division of the Department of Surgery, University of Virginia Medical Center, Charlottesville, speaks of solutions "based on the circumstances of each case rather than by means of a dogmatic formula approach." Are these really the only options available to us? Shaw's statement makes it appear that the ethical alternatives are narrowed to dogmatism (which imposes a formula that prescinds from circumstances) and pure concretism (which denies the possibility or usefulness of any guidelines).

Are Guidelines Possible?

Such either-or extremism is understandable. It is easy for the medical profession, in its fully justified concern with the terrible concreteness of these problems and with the issue of who makes these decisions, to trend away from any substantive guidelines. As *Time* remarked in reporting these instances: "Few, if any, doctors are willing to establish guidelines for determining which babies should receive lifesaving surgery or treatment and which should not" (March 25, 1974). On the other hand, moral theologians, in their fully justified concern to avoid total normlessness and arbitrariness wherein the right is "discovered," or really "created," only in and by brute decision, can easily be insensitive to the moral relevance of the raw experience, of the conflicting tensions and concerns provoked through direct cradleside contact with human events and persons.

But is there no middle course between sheer concretism and dogmatism? I believe there is. Dr. Franz J. Ingelfinger, editor of the *New England Journal of Medicine*, in an editorial on the Duff-Campbell-Shaw articles, concluded, even if somewhat reluctantly: "Society, ethics, institutional attitudes, and committees can provide the broad guidelines, but the onus of decision making ultimately falls on the doctor in whose care the child has been put" (1973). Similarly, Frederick Carney of Southern Methodist University, Dallas, and the Kennedy Center for Bioethics stated of these cases: "What is obviously needed is the development of substantive standards to inform parents and physicians who must make such decisions" (Washington *Post*, March 20, 1974).

"Broad guidelines," "substantive standards." There is the middle course, and it is the task of a community broader than the medical community. A guideline is not a slide rule that makes the decision. It is far less than that. But it is far more than the concrete decision of the parents and physician, however seriously and conscientiously this is made. It is more like a light in a room, a light that allows the individual objects to be seen in the fullness of their context. Concretely, if there are certain infants that we agree ought to be saved in spite of illness or deformity, and if there are certain infants that we agree should be allowed to die, then there is a line to be drawn. And if there is a line to be drawn, there ought to be some criteria, even if very general, for doing this. Thus, if nearly every commentator has disagreed with the Hopkins decision, should we not be able to distill from such consensus some general wisdom that will inform and guide future decisions? I think so.

This task is not easy. Indeed, it is so harrowing that the really tempting thing is to run from it. The most sensitive, balanced, and penetrating study of the Hopkins case that I have seen is that of the University of Chicago's James Gustafson (1973). Gustafson disagreed with the decision of the Hopkins physicians to deny surgery to the mongoloid infant. In summarizing his dissent, he notes: "Why would I draw the line on a different side of mongolism than the physicians did? While reasons can be given, one must recognize that there are intuitive elements, grounded in beliefs and profound feelings, that enter into particular judgments of this sort." He goes on to criticize the assessment made of the child's intelligence as too simplistic, and he proposes a much broader perspective on the meaning of suffering than seemed to have operated in the Hopkins decision. I am in full agreement with Gustafson's reflections and conclusions. But ultimately, he does not tell us where he would draw the line or why, only where he would *not*, and why.

This is very helpful already, and perhaps it is all that can be done. Dare we take the next step, the combination and analysis of such negative judgments to extract from them the positive criterion or criteria inescapably operative in them? Or more startlingly, dare we *not* if these decisions are already being made? Gustafson is certainly right in saying that we cannot always establish perfectly rational accounts and norms for our decisions. But I believe we must never cease trying, in fear and trembling to be sure. Otherwise, we have exempted these decisions in principle from the one critique and control that protects against abuse. Exemption of this sort is the root of all exploitation, whether personal or political. Briefly, if we must face the frightening task of making quality-of-life judgments—and we must—then we must face the difficult task of building criteria for these judgments.

Facing Responsibility

What has brought us to this position of awesome responsibility? Very simply, the sophistication of modern medicine. Contemporary resuscitation and life-sustaining devices have brought a remarkable change in the state of the question. Our duties toward the care and preservation of life have been traditionally stated in terms of the use of ordinary and extraordinary means. For the moment and for purposes of brevity, we may say that, morally speaking, ordinary means are those whose use does not entail grave hardships to the patient. Those that would involve such hardships are extraordinary. Granted the relativity of these terms and the frequent difficulty of their application, still the distinction has had an honored place in medical ethics and medical practice. Indeed, the distinction was recently reiterated by the

House of Delegates of the American Medical Association in a policy statement. After disowning intentional killing (mercy killing), the AMA statement continues:

> The cessation of the employment of extraordinary means to prolong the life of the body when there is irrefutable evidence that biological death is imminent is the decision of the patient and/or his immediate family. The advice and judgment of the physician should be freely available to the patient and/or his immediate family. (JAMA 227[1974]:728)

This distinction can take us just so far—and thus the change in the state of the question. The contemporary problem is precisely that the question no longer concerns only those for whom "biological death is imminent" in the sense of the AMA statement. Many infants who would have died a decade ago, whose "biological death was imminent," can be saved. Yesterday's failures are today's successes. Contemporary medicine with its team approaches, staged surgical techniques, monitoring capabilities, ventilatory support systems, and other methods, can keep almost anyone alive. This has tended gradually to shift the problem from the means to reverse the dying process to the quality of the life sustained and preserved. The questions, "Is this means too hazardous or difficult to use" and "Does this measure only prolong the patient's dying," while still useful and valid, now often become "Granted that we can easily save the life, what kind of life are we saying?" This is a quality-of-life judgment. And we fear it. And certainly we should. But with increased power goes increased responsibility. Since we have the power, we must face the responsibility.

A Relative Good

In the past, the Judeo-Christian tradition has attempted to walk a balanced middle path between medical vitalism (that preserves life at any cost) and medical pessimism (that kills when life seems frustrating, burdensome, "useless"). Both of these extremes root in an identical idolatry of life—an attitude that, at least by inference, views death as an unmitigated, absolute evil, and life as the absolute good. The middle course that has structured Judeo-Christian attitudes is that life is indeed a basic and precious good, but a good to be preserved precisely as the condition of other values. It is these other values and possibilities that found the duty to preserve physical life and also dictate the limits of this duty. In other words, life is a relative good, and the duty to preserve it a limited one. These limits have always been stated in terms of the *means* required to sustain life. But if the implications of this middle position are unpacked a bit, they will allow us, perhaps, to adapt to the type of quality-of-life judgment we are now called on to make without tumbling into vitalism or a utilitarian pessimism.

A beginning can be made with a statement of Pope Pius XII in an allocution to physicians delivered November 24, 1957. After noting that we are normally obliged to use only ordinary means to preserve life, the Pontiff stated: "A more strict obligation would be too burdensome for most men and would render the attainment of the higher, more important good too difficult. Life, death, all temporal activities are in fact subordinated to spiritual ends." Here it would be helpful to ask two questions. First, what are these spiritual ends, this "higher, more important good"? Second, how is its attainment rendered too difficult by insisting on the use of extraordinary means to preserve life?

The first question must be answered in terms of love of God and neighbor. This sums up briefly the meaning, substance, and consummation of life from a Judeo-Christian perspective. What is or can easily be missed is that these two loves are not separable. St. John wrote: "If any man says I love God and hates his brother he is a liar. For he who loves not his brother, whom he sees, how can he love God whom he does not see?" (1 John 4 : 20–21). This means that our love of neighbor is in some very real sense our love of God. The good our love wants to do Him and to which He enables us, can be done only for the neighbor, as Karl Rahner has so forcefully argued. It is in others that God demands to be recognized and loved. If this is true, it means that, in Judeo-Christian perspective, the meaning, substance, and consummation of life is found in human relationships, and the qualities of justice, respect, concern, compassion, and support that surround them.

Second, how is the attainment of this "higher, more important (than life) good" rendered "too difficult" by life-supports that are gravely burdensome? One who must support his life with disproportionate effort focuses the time, attention, energy, and resources of himself and others not precisely on relationships, but on maintaining the condition of relationships. Such concentration easily becomes overconcentration and distorts one's view of and weakens one's pursuit of the very relational goods that define our growth and flourishing. The importance of relationships gets lost in the struggle for survival. The very Judeo-Christian meaning of life is seriously jeopardized when undue and unending effort must go into its maintenance.

I believe an analysis similar to this is implied in traditional treatises on preserving life. The illustrations of grave hardship (rendering the means to preserve life extraordinary and nonobligatory) are instructive, even if they are outdated in some of their particulars. Older moralists often referred to the hardship of moving to another climate or country. As the late Gerald Kelly (1958) noted of this instance: "They (the classical moral theologians) spoke of other inconveniences, too: e.g., of moving to another climate or another country to preserve one's life. For people whose lives were, so to speak, rooted in the land, and whose native town or village was as dear as life itself, and for whom, moreover, travel was always difficult and often dangerous—for such people, moving to another country or climate was a truly great hardship, and more than God would demand as a 'reasonable' means of preserving one's health and life."

Similarly, if the financial cost of life-preserving care was crushing, that is, if it would create grave hardships for oneself or one's family, it was considered extraordinary and nonobligatory. Or again, the grave inconvenience of living with a badly mutilated body was viewed, along with other factors (such as pain in preanesthetic days, uncertainty of success), as constituting the means extraordinary. Even now, the contemporary moralist, M. Zalba (1957) states that no one is obliged to preserve his life when the cost is "a most oppressive convalescence" (*molestissima convalescentia*).

The Quality of Life

In all of these instances—instances where the life could be saved—the discussion is couched in terms of the means necessary to preserve life. But often enough it is the kind of, the quality of life thus saved (painful, poverty-stricken and deprived, away from home and friends, oppressive) that establishes the means as extraordinary. *That* type of life would be an excessive hardship for the individual. It would distort and jeopardize his grasp on the overall meaning of life. Why? Because, it can be argued, human relationships—which are the very possibility of growth in love of God and neighbor—would be so threatened, strained, or submerged that they would no longer function as the heart and meaning of the individual's life as they should. Something other than the "higher, more important good" would occupy first place. Life, the condition of other values and achievements, would usurp the place of these and become itself the ultimate value. When that happens, the value of human life has been distorted out of context.

In his *Morals in Medicine*, Thomas O'Donnell (1960) hinted at an analysis similar to this. Noting that life is a relative, not an absolute good, he asks: Relative to what? His answer moves in two steps. First, he argues that life is the fundamental natural good God has given to man, "the fundamental context in which all other goods which God has given man as means to an end proposed to him, must be exercised." Second, since this is so, the relativity of the good of life consists in the effort required to preserve this fundamental context and "the potentialities of the other goods that still remain to be worked out within that context."

Can these reflections be brought to bear on the grossly malformed infant? I believe so. Obviously there is a difference between having a terribly mutilated body as the result of surgery, and having a terribly mutilated body from birth. There is also a difference between a long, painful, oppressive convalescence resulting from surgery, and a life that is from birth one long, painful, oppressive convalescence. Similarly, there is a difference between being plunged into poverty by medical expenses and being poor without ever incurring such expenses. However, is there not also a similarity? Can not these conditions, whether caused by medical intervention or not, equally absorb attention and energies to the point where the "higher, more important good" is simply too difficult to attain? It would appear so. Indeed, is this not precisely why abject poverty (and the systems that support it) is such an enormous moral challenge to us? It simply dehumanizes.

Life's potentiality for other values is dependent on two factors, those external to the individual, and the very condition of the individual. The former we can and must change to maximize individual potential. That is what social justice is all about. The latter we sometimes cannot alter. It is neither inhuman nor un-Christian to say that there comes a point where an individual's condition itself represents the negation of any truly human—i.e., relational—potential. When that point is reached, is not the best treatment no treatment? I believe that the *implications* of the traditional distinction between ordinary and extraordinary means point in this direction.

In this tradition, life is not a value to be preserved in and for itself. To maintain that would commit us to a form of medical vitalism that makes no human or Judeo-Christian sense. It is a value to be preserved precisely as a condition for other values, and therefore insofar as these other values remain attainable. Since these other values cluster around and are rooted in human relationships, it seems to follow that life is a value to be preserved only insofar as it contains some potentiality for human relationships. When in human judgment this potentiality is totally absent or would be, because of the condition of the individual, totally subordinated to the mere effort for survival, that life can be said to have achieved its potential.

Human Relationships

If these reflections are valid, they point in the direction of a guideline that may help in decisions about sustaining the lives of grossly deformed and deprived infants. That guideline is the potential for human relationships associated with the infant's condition. If that potential is simply nonexistent or would be utterly submerged and undeveloped in the mere struggle to survive, that life has achieved its potential. There are those who will want to continue to say that some terribly deformed infants may be allowed to die *because* no extraordinary means need be used. Fair enough. But they should realize that the term "extraordinary" has been so relativized to the condition of the patient that it is this condition that is decisive. The means is extraordinary because the infant's condition is extraordinary. And if that is so, we must face this fact head-on—and discover the substantive standard that allows us to say this of some infants, but not of others.

Here several caveats are in order. First, this guideline is not a detailed rule that preempts decisions; for relational capacity is not subject to mathematical analysis but to human judgment. However, it is the task of physicians to provide some more concrete categories or presumptive biological symptoms for this human judgment. For instance, nearly all would very likely agree that the anencephalic infant is without relational potential. On the other hand, the same cannot be said of the mongoloid infant. The task ahead is to attach relational potential to presumptive biological symptoms for the gray area between such extremes. In other words, individual decisions will remain the anguishing onus of parents in consultation with physicians.

Second, because this guideline is precisely that, mistakes will be made. Some infants will be judged in all sincerity to be devoid of any meaningful relational potential when that is actually not quite the case. This risk of error should not lead to abandonment of decisions; for that is to walk away from the human scene. Risk of error means only that we must proceed with great humility, caution, and tentativeness. Concretely, it means that if err we must at times, it is better to err on the side of life—and therefore to tilt in that direction.

Third, it must be emphasized that allowing some infants to die does not imply that "some lives are valuable, others not" or that "there is such a thing as a life not worth living." Every human being, regardless of age or condition, is of incalculable worth. The point is not, therefore, whether this or that individual has value. Of course he has, or rather *is* a value. The only point is whether this undoubted value has any potential at all, in continuing physical survival, for attaining a share, even if reduced, in the "higher, more important good." This is not a question about the inherent value of the individual. It is a question about whether this worldly existence will offer such a valued individual any hope of sharing those values for which physical life is the fundamental condition. Is not the only alternative an attitude that supports mere physical life as long as possible with every means?

Fourth, this whole matter is further complicated by the fact that this decision is being made for someone else. Should not the decision on whether life is to be supported or not be left to the individual? Obviously, wherever possible. But there is nothing inherently objectionable in the fact that parents with physicians must make this decision at some point for infants. Parents must make many crucial decisions for children. The only concern is that the decision not be shaped out of the utilitarian perspectives so deeply sunk into the consciousness of the contemporary world. In a highly technological culture, an individual is always in danger of being valued for his function, what he can do, rather than for who he is.

It remains, then, only to emphasize that these decisions must be made in terms of the child's good, this alone. But that good, as fundamentally a relational good, has many dimensions. Pius XII, in speaking of the duty to preserve life, noted that this duty "derives from well-ordered charity, from submission to the Creator, from social justice, as well as from devotion toward his family." All of these considerations pertain to that "higher, more important good." If that is the case with the duty to preserve life, then the decision not to preserve life must likewise take all of these into account in determining what is for the child's good.

Any discussion of this problem would be incomplete if it did not repeatedly stress that it is the pride of Judeo-Christian tradition that the weak and defenseless, the powerless and unwanted, those whose grasp on the goods of life is most fragile—that is, those whose potential is real but reduced—are cherished and protected as our neighbor in greatest need. Any application of a general guideline that forgets this is but a racism of the adult world profoundly at adds with the gospel, and eventually corrosive of the humanity of those who ought to be caring and supporting as long as that care and support has human meaning. It has meaning as long as there is hope that the infant will, in relative comfort, be able to experience our caring and love. For when this happens, both we and the child are sharing in that "greater, more important good."

Were not those who disagreed with the Hopkins decision saying, in effect, that for the infant, involved human relationships were still within reach and would not be totally submerged by survival? If that is the case, it is potential for relationships that is at the heart of these agonizing decisions.

References

Duff, Raymond S., and A. G. M. Campbell. "Moral and Ethical Dilemmas in the Special-care Nursery." *New England Journal of Medicine* 289 (October 25, 1973): 890–94.

Gustafson, James M. "Mongolism, Parental Desires, and the Right to Life." *Perspectives in Biology and Medicine* 16 (Summer 1973): 529–57.

Ingelfinger, Franz J. "Bedside Ethics for the Hopeless Case." *New England Journal of Medicine* 289 (October 25, 1973): 914–15.

Kelly, Gerald. *Medico-Moral Problems.* St. Louis: Catholic Hospital Association, 1958.

O'Donnell, Thomas. *Morals in Medicine.* Westminster, Md.: Newman Press, 1960.

Shaw, Anthony. "Dilemmas of 'Informed Consent' in Children." *New England Journal of Medicine* 289 (October 25, 1973): 885–90.

Zalba, M. *Theologiae Moralis Summa.* Madrid: La Editorial Catolica, 1957.

14

Maine Medical Center v. Houle

❧❧❧❧❧

Superior Court of the State of Maine

Maine Medical Center and
Martin A. Barron, Jr., M.D.,
      Petitioners,
       vs.
Lorraine Marie Houle and   No. 74-145
Robert B. T. Houle,   opinion
      Respondents.   and
               order

THE complaint herein seeks the intervention of the court between the
parents of a newborn child and the hospital and attending physician concerning parental decision as to the future course of treatment. The existence
of the child herein gives the court equitable jurisdiction to fulfill the responsibility of government in its character as parens patriae to care for infants
and protect them from neglect. This power has been historically exercised
by courts of chancery, and the existence of statutory jurisdiction in the
Probate Court and District Court does not divest this court of its equity powers.

 The testimony herein indicates that a male child was born to the defendants on February 9, 1974, at the Maine Medical Center. Medical examination by the hospital staff revealed the absence of a left eye, a rudimentary
left ear with no ear canal, a malformed left thumb and a tracheal esophageal
fistula. The latter condition prevented the ingestion of nourishment, neces-
sitated intravenous feeding, and allowed the entry of fluids into the infant's

lungs leading to the development of pneumonia and other complications. The recommended medical treatment was surgical repair of the tracheal esophageal fistula to allow normal feeding and respiration. Prior to February 11, 1974, the child's father directed the attending physician not to conduct surgical repair of the fistula and to cease intravenous feeding. . . .

Quite literally the court must make a decision concerning the life or death of a newborn infant. Recent decisions concerning the right of the state to intervene with the medical and moral judgments of a prospective parent and attending physician may have cast doubts upon the legal rights of an unborn child; but at the moment of live birth there does exist a human being entitled to the fullest protection of the law. The most basic right enjoyed by every human being is the right to life itself.

Where the condition of a child does not involve serious risk of life and where treatment involves a considerable risk, parents as the natural guardians have a considerable degree of discretion and the courts ought not intervene. The measures proposed in this case are not in any sense heroic measures except for the doctor's opinion that probable brain damage has rendered life not worth preserving. Were it his opinion that life itself could not be preserved, heroic measures ought not be required. However, the doctor's qualitative evaluation of the value of the life to be preserved is not legally within the scope of his expertise.

In the court's opinion the issue before the court is not the prospective quality of the life to be preserved, but the medical feasibility of the proposed treatment compared with the almost certain risk of death should treatment be withheld. Being satisfied that corrective surgery is medically necessary and medically feasible, the court finds that the defendant's herein have no right to withhold such treatment and that to do so constitutes neglect in the legal sense. Therefore, the court will authorize the guardian ad litem to consent to the surgical correction of the tracheal esophageal fistula and such other normal life supportive measures as may be medically required in the immediate future. It is further ordered that Respondents are hereby enjoined until further order of this court from issuing any orders to Petitioners or their employees which, in the opinion of the attending physicians or surgeons, would be injurious to the medical condition of the child. . . .

David G. Roberts
Justice of the Superior Court
February 14, 1974

adults

15

On (Only) Caring for the Dying

PAUL RAMSEY

The wish to have a death of one's own is growing ever rarer. Only a while yet, and it will be just as rare to have a death of one's own as it is already to have a life of one's own.

Rainer Maria Rilke

The Problem

Shall a patient suffering from terminal illness be given life-sustaining procedures? Should he be placed on a respirator, and is there reason for ever turning off the respirator if such treatment was hopefully begun? Is there any moral difference between not starting the respirator, compared to turning it off once started? Are we bound to begin and continue the use of the intravenous drip because it is so standard a procedure? The "essentially isolated heart" can be kept beating for weeks; should this be begun or continued? Alternatively, the heart can be stopped for surgery or transplantation, while circulation of the blood is shunted around the heart and maintained, along with artificial respiration, by a heart-lung machine: are we obliged to use these means, and, if sometimes not, when not? Should a hopelessly paralyzed person be placed in an iron lung for the rest of his life? Must a terminal cancer patient be urged to undergo major

Reprinted from *The Patient as Person.* pp. 114–41, 144–53, and 157–64, with the permission of the author and Yale University Press. Copyright © 1970 by Yale University. Some footnotes omitted.

surgery for the sake of a few months' palliation? What of fragmented creatures in deep and prolonged coma from severe brain damage, whose spontaneous cerebral activities have been reduced to those arising from the brain-stem (diencephalon, mesencephalon, pons, and medulla) but who can be maintained "alive" for years by a combination of artificial activators and by nourishment? How much blood are we going to give a terminal patient, or how many successive organ transplants? Should transfusions for the treatment of hemorrhage from a gastrointestinal cancer be discontinued, when an operation to relieve this condition is not contemplated or feasible? Is there no end to the doctor's vocation to maintain life until the matter is taken out of his hands?

Alternatively expressed, ought there to be any relief for the dying from a physician's search for exquisite triumphs over death in a sort of salvation by works? Is a quadruple amputee absolutely obliged to choose existence on such terms? If not, what right has a doctor to save his life forcibly (apart from the general benefit of pushing back the frontiers of medical science); and then by what right should medical practice advance through achieving this success by means of him? Should cardiac surgery be performed to remove the lesions that are part of the picture in cases of mongolism, from which many mercifully died before the brilliant developments of recent years?

The same sort of question can be raised about many quite standard or routine procedures. Suppose that a diabetic patient long accustomed to self-administration of insulin falls victim to terminal cancer, or suppose that a terminal cancer patient suddenly develops diabetes. Is he in the first case obliged to continue, and in the second case obliged to begin, insulin treatment and die painfully of cancer, or in either or both cases may the patient choose rather to pass into diabetic coma and an earlier death? The same question can be raised in case of the onset of diabetes in a patient who has lived to old age in an institution for the severely retarded. What of the conscious patient suffering from painful incurable disease who suddenly gets pneumonia? Or an old man slowly deteriorating who from simply being inactive and recumbent gets pneumonia: are we to use antibiotics in a likely successful attack upon this disease which from time immemorial has been called "the old man's friend"? If this is the judgment to be made in regard to the aged, what shall we say of an infant who has hydrocephalus and develops pneumonia which could cause death in a short time? Should a baby born with serious congenital defect be respirated and saved from normal dying by advanced incubator procedures, or protected from the compensating abnormality which nature has somehow provided in the form of lower resistance to ordinary infections? Shall the child who is gravely impaired by mongolism be saved by a simple treatment from an infection that could cause his death?

The question whether it is right to withhold routine procedures in these cases may remain to haunt us even if we agree with Dr. Edward Rynearson (1959) that a combination of the heroic measures that are now possible may deprive many a patient of a fulfillment of the wish to have a death of one's own. The scene Dr. Rynearson describes is one of patients with an "untreatable" disease being "kept alive indefinitely by means of tubes inserted into their stomachs, or into their veins, or into their bladders, or into their rectums—and the whole sad scene thus created is encompassed within a cocoon of oxygen which is the next thing to a shroud"—separated from family, from friends, and from themselves—the victims, this physician believes, of massive and unwarranted medical interventions upon their own particular death that has seized them.

One cannot hope to resolve the legitimate disagreement of conscientious men over every one of these questions. These cases suffice to show the importance of the problem raised by asking whether, beyond many present-day efforts to rescue the perishing, there does not arise a medical duty to (only) care for the dying. But this much can be said at the outset. These questions should be resolved one way or the other as *patient*-policy questions and not as public-policy questions because of the scarcity of beds and other hospital resources. Unless we give an ethically valid, patient-centered answer to them, medically advanced societies will move more and more to decisions based on the numbers and needs that can be accommodated.

The public-policy or hospital-policy question is already enormous. Are we not in modern medicine, a doctor (Long 1960) asks, "piling up one Pyrrhic victory after the other, while gradually losing the war?" The public-policy question in regard to relentlessly prolonging life is a serious one. "Inevitably," writes Dr. Henry K. Beecher (1970), "with increasingly bold, venturesome, and commendable attempts to rescue the dying, there will be an accumulation of individuals in hospitals who can be kept 'alive' only by extraordinary means despite the fact that there is no hope of recovery of consciousness, let alone recovery to a functioning, pleasurable existence—all this at a cost of $25,000 to $30,000 per year." Another way to state the cost that others are paying for these "heroic" procedures is that a single irretrievably unconscious patient, or incurable patient in great pain and indignity, occupies space that could have been used by 26 other patients staying on the average of two weeks in the hospital. This suggests that not only in the "disaster medicine" practiced in case of natural disasters, such as the typhoons on the Texas coast a few years ago, or designed to be used in case of nuclear attack upon cities (probably administered from the "dog and cat" hospitals left standing in the outskirts), may some form of triage become necessary. Triage sets aside the more serious casualties (as "expectants"), on whom great and lengthy effort by teams of doctors and nurses would have to be expended to save their lives, for the sake of the greater healing of a greater number. Are we coming into a time when, because of the unlimited application of more and more extraordinary means of saving life, we will be tempted to apply the principles of triage under normal circumstances? There would be something unsavory about doing this in regard to the treatment of the dying (because his bed is needed), just as it is an unsavory fact that we recently began to think seriously about updating the definition of clinical death, not for the sake of the patient, but when potential recipients of his organs came into view.

We need rather to discover the moral limits properly surrounding efforts to save life. We need to recover the meaning of only caring for the dying, and the justification—indeed the obligation—of intervening against many a medical intervention that is possible today. This is what I mean by a *patient*-centered answer to the foregoing questions. I also suggest that a culture that defines death as always a disaster will be one that is tempted to resolve these questions in terms of triage—disaster medicine. If we do not deliberately set aside the worst cases as a matter of public or hospital policy, the terminal cases will increasingly be neglected, because, paradoxically, of other demands upon sparse medical resources in a society that knows no other ethics in regard to dying patients than always by every means to keep them "alive."

Ordinary and Extraordinary Means

In any proper discussion of the physician's duty to heal and to save life, there are three interrelated distinctions that must be taken into account.

These are the distinctions (1) between "ordinary" and "extraordinary" means of saving life; (2) between saving life by prolonging the living of it and only prolonging a patient's dying; and (3) between the direct killing under certain conditions of specifiable sorts of "hopeless cases" (called *euthanasia*) and merely allowing a patient to die by stopping or not starting life-sustaining procedures deemed not morally mandatory. By making use of all these concepts, the medical ethics developed in Western Christendom set its face resolutely against the direct killing of terminal patients which it judged to be murder, whatever warrants may be alleged in favor of the practice. At the same time, medical ethics in the centuries before the recent achievements in scientific medicine and technology afforded reasonable grounds for refusing to "war without retreat and without quarter" against almighty God for the last shred of sentient life, worldly value, or physiological existence in the dying man.

It is necessary for us to enter this thicket if we are to gain an adequate comprehension of what is morally required in caring for the dying. This we must do if we are concerned to explore the possible bearing of religious ethics on medical practice.

It is necessary for us to enter the thicket of the several meanings the moralists had in mind for yet another reason. Physicians themselves ponder this question of the care of the dying, and they repeatedly draw a distinction between "ordinary" and "heroic" measures. The generic duty to "save life" which governs medical practice is readied for application in the moral-species terms distinguishing ordinary from extraordinary means. This tells physicians the difference between a mandatory and an elective effort to save life. Therefore, the relativity in the meanings of ordinary and extraordinary procedures is precisely a chief virtue of using this distinction in the practice of medicine. It is not—as often is said—a reason for dismissing the distinction as worthless. This would be the conclusion only from the premise that ethics must deal in absolutes unrelated to practice, or in principles that are inapplicable. Or else dismissal of this distinction is simply a vain effort to eliminate the role of prudence (practical wisdom) in applying moral rules by demanding the certitude of secondary rules for the application of them.

First, we need in preliminary fashion to notice some important differences between the moralist's meaning and the physician's meaning when each uses the terms *ordinary* and *extraordinary*. It is, of course, difficult to generalize, and no doubt there are some doctors who are closer than others to the moralists on the point in question. Still as a general rule—if I have not mistaken the general tenor or emphasis in the medical literature—a doctor's understanding and a moralist's understanding of ordinary and extraordinary means are likely to be different in three important and related respects.

First, the doctor is apt to use the distinction to mean customary as opposed to unusual procedures. Physicians use these terms relative to the state of medical science and the healing art, by reference to whether or not a remedy has become a part of customary medical practice. In contrast, the moralists are somewhat more likely than doctors to use these terms relative to a patient's particular medical condition. While an unusual practice may become customary and the medical imperative change as medicine advances, it is also the case that the medical imperative ought to change according to the patient's condition and its "advances," no matter how usual the remedy may be for other patients or for this patient at other times. The first relativity is to the disease and to what is ordinarily done to remedy it. The second relativity is to the condition of the man who has the disease; these relative meanings lead to a definition of optional remedies in terms of what would be "extraordinary" for this individual.

Apart from what doctors may sometimes or often do in withholding or stopping treatments in particular cases, one observes in medical writings a tendency to define *extraordinary* in terms of "heroic" or unusual efforts. This is not only because doctors may be in danger of malpractice suits if they depart too far from customary medical practice in what they do or omit to do. In general, the doctor's conscience is formed in these terms; his imperative is likely to be to do everything medical science affords as established practice in the saving of life. He will justify refraining from trying some unusual remedy more readily than he can justify stopping or not using a customary procedure. He is likely to feel that the moralist's understanding of "extraordinary" grants him more liberty than either law or a proper medical conscience allow.

Second, for the moralist, a decision to stop "extraordinary" life-sustaining treatments requires no greater and in fact the same moral warrant as a decision not to begin to use them. Again if I have understood the medical literature, a physician can make the decision not to institute such treatments with an easier conscience than he can make the decision to stop them once begun. "I believe that it is of primary importance," writes Dr. Jørgen Voight (1967), "not to get unawares into a situation in which it may be necessary to make a decision regarding the continuation of respirator treatment. Before institution of such treatment, as with every form of therapy [such as palliative interventions in inoperatable cancer patients], a decision must be taken as to whether it is *indicated*." That, of course, is true. But there should be no greater reluctance to judge that continuation of treatments is no longer indicated than to judge that they should not be begun. The moralists would support physicians in this conclusion. Since a trial treatment is often a part of diagnosis of a patient's condition, one might expect there to be greater reluctance on the part of physicians in not starting than in stopping extraordinary efforts to save life. As I understand them, physicians often have the contrary difficulty.

Putting these first two points together in summary, a doctor "is more likely to refrain from giving an antibiotic than he is to direct the withholding of nourishment. He is likely to hesitate longest over switching off the machine for artificial respiration. The reasons for these variations in reactions are probably psychological rather than rational" (Church of England report, 1965).

Of course, there may be no difference between the moralist and the physician on the matter of the weight given to customary medical practice and to individual medical circumstance in defining ordinary (imperative) and elective medical care of the fatally ill, or in the matter of stopping or not starting heroic efforts to save life. If no disagreement is to be found on these two points, one is likely to arise on the third.

Third, moralists almost always understand the distinction between ordinary and extraordinary procedures to refer decisively to morally relevant, nonmedical features of a particular patient's care: his "domestic economy," his familial obligations, the neighborhood that has become a part of his human existence, the person and the common good, and whether a man's fiduciary relations with God and with his fellow man have been settled. The difference between an imperative and an elective effort to save life will vary according to evaluations of these features of a human life, and a moralist's terms for expressing this final verdict are *ordinary* and *extraordinary*.

Thus, the standard definition reads as follows: "*Ordinary* means of preserving life are all medicines, treatments, and operations, which offer a reasonable hope of benefit for the patient and which can be obtained and used without excessive expense, pain, or other inconvenience. . . . *Extraordinary* means of preserving life . . . mean all medicines, treatments, and operations, which cannot be obtained without excessive expense, pain or other inconvenience, or which, if used, would not offer a reasonable hope of benefit" (Kelly 1958). In explanation of the moral judgment that "one may, but need not, use extraordinary means to preserve life," another writer sums up the morally relevant factors that go into determining the meaning of this by saying, "We may define as an extraordinary means whatever here and now is very *costly* or very *unusual* or very *painful* or very *difficult* or very *dangerous*, or if the good effects that can be expected from its use are not proportionate to the difficulty and inconvenience that are entailed" (Healy 1956). It is evident that theologians mean to counsel first the patient and his family and then the physician that, in deciding concerning an elective effort to save life or elective death, it is quite proper to make a balancing judgment involving decisive reference to a number of human (nonmedical) factors that constituted the worth for which that life was lived and that may discharge it from imperative continuation. Speaking as men who are doctors and in their practice, physicians may also say the same; but it is not strictly a medical judgment to say this. This is certainly not what a physician usually means when he distinguishes between ordinary and extraordinary procedures for saving life.

It may be that medical ethics will approach the position staked out by the theological moralists if it takes seriously the banner unfurled by the World Health Organization's positive definition of *health* as general human *well-being*. An erratic application of this extensive and liberal construction of a medical judgment, however, would not suffice. It would not suffice for the medical profession to invoke the psychosocial well-being of the woman as a justification for abortion while limiting professional judgment to strictly bodily considerations in caring for the hopelessly dying. That broad definition of health will either have to be withdrawn or else consistently applied. The latter would mean that professional medical judgments assume responsibility for the full range of human moral considerations. This would be to locate medical considerations in direct lineage with all of man's moral reflection upon the meaning of *eudaimonia* (well-being, happiness) since Aristotle!

This, I rather think is an alarming suggestion from which the medical profession should draw back in the direction of a stricter construction of medical judgments as such. The oddity is that the medical profession seems to have adopted a comprehensive definition of health precisely in a period in which we are undertaking to conceive that inconceivable thing: a society that itself has no moral philosophy and no common assumptions as to the good or well-being of man which medicine sporadically invokes. Increasingly, the medical profession—if it moves from a strictly medical to a more extensive definition of health—would have to find the sources of its medical ethics not in the culture generally but by developing within its own community a moral ethos representative of mankind's general well-being. In this respect, medical ethics would be not unlike the ethics of church and synagogue. The ethics of no group today floats upon a sea of social ethics or upon a received moral philosophy or an understanding of man's well-being or that of society generally.

This being so, it would seem wise for the medical profession to hesitate before assuming, along with social scientific judgments, also the tasks of an entire moral philosophy under a definition of health as general human well-being. For this reason, in the sequel I shall sometimes speak of *the medical imperative*, at other times of *the moral imperative* in dealing with the dying. These, of course, cannot be entirely separated, because the doctor is both a physician and a man. But this does suggest a distinction between the physician *qua* physician and whatever authority or role he may have as a man in relation to the well-being of the man who is his patient. It suggests a continuing distinction between the medical meaning and the theological-moral or humanistic meaning of imperative and elective procedures for saving life. This would require that the doctor lean against his understanding of the medical imperative in order to keep it optional for his patients; and that, as a man who happens also to be a doctor, he should make room for the primacy of human moral judgment on the part of the men who are his patients, the relatives of his patients, and their spiritual counselors to elect life-sustaining remedies or to elect them not. His may be the task of only caring for the dying for reasons that are not within his special competence to determine.

The Morality of (Only) Caring for the Dying

In discussions of ordinary and extraordinary means it is commonly assumed by physicians and moralists alike that the use of all "ordinary" remedies is morally required of everyone, and that the failure to provide or use ordinary means of preserving life is the equivalent of euthanasia. The crucial question to be asked of traditional medical ethics is whether ordinary, imperative procedures can, in a proper moral judgment, become "extraordinary" and elective only. Can a patient morally refuse ordinary remedies? Can a physician morally fail to supply them or fail to continue ordinary remedies in use?

This is an unavoidable question, and one that goes to the heart of the morality of *caring*, but *only* caring, for the dying. Whoever raises this question lightly, or with a concern to disprove or dismiss past moral reflection, can only deny himself one possible source of helpful insights. Our inquiry shall concern whether and in what sense traditional medical ethical concepts and distinctions should be ethically regulative of present-day medical practice in regard to the fatally ill and the dying. During this brief journey into the meanings of the moralists, our "method" of doing medical ethics will not be to propose *replacing* definitions. Instead, our search will be for an understanding of past moral wisdom, and in this to locate places at which a *reforming* definition of one or another relevent moral concept suggests itself. In this section two such important qualifications or creative lines of development will be brought into focus which are needed to complete an ethics of caring for the dying. Then in the following section, we shall ask whether, understood in terms of these reforming definitions, the ancient distinctions between ordinary and extraordinary (as a way of telling the difference between mandatory and elective efforts to save life) do not in sum reduce to the obligation to determine when a person has begun to undergo irreversibly the process of his own particular dying; and whether with *the process of dying* (all other terms aside) there does not arise the duty only to care for the dying, simply to comfort and company with them, to be present to them. This is the positive object of our search.

Then, in subsequent sections, we shall have to ask whether, over and above only caring for the dying, there is significant meaning still remaining in the distinction between ordinary and extraordinary means as specifications of our human obligation to continue or to discontinue life-sustaining procedures in the case of persons seriously or perhaps fatally ill, but not yet irreversibly dying. In addition to positing or enforcing the duty to respect with simple acceptance the dying process of a fellow man, the question then will be: Do these terms have any relevance for the medical care of persons not yet seized by their own dying?

A good place to cut into the moralists' analysis of the question whether "ordinary" medical procedures are always imperative is with the publication of two articles by Gerald Kelly in *Theological Studies* in 1950 and 1951. Here we can plainly see how far traditional medical morality was willing to go in limiting the active use even of so-called ordinary means of sustaining life. The title of Kelley's 1950 article ("The Duty of Using Artificial Means of Preserving Life") suggests that he answered the question just raised by distinguishing between "natural" and "artificial" among the ordinary means of preserving life. Closer examination will show that there is more to it than that; and that in fact Kelly has himself already elaborated good reasons for dispensing from ordinary natural no less than from ordinary artificial means of preserving life.

Kelly makes it quite clear that he is willing to remove "ordinary" means under certain circumstances from the class of morally or medically imperative means. Agreeing with those moralists who regard intravenous feeding as in itself an ordinary means (and who *therefore* judged it to be imperative), Kelly says instead that "even granted that it is ordinary one may not immediately conclude that it is obligatory." An ordinary means may be out of place because of the condition of a patient—as out of place as unusual or heroic procedures. In regard to the usual use of a stimulant to prolong life for only a short time, Kelly calls that also an ordinary means. In this instance he gives two reasons for dispensing with the stimulant: "since it is artificial and since it has practically no remedial value in the circumstances, the patient is not obliged to use it." It is evident, however, that in Kelly's argument the latter reason is far more important than the former. His argument is quite sufficient to make it unnecessary to distinguish between natural and artificial remedies in morally evaluating whether they should be used or not.

The argument revolves around whether the means used are really *remedies* or not. One is excused from using a proposed "remedy" if it does not offer a reasonable hope of success; it is then not a remedy. Kelly is simply intent on establishing that ordinary means may be omitted. His warrant for this is "the fine distinction between omitting an ordinary means and omitting a useless ordinary means." The uselessness of it is decisive; and it is hard to see why this does not afford us another "fine distinction," namely, that between omitting a natural means and omitting a *useless* natural means—if there is ever any need to invoke this principle in actual practice. In any case, the artificiality of the ordinary means which may be omitted Kelly puts decisively aside. Simply the fact that they are no longer *remedies* or are no longer useful in saving the life of a patient alone warrants the omission of efforts to save life. The means would have to be means-full—of use to a human life. There is no obligation to do anything that is useless.

I suppose that the point in drawing attention to the fact that this argument encompasses "natural" no less than "artificial" means is simply to demonstrate how far traditionally minded moralists were in principle willing to go in ordering means to the human life they are supposed to serve. Physicians should observe this, if they are inclined in conscience to continue beyond genuine usefulness the use of means that in the course of medical progress have become "usual" or "customary," and if they are any more ready for reasons relative to the patient to omit only their spectacular or "heroic" efforts.

The present writer has removed Kelly's delaying reference to the "artificiality" of the *useless* means that may be dispensed, He not I, embraces also "natural" means—not alone in the logic of his argument but in specific cases as well. This happened in his apparent approval of the solution of two cases by Cardinal De Lugo. If a man, about to be burned to death by his enemies, has only a few buckets of water, he is obliged to use the available water if he can prevent his death; but if the use of the water would only delay the inevitable he is not bound to use it. Water would seem to be a "natural" means of putting out fire, if anything is. If anyone doubts this, the second case settles the matter. Is a starving man bound to eat food brought to him by his friends? Yes, if he can get food regularly enough to ward off death. No, if by eating he only postpones his death by starvation. In sum, a prolongation of life that "may be normally considered as nothing" is *never* imperative whether the means are "natural" or "artificial," "ordinary" or "extraordinary" (1950).

Several times in the foregoing paragraphs I have suggested that in an era of scientific and technical medicine, and since few people are likely to try suicide by ceasing to eat, to talk about the moral dispensability of "natural" means of saving life may be a moot question. This is not so, since so-called "natural" means (and also artificial means) have other uses than as *remedies* (or as "means" to any future). These are things done for no purpose except to care. To give a cup of cold water to a man who has entered upon the course of his own particular dying is to slack the thirst of a man who will soon thirst again, and thirst unto death. When a man is irreversibly in the process of dying, to feed him and to give him drink, to ease him and keep him comfortable—these are no longer given as means of preserving life. The use of glucose drip should often be understood in this way. This keeps a patient who cannot swallow from feeling dehydrated, and is often the only remaining "means" by which we can express our present faithfulness to him during his dying (since to give him water intravenously would destroy his red blood cells and directly weaken and kill him). If a glucose drip prolongs this patient's dying because of the calories that are also introduced into his system, it is not done for that purpose or as a means in a continuing useless effort to save his life.

The administration of increased dosages of pain-killing drugs in the care of the dying is, as it were, the "mirror image" of the glucose drip: these drugs are judged to be life-shortening (to an immeasurable degree, because to suffer extreme pain would also be debilitating), but they are properly to be given in order to keep the patient as comfortable as possible, to show that we understand his need for succor, and not as a "useful" means to push him beyond our love and care. All these procedures, some "natural," others "artificial," are appropriate means—if "means" they should be called—of only caring for the dying, of physically companying with the dying. They are the embodied and effective gestures of soul to soul. As such, these acknowledgments of solidarity in morality are due to the dying man from any of us who also bear flesh. Thus do men give answer by their presence and comfort to the faithfulness-claims of persons who are passing through the acceptable death of all flesh. If death should be accepted and treatment can no longer affect it, one might even raise the question whether *glucose* water should be used to keep the dying patient comfortable. I understand that there are certain sugars which it might be possible to use to give water for hydration without metabolizing calories and prolonging the dying process.

A second place at which a liberalizing definition of our obligation to care for the dying begins to suggest itself is in Kelly's answer to the question, "Is a person who suffers from two lethal diseases obliged to take ordinary means of checking one of them when there is no hope of checking the other?" The question at issue is whether a person suffering from incurable cancer who develops diabetes is obliged to begin insulin treatment, or a diabetic who develops an incurable cancer obliged to continue on insulin, and die slowly of the cancer instead of sooner in coma. Other moralists had answered that the patient must use the insulin since that is an "ordinary" means of checking the *disease* diabetes. Kelly doubts whether a patient is bound to "prescind from the cancer in determining her obligation of using the insulin." The latter depends on two factors: that it is an ordinary means and that it offers a reasonable hope of success. The simultaneous presence of cancer throws doubt on the second stipulation. But then Kelly observes: "I think the doubt would be even stronger were there some connection between the two diseases." An illustration of this would be the need for intravenous feeding *connected with* the fatal disease from which a patient is dying. Presumably Kelly would be more certain about the judgment that it is permissible to withdraw intravenous feeding in this case, although nowadays a drip is surely per se an ordinary procedure for sustaining life. Thus, in assessing mandatory and only elective remedies, Kelly moves away from judging this in terms of *single* diseases only, to connected diseases, and only hesitantly beyond that. His reasoning should be faulted only for this hesitation.

The patient is not exhaustively characterized by one disease, two separate diseases, or the interconnected diseases from which he may be suffering, both incurable, one involving prolonged dying. Ideally, Kelly wanted the description of the human act of caring for this patient to terminate in a texture of related diseases. But a proper description of the human acts of caring for mortal man terminates in that man. He is the unity of the diseases he suffers when one his quietus makes. Doctors do not treat diseases, though often they conquer them. They treat patients, and here finally all fail. If a diabetic patient need not prescind from the cancer in determining her obligation to start or to continue to use insulin, the reason is that she is the one flesh in which both diseases inhere. If to use insulin is for her quite useless, it is surely contraindicated. To move beyond the interrelation of the ills to which all flesh is heir requires that we move to *the flesh* that is heir to all its ills, indifferent to whether these ills are themselves connected or physiologically unrelated. It is this flesh, and not diseases one by one, that is the subject of medical treatment. This truth is enough to undercut the bondage of conscience to the imperativeness of "customary" or "usual" procedures for treating single diseases.

We need to ponder one further possible entailment of the reforming definition of only caring for the dying at which we have arrived. If the unity of the person in whom the diseases inhere is the important point, and not a texture of interrelated diseases, this concept has important bearing on the treatment of infants with serious congenital defects. The argument cannot always be, as Kelly seems still to contend, that "the determination of ordinary and extraordinary means begin with the mentally normal" and this be then applied without qualification to the congenitally abnormal. That requirement may hold true for the chronically defective, like infants afflicted with mongolism, who often have a satisfactory degree of human existence that is only a burden, sometimes rewarding, to others.

The theologian who recently judged that "a Downs is not a person" uttered a scandalous untruth; and the fact that our advanced societies are now launching out upon the practice of allowing to be killed in utero all who are likely to be born mentally or physically defective shows, in the prismatic case of the most vulnerable, what we are coming to think of mankind's needy and helpless life in general. Nevertheless, the "abnormal" have, at the first of life, often been sized by their particular process of dying unless medical science relentlessly intervenes. Here there are even related defects any one of which will be mortal unless we intervene to stop them in course. Since we ought not to absolutize the distinction between "usual" and "heroic" treatment of newborn babies, not to place "a monstrosity in a heating bassinet" or to stop opposing the infection to which it is prone cannot be declared morally wrong while an operation is said to be optional to provide a child who was born with congenital atresia with an artificial or implanted esophagus.

"Ordinary" or imperative, and "extraordinary" or only elective treatments are, as we have seen, not fixed categories. The feeling that infants should be given the greatest protection does not alone settle what we ought to do. Life in the first of it and life in the last of it are both prismatic cases of human helplessness. The question is, What does loyalty to the newborn and to the dying require of us? Consistently, we could say that both should unqualifiedly be given every effort that might save or prolong their existence. But if a balancing judgment is permitted—even morally mandatory—concerning whether proposed remedies will be beneficial to the adult dying, the same reasoning cannot be preemptorially excluded from our care of the newborn.

If in the case of terminal patients the quality of life they can expect enters into the determination of whether even ordinary or customary measures would be beneficial and should or should not be used, cannot the same be said of infants? It is not obvious that an anencephaletic baby should be respirated while a grown man in prolonged coma should no longer be helped to breathe. In the first of life, a human being may be seized by his own unique dying. Indeed, far from taking the death of the aged and the enormous death rate of zygotes and miscarriages to be a part of the problem of evil, a religious man is likely to take this as a sign that the Lord of life has beset us behind and before in this dying life we are called to live and celebrate. There is an acceptable death of the life of all flesh no less in the first than in the last of it. An ethical man may always gird himself to oppose this enemy, but not the religious ethical man.

The Process of Dying

In the foregoing analysis we have drawn two pivotal conclusions: (1) that there is no duty to use useless means, however natural or ordinary or customary in practice; and (2) that the description of human acts of caring for the dying (or caring for the not yet dying) terminates in the man who is the patient of these ministrations and not in the disease or diseases he has. These are related points: in judging whether to try a given treatment one has to estimate whether there is a reasonable hope of success in saving the man's life.

A recent essay (Nolan 1968) reviewing the distinction of extraordinary from ordinary means, and the different ways in which particular cases have been judged by traditional moralists, concludes that in the final analysis "the one general positive guideline from the past that will remain" may prove to be the directive that "the use of any means should be based on what is commonly termed a 'reasonable hope of success.' " The residue of the distinctions we have reviewed, this author seems to suggest, is the test of usefulness. If so, the moral meaning of dispensable means would seem to reduce without remainder to a determination of an irreversible "process of dying."

This is certainly a pincipal component of the medical-moral imperative. It can certainly be said that our duties to the dying differ radically from our duties to the living or to the potentially still living. Just as it would be negligence to the sick to treat them as if they were about to die, so it is another sort of "negligence" to treat the dying as if they are going to get well or might get well. The right medical practice will provide those who may get well with the assistance they need, and it will provide those who are dying with the care and assistance they need in their final passage. To fail to distinguish between these two sorts of medical practice would be to fail to act in accord with the facts. It would be to act in accord with some rule-book medicine. It would be to act without responsivity to those who have no longer any responsivity or recuperative powers.

Thus would we fail to care for them as the dying men they are, just as surely as if we failed to take account of the responsivity that the living sick or the not yet dying still have. Only a physician can determine the onset of the process of dying. For all the uncertainty, he must surely make this determination. He is bound to distinguish so far as he can between that time span in which his treatment of a patient is still a part of diagnosis and treatment—diagnosis and treatment not of the disease but of a patient's particular responsivity—and a subsequent time in which the patient is irreversibly doing his own dying. The "treatment" for that is care, not struggle. The claims of the "suffering-*dying*" (Nolan) upon the human community are quite different from the claims of those who, though suffering, still may live, or who are incurably ill but not yet dying.

In connection with all that has just been said we should not have in mind only those patients who are in deep and prolonged coma. A conscious patient as well may have begun irreversibly the process of his particular dying; and, precisely because conscious, his claims are strong upon the human community that only care and comfort and company be given him and that pretended remedies or investigative trials or palliative operations be not visited upon him as if these were hopeful therapy. Therefore, to all of the foregoing the words of David Daube, Professor of Law at Oxford University, are pertinent. "The question of at what moment it is in order to discontinue extraordinary—or even ordinary—measures to keep a person alive," Professor Daube (1966) writes, "should not be confused with the question of what moment a man is dead" or with the question whether he is conscious or unconscious. "Discontinuation of such measures is often justifiable even while the patient is conscious."

This risk-filled decision concerning the onset of a man's own process of dying can be and is made by physicians. The problem is to find the courage (and perhaps legal protection) to act upon it. Dr. John R. Cavanagh (1963) defines the "dying process" as "the time in the course of an irreversible illness when treatment will no longer influence it." The patient has entered a covenant with the physician for his complete *care*, not for continuing useless efforts to *cure*. Therefore, Dr. H. P. Wasserman (1967) calls for "a program of 'premortem care,' " and for the training of doctors in this, and in the diverse ways in which they may fulfill their vocation to cure sometimes, to relieve often, and to comfort always.

If the sting of death is sin, the sting of dying is solitude. What doctors should do in the presence of the process of dying is only a special case of what should be done to make a human presence felt to the dying. Desertion is more choking than death, and more feared. The chief problem of the dying is how not to die alone. To care, if only to care, for the dying is, therefore, a medical-moral imperative; it is a requirement of us all in exhibiting faithfulness to all who bear a human countenance. In an extraordinary article, Dr. Charles D. Aring (1968) says flatly that "it is not to be surmised that under the most adverse circumstances the patient is not aware." That may be to say too much, but it strongly suggests that the sound of human voices and the clasp of the hand may be as important in keeping company with the dying as the glucose-drip "drink of cool water" or relieving their pain.

Dr. Aring tells of the case of a man who, under continuing exotic treatments, kept asking to be returned to his ward and to within the presence of his three ward companions. Instead, "he died alone, denied what he most wanted, the unspoken comfort of people—any people—around him." This physician's judgment is that this man's "want of his friends and familiar surroundings, new though they were, should have been an imperative and taken precedence over any and all technical matters." That would have been proper "premortem care" of the dying. To do this, the physician needs to become aware of his own feelings about death, and to lean against his possible proneness to visit cursorily or to pass hurriedly by the room in which lies one of his "failures." And all of us in the "age of the enlightenment" need to recognize "death's growing remoteness and unfamiliarity," the masks by which it is suppressed, the fantastic rituals by which we keep the presence of death at bay and our own presence from the dying, the inferiority assigned to the dying because it would be a human accomplishment not to do so, the ubiquity of the fear of dying that is one sure product of a secular age.

There is a final entailment of caring for the dying that is required of priests, ministers, rabbis, and every one of us, and not only or not even mainly of the medical profession. "The process of dying" needs to be got out of the hopsitals and back into the home and in the midst of family, neighborhood, and friends. This would be a "systemic change" in our present institutions for caring for the dying as difficult to bring about as some fundamental change in foreign policy or the nation-state system. Still, any doctor will tell you that by no means does everyone need to die in a hospital who today does so. They are there because families want them there, or because neighbors might think not everything was done in efforts to save them. They are there because hospitals are well equipped to "manage death," and families are ill equipped to do so.

If the "systemic change" here proposed in caring for the dying were actually brought about, ministers, priests, and rabbis would have on their hands a great many shattered families and relatives. But for once they would be shattered by confrontation with reality, by the claims of the dying not to be deserted, not to be pushed from the circle that specially owes them love and care, not to be denied human presence with them. Then God might not be as dead as lately He is supposed to be. The "sealing up of metaphysical concerns," Peter Berger recently pointed out, is one of the baneful results of a "happy" childhood—a childhood unhappily sheltered from the dying in all our advanced societies (New York *Times*, March 26, 1969).

Caring for the Seriously Ill and the Irreversibly Ill

Nevertheless, it would not be correct to suggest that the distinction of extraordinary from ordinary treatments—of elective from imperative remedies—and the subtle ethical judgments falling under these heads can be reduced without significant remainder to the twin concepts of "reasonable hope of success" (usefulness) and "the process of dying." That, as we have seen, is an important component. It is, in fact, the component encompassing the duty of only caring for the dying. In this respect, the moral imperative and the medical imperative are the same. For medicine to do more or otherwise would be blameworthy. But this is not all the meaning of ordinary-extraordinary—of imperative and only elective efforts to save life.

In the remaining meaning of these concepts, the moral imperative may be more extensive than the medical imperative. The "process of dying" is not the only condition for stopping the use of medical means, although when present it is a sufficient and a morally obliging condition. Other conditions can make it morally right to stop the use of medical means, although the decision to do so may not be a strictly medical judgment. "No reasonable hope of success" (uselessness) is not the only warrant for stopping the use of medical means, although where present it is a sufficient and a morally obliging condition. Other grounds than hopelessness can make it morally right to stop the use of medical means, although the decision to cease using them is not a strictly medical judgment. Kelly (1950) speaks of "the recognized principle that an extraordinary means is not per se obligatory even when success would be certain." The true humanity of moralists of the past led them unanimously to say that there are conditions that could make efforts to save life only elective even if they are certain to be successful. When a physician yields or—better still—himself makes room for these more extensive moral and human judgments, he likely does so as a man who is a doctor, by an exercise of the moral authority he has acquired in relation to the man who is his patient and to his family, and not by virtue of his medical expertise.

Even when he could succeed, a doctor may and sometimes should allow his medical judgment to defer to a patient's estimate of the higher importance of the worth and the relations for which his life was lived. In doing so the doctor acts the more as a man than as a medical expert, acknowledging the preeminence of the human relations in which he stands with these and all other men, rather than solely in his capacity as a scientist or as a healer.

In this age of scientific medicine and of the authority figure in a white coat, it is salutary to remind ourselves of some of the measures which, until not so long ago, no one needed to use to save his life. Kelly lists the following examples: "Leaving one's home to go to a more healthful climate; the maiden's repugnance to being treated by a (male) physician or surgeon; the amputation of a limb; other major operations, especially those involving the opening of the abdomen; and all very costly treatments." Thomas J. O'Donnell (1960) has roundly criticized these out-of-date cases and his fellow moralists for not keeping up with advancements in medical practice. Still, we should notice the humane wisdom contained in some of these illustrations, a sensitivity to human factors that is too likely to be evacuated in this age of technology. We should notice the good moral reasons that could be adduced for formerly deeming only elective certain of the medical practices that have become established practices with the advancement of the science and art of medicine. Thus to accent the morally relevant features of practices and patients that made it right to elect death will be to indicate precisely those morally relevant features that had to be overridden by medical progress, and that have always to be removed or otherwise cared for if saving life under certain conditions is to be pronounced always imperative.

Leaving Home.

This may no longer be a test in the age of the jet airplane and the mobility of populations. Still, to say this is in a sense to call attention to the human and familial and neighborly values which have in part been destroyed by the very same achievements of a technical civilization that now make imperative many a lifesaving procedure that formerly was likely not choiceworthy. It is at least still arguable that the New York state legislator who went from Queens to Houston to wait for and receive a heart transplant, and there to die, need not have done so. Houston may be a far more beautiful city than Queens, but Queens was his own hometown! There were the people and relationships that made up the fabric of his human existence, and among them he might well have chosen to die.

Repugnance

Slight support can now be given for a "maiden's" repugnance to be treated by a male physician. But repugnance in general cannot be so easily set aside as one of the right-making or wrong-making features important in deciding to submit to or not to use medical procedures. The personal repugnance of a member of the religious sect of Jehovah's Witnesses to having his life saved by a transfusion of the blood (the "life") of another human being is surely grounds for his right to be allowed to die—even if we do not, and the medical profession does not, believe that this can be "reasonably requested." This "makes the transfusion for him an extraordinary means of preserving life" (Ford 1955). Moreover, a more well-founded repugnance is still a factor in assessing what the moralists used to call "notable operations." If plastic and other corrective surgery not actually needed for life or health can be justified because of the human difficulty of living with grotesque deformities or facial disfigurement, then such like consequences of surgery that alone can save life may be grounds for not choosing life under those conditions. The medical-moral imperative is not first to save the life, and then to seek over the course of future progress to provide the ancillary remedies for those human consequences. It works the other way round: as medical progress removes or lessens the consequences that are repugnant, its elective extraordinary procedures that succeed in saving life only at the cost of "notable" and repugnant consequences may become imperative.

Very Costly Treatments

One moralist (Healy 1956) declared only a few years ago that in normal times $2,000 or more would constitute too great a sum for the average man; and that, if the treatment would cost that amount or more, one would not be obliged to seek treatment! To say that this statement attempts to turn ethics into an exact, monetary science would—while true—not be a proper response. That statement rests rather upon a regard for the average man; and, in estimating the human burden of costly treatment, it rightly takes account of the fabric of personal relationships and values which constituted the worth for which the terminal patient has lived. Here again, the medical-moral imperative is not first to save life at these costs, and then seek by some future course of action to remedy the human costs of warding off death. It works the other way round: the social distribution of medical care, removing or lessening these human costs, can alone transform presently elective (because costly) procedures into imperative ones.

Amputations

This, of course, is the classic example of how an operation may become "ordinary" through the advancement of medical science. Not too many decades ago every Christian moralist characterized the amputation of an arm or a leg as an extraordinary operation which no man had the affirmative obligation to endure. That was before there were anaesthetics to remove the terrible pain, or disinfectants to ward off the high probability of infection. Today, the amputation of an arm or a leg is clearly an ordinary and morally imperative means of saving life. Nevertheless, it is noteworthy that the physical pain or the physical danger of infection were not the only reasons adduced for this judgment upon amputations. Even in regard to removing pain, one moralist declared at the beginning of this century that a general anaesthetic is itself an extraordinary means becuase it takes away reason for a time. A man might choose to do his own dying with reason and self-consciousness in exercise. Whatever we may think of that suggestion, the moralists who judged amputations to be morally dispensable were chiefly concerned to hold open the possibility that a man might not judge life to be worth living without an arm or leg. In regard to this more human and enduring disadvantage in the balancing judgment about amputations, it is the development and provisioning of subtle artificial limbs that has done most to render these operations morally choiceworthy or imperative as a means of saving life.

We should also observe that, while the advancement of the science and art of medicine may suffice to shift a means from the elective to the imperative category, this shift does not automatically take place. Not every means for prolonging life, once it is successful and made available—even "customary" medical practice—becomes thereby ordinary and mandatory upon both patient and doctor. There are always broader human factors to be taken into account, and these always in Christian medical ethics kept the saving of life from being made an absolute and inflexible norm, a hardship inhumanly applied. Medical progress may be described as a process of constantly creating ordinary means out of extraordinary ones, but also as a process of constantly creating more and more extraordinary means that need not be used and perhaps ought not to be chosen. . . .

The Same Objection from Two Opposite Extremes

There are physicians, of course, who entirely agree with the moralists' distinction ethically between direct killing (euthanasia) and allowing to die, and who also affirm the importance of this distinction for medical ethics. Dr. J. Russell Elkinton (1968) of the University of Pennsylvania School of Medicine, for example, calls upon his fellow physicians to attend, in addition to their obligation to save life, to their "other obligation" to allow the patient, if he is to die, to die with comfort and dignity. He acknowledges that if an extraordinary treatment (such as use of a respirator) is stopped, that is *an action,* but it is "an 'invisible act' of omission." Morally, it is decisive that "the patient dies not from that act but from the underlying disease or injury." The physician stands aside.

For Elkinton also, in caring for the dying, it is a matter of indifference whether usual or rare and untried or new treatments are at issue. "More than 20 years ago," he writes, "I was responsible for the care of a young woman in the end state of multiple sclerosis. She was in great pain and had widespread ulcerations over the surface of her body from which she developed a septicemia (infection of her bloodstream). At that time a new antibiotic, penicillin, had just become available. With the agreement of the patient's family I withheld the penicillin and the patient died quickly—her suffering was relieved. Penicillin is an ordinary treatment today but I would still make the same decision." Thus, the advancement of medical science and practice is not alone sufficient to transform elective into morally imperative treatments. So also said Dr. G. B. Giertz (1966) in the Ciba Symposium: "No step is taken with the object of killing the patient. We refrain from treatment because it does not serve any purpose. . . . I cannot regard this as killing by medical means: death has already won, despite the fight we have put up, and we must accept the fact."

This is also the medical care that small children deserve. "I will fight for every day," writes Dr. Rudolf Toch (1964) of the Pediatric Tumor Clinic at Massachusetts General Hospital, "if I have even the slightest chance of doing something more than just gaining one more day. . . . On the other hand, I recall a youngster whom we recently had on the ward with osteogenic sarcoma, the lungs completely riddled with tumor, who had not responded at all to the most potent chemotherapy and for whom we really had nothing further to offer. I did not feel any compunction at all about not doing thoracenteses daily, keeping intravenous therapy going, etc. All we did was give her adequate sedation, and I think she rather peacefully slept away." In saying this, Dr. Toch expressed the general and continuous consensus of Western medical ethics.

However, the ethics of only caring for the dying which, as we have seen, was our traditional medical ethics, and which is still promulgated by theological moralists and many doctors, will be opposed, trivialized, and ridiculed by two opposite extremes. One of these extremes is the medical and moral opinion that there is never any reason not to use or to stop using any and all available life-sustaining procedures. The other extreme is that of those, including a few theological ethicists, who favor the adoption of active schemes of positive euthanasia which justify, under certain circumstances, the direct killing of terminal patients. The case for either of these points of view can be made only by discounting and rejecting the arguments for saving life qualifiedly but not always. In both cases, an ethics of only caring for the dying is reduced to the moral equivalent of euthanasia—in the one case, to oppose this ever; in the other case, to endorse it. Thus, the extremes meet, both medical scrupulosity and euthanasia, in rejecting the discriminating concepts of traditional medical ethics.

Proponents of euthanasia agree with advocates of relentless efforts to save life in reducing an ethics of omitting life-sustaining treatments to a distinction without a difference from directly killing the dying. Thus D. C. S. Cameron (1956), former Medical and Scientific Director of the American Cancer Society, writes that "actually the difference between euthanasia and letting the patient die by omitting life-sustaining treatment is a moral quibble." Dr. David A. Karnofsky (1960), of the Sloan-Kettering Institute for Cancer Research, also vigorously defends continuous "aggressive or extraordinary means of treatment" to prolong life. Karnofsky acknowledges that "the state of dying" may often be protracted only by "expensive and desperate supportive measures," and that the patient may be "rescued from one life-threatening situation only to face another." He has heard the pleas of those who, "contemplating this dismal scene," beg the doctor to "let the patient go quickly, with dignity and without pain." This strikes him as the same as getting rid of the dying by any means: "Withholding of aggressive or extraordinary treatment can be urged and supported by state planners, efficiency experts, social workers, philosophers, theologians, economists, and humanitarians. For here is one means of ensuring an efficient, productive, orderly and pain-free society, by sweeping out each day the inevitable debris of life."

The medical imperative, in Karnofsky's opinion, is to apply one temporary relief after another, stretching the life of a patient with cancer of the large bowel to ten months, who would have died within weeks if any one massive remedy had not been used. To the question, "When should the physician stop treating the patient?" there can be but one answer: "He must carry on until the issue is taken out of his hands." From the point of view of this medical ethics of univocal and relentless life prolonging, the moralists' notion of imperative and elective means is bound to seem a moral quibble, and such an outlook will be exceedingly suspicious of all talk of allowing patients to die and only caring for them. There are moralists who agree with this point of view, and who, in order to protect human life at all costs, would be very suspicious of vesting physicians with the right to make the balancing sorts of medical and moral judgments expounded in this chapter.

On the other hand, precisely the same objection will be brought against the flexibly wise categories of traditional medical ethics from the opposite quarter. This time the objection is raised by proponents of schemes of euthanasia or the direct killing of dying or of untreatable patients. Tribute should be paid to Professor Joseph Fletcher for in season and out of season having kept open the question of allowing to die in the minds and consciences of the public beyond the limits of the medical profession. Still, the fact that he is himself a proponent of euthanasia—he "almost" says "honest" or "straightforward" euthanasia—has meant on his part a serious misunderstanding of the ethics of only attending the dying (1968). He subscribes to this ethics, of course, in moments when he seems compelled to acknowledge that euthanasia is a nonproblem in our present society, and when he wants provisionally to endorse the more commonly shared ethics of allowing to die. But because this is for him a halfway house, he seriously misunderstands the positive quality of the nonconsequential "action" put forth in attending and caring for the dying, and he introduces some confusion by his use of the carefully wrought categories of this ethics.

There is a terminological problem to be settled one way or another at the outset. It is possible to use the term *euthanasia* with the meaning of the two Greek words of which it is composed: a "good death." Dr. Wasserman (1967) uses the word in this sense when he says, "The inevitability of death suggests that medicine's greatest gift to mankind could be that of euthanasia in its literal meaning, i.e., death without suffering." By this he meant the practice of only caring for the dying, and he proposed the establishment of a program of "premortem care," and training medical students not only as invincible conquerers who unhappily fail, but also in this positive aspect of their profession. While this is the literal and the original meaning of the term *euthanasia*, it has since and in modern times acquired a quite different meaning. This meaning, I suggest, is now unreformably the meaning or part of the meaning the term will have in current usage. It is better to invent terms of art such as *agathanasia* or *bene mori* (Cavanaugh) or *premortem care* to convey the ethics and practice of only caring for the dying, if this is what is meant.

Of course, we can agree to use either convention. But there is evidence that efforts to use the term *euthanasia* with any other sense than the one it has in current usage, i.e., direct killing, do not fully succeed. If this is true, our terminological problem has substantive import for ethical analysis and the moral life. The writings of Joseph Fletcher are an instance. He wishes to subscribe both to an ethics of caring, but only caring, for the dying, and to euthanasia in its current meaning. He calls both these practices by the name of euthanasia. He then must attach to the term qualifying predicates. This leads to confusion and inaccuracy in his use of the carefully wrought categories of traditional medical ethics, which he uses as these qualifiers, and to a failure to grasp the positive quality of only caring for the dying.

Thus Fletcher permits himself to speak of a decision to only care for the dying as *indirect euthanasia*. We cannot move forward without flatly denying this concept to be true. There is only one procedure in caring for the dying that need invoke what moralists call the "indirectly voluntary." This is the use of pain-relieving drugs that may also debilitate a patient's strength and shorten his life, or his dying. In this case, the justification is that relief of his pain is the "directly voluntary" action, while the administration of the drug shortens the dying process in only an "indirectly voluntary" way. What one does directly and immediately is to help the patient in his insufferable pain. That he dies sooner is not the primary result. This case is a prism in which we can see the ingredients that must be present in a case for which the language of "direct" or "indirect" is at all appropriate. There must be two effects caused by the same action, whether these effects are relieving pain and shortening life, or, in conflict-of-life cases, unavoidably and fore-knowingly causing the death of a fetus as the "indirectly voluntary" effect of action whose directly voluntary end is the saving of a mother's life.

Incidentally, the life-shortening effect of using pain-relieving drugs is not quite as clear as moralists sometimes assert. Prolonged suffering from extreme pain is also exceedingly debilitating; and it is not always clear whether to keep pain at bay or not to do so would be more effective in hastening the dying man to realms beyond our love and care. In any case, drugs are not given for that consequence. They rather express in objective service to the dying that we still care for them, and are affirmatively doing so.

It may be entirely appropriate to use the expression *indirect euthanasia* in the case of death-hastening pain-killers. But it is not at all appropriate to use these words to describe cases of ceasing treatments that prolong the patient's life, or withholding life-sustaining treatments altogether, which Fletcher (1967) lumps together under this rubric with positive acts of administering drugs which cause the double effect we have described. This he does on the grounds that in these cases "death occurs through omission rather than directly by commission"; it is "not induced but only permitted." Fletcher calls this concept *"indirect euthanasia"* and his warrant for doing so, he says, is because "in some kinds of Christian ethics and moral theology, an action of this kind is called 'indirect voluntary.' " This usage is entirely mistaken. Fletcher's use is a *persuasive* use of language, not a convincing one. Writing primarily as a proponent of euthanasia (current usage), he subscribes along the way to an ethics of only caring for the dying. By calling the latter "indirect euthanasia" his words, at least, gain the force of suggesting that this point of view is not quite as honest or forthright as "direct" euthanasia.

To insist that this usage confuses the carefully fashioned categories of medical ethics is no mere logomachy, since it is of first importance, in the characterization or description of actions to be morally evaluated, to make clear precisely this distinction between acts of omission and acts of commission. The difference between only caring for the dying and acts of euthanasia is not a choice between indirectly and directly willing and doing something. It is rather the important choice between doing something and doing nothing, or (better said) ceasing to do something that was begun in order to do something that is better because now more fitting. In omission no human agent causes the patient's death, directly or indirectly. He dies his own death from causes that it is no longer merciful or reasonable to fight by means of possible medical interventions. Indeed, it is not quite right to say that we only care for the dying by an omission, by "doing nothing" directly or indirectly. Instead, we cease doing what was once called for and begin to do precisely what is called for now. We attend and company with him in this, his very own dying, rendering it as comfortable and dignified as possible.

In any case, doing something and omitting something in order to do something else are different sorts of acts. To do or not to do something may, then, be subject to different moral evaluations. One may be wrong and the other may be right, even if these decisions and actions are followed by the same end result, namely, the death of a patient. One need not deny that in the moral life commission and omission may sometimes be morally equivalent. Still, before we reach the individual case or the sort of cases in which to do and not to do are judged to be the same, we need to explore the possibility that to omit and to do may not at all be equivalent actions, and to ascertain the pertinence of this possibility for medical practice.

What Fletcher has gained by an improper characterization of actions that allow a patient to die while caring for him—by calling them indirect voluntary euthanasia—is that, without abandoning the case he and many other moralists have made for only caring for the dying, he can the more readily succeed in apparently reducing the warrants for omitting medical interventions to the moral equivalent of the alleged warrants for acts of direct euthanasia. Here it is that he mounts the very same objection against an ethics of only caring for the dying as the one affirmed by defenders of medical scrupulosity in the unending use of all available means. Many teachers, Fletcher writes, Roman Catholics and others, "claim to see a moral difference between deciding to end a life by deliberately doing something and deciding to end a life by deliberately *not* doing something." This, Fletcher writes, "seems a very cloudy distinction"; and he asks rhetorically, "What, morally, is the difference between doing nothing to keep a patient alive and giving a fatal dose of a pain-killing or other lethal drug?" Of course, as Fletcher goes on to say, the decision to do or not to do are both "morally deliberate." Who ever said they were not? Of course, "the intention is the same, either way"—meaning the end in view (and not bothering here to introduce the usage of the word "intention" in a considerable number of ethical writings where its meaning is *not* restricted to the end in view). Fletcher's whole case depends, then, on his next statement: "As Kant said, if we will the end we will the means."

That, I suppose, is a statement from Kant's analysis of hypothetical imperatives, which are dependent on consequences; and it might be pointed out that Kant did not believe conditional imperatives to be at all constitutive of a truly moral life. One could argue that if one wills the end he wills the means—but not just any old means. One could argue that it is ethical to will the end we have here in mind; for the strictest religious ethics "the desire for death can be licit" (Kelly 1950). One could say that there are different means—and differences between action and omissions that make room for properly caring actions—that may let the patient have the death he not improperly or even quite rightly desires. While it might be argued that the Kantian maxim applies to means necessary to secure a desired and desirable end, still where there are more than one means to this same end, to will that end leaves open the choice among means. A means may be right, another wrong, to the same end.

But to respond in this way would exhibit a considerable misunderstanding of the positive quality and proper purpose intended in only caring for the dying. It is true that death is now accepted; and it is no longer opposed. This makes room for appropriate caring actions which are means to no future consequence. These actions are fulfillments of the *categorical* imperative: Never abandon care! Perhaps they should not be called means at all, since they effectuate or hasten the coming of no end at all. Upon ceasing to try to rescue the perishing, one then is free to care for the dying. Acts of caring for the dying are deeds done bodily for them which serve solely to manifest that they are not lost from human attention, that they are not alone, that mankind generally and their loved ones take note of their dying and mean to company with them in accepting this unique instance of the acceptable death of all flesh. An attitude toward the dying premised upon mature and profoundly religious convictions will display an indefectable charity that never ceases to go about the business of caring for the dying neighbor. If we seriously mean to align our wills with God's care here and now for them, there can never be any reason to hasten them from the here and now in which they still claim a faithful presence from us—into the there and then in which they, of course, cannot pass beyond God's love and care. This is the ultimate ground for saying that a religious outlook that goes with grace among the dying can never be compatible with euthanasiac acts or sentiments. . . .

Two Possible Qualifications of Our Duty Always to Care for the Dying

A number of contemporary moralists have recently raised the question whether to assist a patient through his own "process of dying" may be justifiable. (Even liberal Catholics seem to have an aptitude for coming up with ideas like that!) We need now to examine these suggestions, and finally ourselves to ask whether there are any further possible qualifications or proper exceptions to our duty always to care for the dying.

Kieran Nolan (1968) ponders whether, "if to use expensive means to add a few hours of life to a terminal patient is not in keeping with Christian charity, [it is] in keeping with Christian charity to allow a terminal patient to continue for months in such a condition without providing some positive assistance to the dying process." Nolan puts this forward as a question needing further exploration. He anticipates, however, that future serious moral reflection may eventually make "somewhat clearer how positive assistance to the suffering-*dying* is a matter quite different from euthanasia as the merciful relief of suffering when one is not dying."

In a wide-ranging discussion with Dr. Robert White, neurosurgeon at the Cleveland Metropolitan General Hospital, the Rev. Charles E. Curran (1968) puzzled: "In the past, we have definitely placed great stress on the distinction between acts of omission and acts of commission. . . . Let me ask you, doctor, is there such a thing as the dying *process*? . . . Maybe death isn't an instantaneous thing. And if all you do is *hasten* the dying process, is this 'interfering with nature'? I'm not suggesting that we can justify such a procedure here and now, but we're not being true to our profession if we're afraid to ask questions." Curran might better have asked: If all we do is *hasten* the dying process, is this not morally equivalent to no longer opposing the process of dying?

Thomas A. Wassmer (1968) writes that "it can plausibly be asked just where the difference lies in accelerating the dying process by acts of commission as well as by acts of omission." And concerning the use of pain-relieving, life-shortening drugs, Wassmer states his opinion that "it is hard to see at times how the effect of death is not involved in the very intentionality of the administrator. It seems somewhat unreasonable to assert that a patient who is given such drugs in order to eliminate pain, although the process of death is going to be accelerated, is always unaware of this combined intentionality in the minds of his physician and family."

The entire argument of this chapter affords some response to these suggestions.

1. Reference to the fact that, in keeping a patient comfortable by the use of pain-relieving drugs, shortening his life may be the meaning held and conveyed to him (because of the double intentionality in the act accompanying the double effect of the drugs) is surely a contingent possibility and not a really fundamental argument. One could as well say that in caring for the dying by giving the patient a glucose-drip "cup of cool water," he may get the idea that the physician is officiously trying to prolong his dying by the input of calories. If a patient knows enough about these procedures, or if he does not, he will likely receive them as *care*. The administrator of them knows they are objectively needed primarily for the patient's comfort, and subjectively it is easy enough for him to tell whether in the one case he is trying to kill or to hasten death (instead of giving a patient relief from pain) and whether in the other he is trying uselessly to prolong a patient's dying process (instead of caring for him in his dying).

2. Each of these authors addresses himself solely to the span of end-time described by the words "the process of dying" and to which the moral judgment "the dispensability of any and all efforts to save life" is applicable. If during this span of end-time there is no significant moral distinction to be made between omitting life-sustaining treatments in order to make room for caring and only caring for the dying, on the one hand, and, on the other, injecting a small bubble of air in his veins in order to kill him or hasten his dying or assist him in the process, then no such distinction can validly be drawn earlier in the case of the "living sick" (the seriously ill and the incurably ill not yet doing their own dying) who also may elect death. This, we

have seen, is the meaning of nonimperative efforts to save life over and above omitting such means in order to make room for caring for the dying. In suggesting the possible collapse of the moral difference between omission and commission, none of these authors takes up the question of the patient who is "not bound to accept excessively burdensome means of prolonging his life unless the foreseen consequences of his dying are such as to make it his duty to live on" (Church of England report 1965). When these authors do take up the question, they are likely to find that if the distinction between omission and commission is abrogated (or if the grounds for this in *care* is forgotten) in the case of patients in process of dying, it cannot be maintained in the case of the ill who are not yet dying.

3. In simply exploring and pondering the question whether in extending medical care to the dying there may be no significant moral difference between acts of omission and acts of commission to assist in the dying process, these authors are lost in the forest of the technical terminology of past moral reflection, and they neglect to stress what the omission was for. They have lost firm grip on the positive quality of an ethics of caring for the dying, and so their discussion of omission-commission turns out to be rather like that of proponents of medical scrupulosity who would extend unending efforts to save life, or that of proponents of euthanasia, when they undertake from either extreme to reduce the flexibly wise and grace-full categories of past medical ethics to a moral quibble. In caring for the dying, *we cease doing what was once called for and begin to do what is called for now.* The omission is only incidentally a "not doing," in order positively to care, to comfort, to be humanly present with the dying. The call cannot go forth: abandon care!

It would be a defection from the faithfulness-claims of a fellow human being that his very own dying be blessed as an event in the human community to which we attend if the dying are hastened beyond the reach of our love and care. To "assist" the process of dying would itself be a sort of abandonment: an affirmative abandonment of the dying solely to God's care in *separation* from ours, a self-contradiction at the heart of Christian charity ceasing, by this act, from its works before released from the claims and needs of a still living fellow man.

Still, there may be possible qualifications of our duty to care for the dying even if, as I argue, the general moral species-term "to assist the dying process" is not one of them, or is too sweeping as a stipulation. This final question must now be addressed. There can be justifiable modifications of moral principles and rules, whether these are based on justice or fairness- or faithfulness-claims or on the moral importance of the consequences of actions. These qualifications or modifications, if there is good reason for introducing them, may be called "exceptions" to the principles or moral rules first subscribed to—since the word "except" or "unless" is usually used in formulating such modifications. A proper exception or "unlessment" specifies a type or class of actions having universalizable right-making features in which similar agents should act similarly. They in no sense weaken the original principle or moral rule governing in all cases except of the type mentioned in the exception. This will be the method of medical ethical analysis to be used in now asking: Are there any specifiable just and charitable qualifications of our duty always to care for the dying?

I suggest that there may be two such qualifications.

1. We may say, Never abandon care of the dying except when they are irretrievably inaccessible to human care. Never hasten the dying process except when it is *entirely indifferent to the patient* whether his dying is accomplished by an intravenous bubble of air or by the withdrawal of useless ordinary natural remedies such as nourishment.

A moralist cannot say whether or not there are cases falling under this justification of direct killing, or assisted dying. This would be for physicians to say. Still there may be actual, or if not there are supposable, sorts of cases in which the duty always to keep caring for the dying is suspended by their inaccessibility to any form of care or comfort. The permanently and deeply unconscious person is, so far as can be known, not suffering at all. An argument that he should be treated "mercifully" by being allowed to die or by being directly killed is misplaced. It is only the suffering of relatives that could be relieved. To do either of these things *for that reason* would be a defect of care for him—*if* this still makes any difference to him.

The proposed justifiable exception depends on the patient's physiological condition which may have placed him utterly beyond reach. If he feels no suffering, he would feel no hunger if nourishment is withheld. He may be alone, but he can feel no presence. If this is a true account of some comatose patients, then in this sort of case we have correctly located the point at which the crucial moral difference between omission and commission as a guide to faithful actions has utterly vanished. The condition of the patient renders it for him a matter of complete indifference whether humankind's final act toward him directly or indirectly allows death to come. He already is beyond our love and care. We must not, as Dr. Karnofsky supposed, carry on our medical efforts to save life until the issue is taken out of our hands. Still we must carry on our ministry of care and comfort and keeping-company with the dying until but only until *that* issue is taken out of our hands. This is not to secure charity's premature release. It would rather be the case that men may, consonant with charity, take note of the fact that they have been released. Can we never say, This man is beyond earthly caring?

The sort of situation that may be covered and resolved by the present proposal in ethical analysis, if it is valid, are the cases of patients in deep and irreversible coma who can be and are maintained alive for many, many years. It has to be acknowledged, of course, that in making a human presence felt to the dying we should not lightly assume that the patient is not aware of the sound of human voices or the touch of a loved one's hand or his breathing nearness. But must it be assumed that this is always so? If there are cases of neglect and defect of care for the dying, there may also be not an excess but a now useless extension of care. Acts of charity or moving with grace among the dying that now communicate no presence or comfort to them are now no longer required. If it is the case that a wife is tragically mistaken when she takes twitches of the eyes to be a sort of language from her husband irreversibly comatose for seven years, or when she takes such reflex actions as the response of the lips to a feeding cup to be evidence of reciprocation and some minimal personal relatedness, then her care is now worthless. Indeed it is no longer care for him. It is no contradiction to withhold what is not capable of being given and received. If caring for the dying should stop, then the basic reason for a significant moral distinction between omission and commission is abrogated. The grounds for that were that we should cease to do something once called for in order to begin to do what is now called for in always only caring for the dying. Now care is no longer called for. Indeed no calls to the dying reach them, and no answering presence to presence. It is then a matter of complete indifference whether death gains the victory over the patient in such impenetrable solitude by direct or indirect action.

2. We might formulate the moral rule governing premortem care so as to include in it a second possibly justifiable stipulation. We could say: Always keep officious treatments away from the dying in order to draw close to them

in companying with them and caring for them; never, therefore, take positive action to usher them out of our presence or to hasten their departure from the human community, *unless* there is a kind of prolonged dying in which it is medically impossible to keep severe pain at bay.

Again, it is not for the moralist to say whether there is this kind of dying. Persons dying from bone cancer may be the sort of case that would fall under this second qualification of the requirement that we always care for the dying and do nothing to place them more quickly beyond our love and care.

One can hardly hold men to be morally blameworthy if in these instances dying is directly accomplished or hastened. The reasons are the same as those advanced in favor of the first stipulation: A patient undergoing deep and prolonged pain, who cannot be relieved by means presently available to use to care for him and make him comfortable, would also be beyond reach of the other ways in which company may be kept with him and he be attended in his dying—as much so, depending on the degree of his undefeatable agony, as the prolonged comatose patient. For the same reasons, this may be another place to locate an abrogation of the good moral reasons for distinguishing between omission and commission in our dealings with the dying.

Suppose that it were agreed that directly death-dealing or death-hastening actions are not inherently or always necessarily wrong. Suppose that it were agreed that, solely in the sort of cases we have discussed, to bring or hasten death would be consonant with caring for the dying. Suppose that it were agreed that the acts described would be no violation of charity; that instead these are qualifications that do no more than extend the meaning of caring for the dying so as to comprehend problematic cases. It would not at once follow that the moral rule of practice governing medical care should include these provisos; that the moral constitution of medical practice should admit these possibly justifiable cases of actively bringing or hastening death.

To say this requires an affirmative answer to the question raised already by an ethics and a practice of allowing to die. Can a doctor, we asked, admit that a patient is incurable while in the ethics of his medical mission never admitting that diseases are incurable? The question now is: Can a doctor and can medicine as a rule of practice admit that a patient is beyond earthly care, inaccessible to care, and so warrant as a practice positive actions that accomplish or hasten his death while not weakening medicine's lifesaving mission? Would the doctors who are the moral agents in these exceptional acts of killing the dying, or acts that allow to die, be corrupted by them, and medicine's impulse to save be weakened? The medical imperative specifying that physicians never cease trying to find the cure or the relief (e.g., to the pain of bone cancer) which future patients need is more extensive and might have to be given preeminence over the humane moral judgments that could warrant bubbles of air for permanently comatose patients and dying patients suffering from undefeatable pain. The question of questions is whether both that imperative and these permissions (with appropriate actions) can dwell together in the same person and calling. Or must one be bartered against the other, and in practice the one weaken the other resolve?

Within the limits of the moral rules for extending care and faithfulness to the dying elaborated in this chapter, and within the strict limits of the "unless" we have appended to the categorical imperative that we keep covenant with them, I do not believe that we need fear any weakening of medicine's impulse to save life. Still no one should forget the judgment of the leading scholar of the Nazi medical cases (Alexander 1949): "Whatever proportion these crimes finally assumed, it became evident to all who investigated them that they had started from small beginnings. . . . It started with the acceptance of the attitude . . . that there is such a thing as life not worthy to be lived . . . its impetus was the attitude toward the nonrehabilitable sick." It is of prime ethical importance that we be concerned about the care and protection of all men in societal and medical practices, and not solely with mercy in individual acts.

References

Alexander, Leo. "Medical Science under Dictatorship." *New England Journal of Medicine* 241 (July 14, 1949); 39–47.

Aring, Charles D. "Intimations of Mortality: An Appreciation of Death and Dying." *Annals of Internal Medicine* 69 (July 1968): 137–52.

Bard, Bernard, and Joseph Fletcher. "The Right to Die." *Atlantic Monthly* 221 (April 1968): 59–64.

Beecher, Henry K. *Research and the Individual.* Boston: Little, Brown, 1970.

Cameron, D. C. S. *The Truth about Cancer.* Englewood Cliffs, N.J.: Prentice-Hall, 1956.

Cavanagh, John R. "Bene Mori: The Right of a Patient to Die with Dignity." *Linacre Quarterly,* May 1963.

Church of England. *Decisions about Life and Death: A Problem in Modern Medicine.* London: Church Information Office, 1965.

Curran, Charles E. "The Morality of Human Transplants." *The Sign,* March 1968.

Daube, David. "Transplantation: Acceptability of Procedures and Their Required Legal Sanctions." In *Ethics in Medical Progress,* edited by E. W. Wolstenholme and Maeve O'Connor. Boston: Little, Brown, 1966.

Elkinton, J. Russell. "The Dying Patient, the Doctor, and the Law." *Villanova Law Review* 13 (Summer 1968): 740–50.

Fletcher, Joseph. *Moral Responsibility.* Philadelphia: Westminster Press, 1967.

Ford, John C. "The Refusal of Blood Transfusions by Jehovah's Witnesses." *Linacre Quarterly* 22 (February 1955): 3–10.

Giertz, G. B. "Ethical Problems in Medical Procedures in Sweden." In *Ethics in Medical Progress,* edited by E. W. Wolstenholme and Maeve O'Connor. Boston: Little, Brown, 1966.

Healy, Edwin F. *Medical Ethics.* Chicago: Loyola University Press, 1956.

Karnofsky, David. "Why Prolong the Life of a Patient with Advanced Cancer?" *Cancer Journal for Clinicians* 10 (January–February 1960): 9–11.

Kelly, Gerald. "The Duty of Using Artificial Means of Preserving Life." *Theological Studies* 11 (June 1950): 203–20.

—— "The Duty to Preserve Life." *Theological Studies* 12 (December 1951): 550–56.

——. *Medico-Moral Problems.* St. Louis: Catholic Hospital Association, 1958.

Long, Perrin H. "On the Quantity and Quality of Life." *Medical Times* 88 (May 1960): 613.

Nolan, Kieran. "The Problem of Care for the Dying." In *Absolutes in Moral Theology?,* edited by Charles E. Curran. Washington, D.C.: Corpus Books, 1968.

O'Donnell, Thomas J. *Morals in Medicine.* Westminster, Md.: Newman, 1960.

Rynearson, Edward H. "You Are Standing at Bedside of Patient Dying of Untreatable Cancer." *CA: A Bulletin of Cancer Progress* 9 (May–June 1959): 85–87.

Toch, Rudolf. "Management of the Child with a Fatal Disease." *Clinical Pediatrics* 3 (July 1964): 418–27.

Voigt, Jorgen. "The Criteria of Death, Particularly in Relation to Transplantation Surgery." *World Medical Journal* 14 (1967): 145–48.

Wasserman, H. P. "Problematic Aspects of the Phenomenon of Death." *World Medical Journal* 14 (1967): 148–49.

Wassmer, Thomas A. "Between Life and Death: Ethical and Moral Issues Involved in Recent Medical Advances." *Villanova Law Review* 13 (Summer 1968): 759–83.

16

Prolonging Life

George P. Fletcher

NEW medical techniques for prolonging life force both the legal and medical professions to reexamine their traditional attitudes toward life and death. New problems emerge from the following recurrent situation: a comatose patient shows no signs of brain activity; according to the best medical judgment, he has an infinitesimal chance of recovery; yet he can be sustained by a mechanical respirator. How long should his physician so keep him alive? And in making his decision, how much weight should the physician give to the wishes of the family, to the financial condition of the family, and to the prospect that his time might be profitably used in caring for patients with a better chance of recovery?

According to one line of thought, the physician's leeway in caring for terminal patients is limited indeed. He may turn off the respirator but only at the risk of prosecution and conviction for murder. The insensitive logic of the law of homicide, disregarding as it does the context of the purpose of the physician's effort, would prompt some to equate the physician's turning off the respirator with a hired gunman's killing in cold blood. The acts of both result in death; the actors intend that death should follow; and in neither case is the killing provoked, excused, or justified. Thus like the gunman, the physician is guilty of first-degree murder.

The approach of equating the physician's turning off a mechanical respi-

Reprinted from the *Washington Law Review* 42 (1967): 999–1016, with the permission of the publisher. Copyright 1967 by the University of Washington. Some footnotes omitted.

rator with the gunman's killing for hire is, to say the least, askew with reality. It totally misses the demands of the medical mission. It means that physicians must use modern devices for sustaining life with trepidation; they must proceed haltingly, unsure of the legal consequences of discontinuing therapy. It is of little solace to the medical practitioner that institutional facts check the cold rigor of the common law. True, his decisions in the operating room are minimally visible; not even the patient's family need learn whether death came "naturally" or upon the disruption of therapy. And even if it should become known to the family and the community that the physician's decision shortened the life span of the patient, it is unlikely that the physician should suffer. Common-law courts have never convicted a medical practitioner either for shortening the life of a suffering, terminal patient or for refusing to render life-sustaining aid. Yet men of goodwill wish to proceed not by predictions of what will befall them but by perceiving and conforming to their legal and moral obligations. . . .

The apparent rigidity of the common law of homicide has evoked demands for reform. The proposals for vesting physicians with greater flexibility in caring for terminal patients is of two strands. The first is a movement toward instituting voluntary euthanasia, which would permit the medically supervised killing of patients who consent to death. These proposals warrant continued discussion and criticism, but they apply only in cases of patients still conscious and able to consent to their own demise. Separate problems adhere to the cases of doomed, unconscious patients who may be kept alive by mechanical means. In the latter area, the movement for reform has stimulated the pursuit of a definition of death that would permit physicians to do what they will with the bodies of hopeless, "legally dead" patients. In France and Sweden as well as in the United States, proponents of reform have urged the cessation of brain activity—as evidence by a flat electroencephalograph (EEG) reading—as the criterion of death. Setting the moment of legal death prior to the stilling of the heart is critical to those pressing for greater legal flexibility in transplanting vital organs from doomed patients to those with greater hopes of recovery. Waiting until the heart fails makes transplanting difficult, if not impossible. At stake in the pursuit of a legal definition of death is the prospect of a vast increase in the supply of kidneys, and, some day, of livers, hearts, and ovaries for the purpose of transplanting. The reliance on the concept of death, however, is a verbal detour. The reformers are concerned about two practical decisions: (1) when can a physician legally discontinue aid to a patient with an infinitesimal chance of recovery; and (2) when can a physician legally remove organs from a terminal patient. To resolve these problems, one need not construct a concept of legal death. Concern for the moment of death presupposes: (1) that both of these decisions should depend on the same criteria; and (2) that the controlling criteria should be medical facts, rather than the host of criteria relating to the patient's financial condition and to the importance of the physician's time and of the machinery used in sustaining life.

Rather than promote either the movement for voluntary euthanasia or the search for a new definition of death, this paper shall propose a third technique for loosening the legal vice currently worrying the medical community. We can furnish practicing physicians at least some flexibility in the operating room by invoking a more sensitive interpretation of the law as it now stands. To loosen the legal vice of the law of homicide, we need only take a closer look at its pinions. We need to question each of the steps leading to the view that the physician's turning off a respirator or a kidney machine is an act subjecting him to tort and criminal liability for homicide.

There are only a few points at which the structure can give. Consider the applicable elements of common-law murder: (1) an act resulting in death, (2) an intent to inflict death, (3) malice aforethought, (4) absence of defenses. Beginning at the end of the list, one is hard pressed to justify or excuse the killing by invoking a recognized defense. If the common-law courts were more amenable to a general defense of necessity in homicide cases, one could argue that if another patient had a superior likelihood of recovery using the machine, the attending physician would be warranted in removing a patient from the machine who was then dependent upon it for his life. A defense of this sort could serve as a welcome guide to those concerned about the legal limits of allocating the use of kidney machines. The appropriate foothold for the defense would be a physician's common-law prerogative to abort a fetus when necessary to save the life of the mother. Yet that defense is premised on the judgment that the life of the mother represents a more worthy interest than that of the unborn child; when it comes to a choice between the two, the mother has a superior right to live. One is advisedly wary of the analogical claim that the patient with the greater likelihood of recovery has a superior right to live. We have lived too long with the notion that all human beings have an equal claim to life.

If the prospects of a defense are questionable, forays on the issues of intent and malice seem hopeless. The aim of the physician's behavior may not be to kill, yet he knows that death is certain to follow if he interrupts therapy to free the respirator for another patient. And knowledge that death is certain to follow is enough to say, at least according to the dictionary of the law, that he "intends" death to result from his conduct. Also, it is too late in the evolution of the common law to make the concept of malice mean what it purports to mean, namely ill will, base motives, and the like. Surely, the man on the street would not say that a physician is malicious in breaking off his care of a fated patient. Indeed, in the interest of saving the family from financial ruin or directing his efforts more profitably, it might be the humane thing to do. Yet the common law long ago betrayed the ordinary English background of its rule that a man must kill "maliciously" to be guilty of murder. The rigors of distinguishing good motives from bad and the elusiveness of motive as an object of prosecutorial proof gave way nearly four centuries ago to the concept of implied malice and thus to the functional demise of malice as a tool for drawing important distinctions in the law of homicide.

It appears that there is only one stage in the structure that might readily yield under analysis. That is the initial claim that the turning off of a mechanical respirator is an act resulting in death. The alternative would be to regard the flipping of the switch as an omission, a forebearance—a classification that would lead to a wholly different track of legal analysis. It seems novel to suggest that flipping a switch should count as an omission. For like the act of the gunman in pulling a trigger, flipping a switch represents an exertion of the will. It is bodily movement, and, for many, that would be enough to say that the behavior constitutes an act, not an omission. Yet as I shall argue in this essay, the turning off of a mechanical respirator should be classified as an omission. It should be regarded on a par with the passivity of that infamous passerby who gleefully watches a stranded child drown in a swimming pool. As we shall see, this view of the problem has vast implications for advising physicians of their legal leeway in rendering therapy to terminal patients.

Much of what follows is an exercise in conceptual analysis. It is an effort to devise a test for determining which of two competitive schemes—that for acts or that for omissions—should apply in analyzing a given question of responsibility for the death of another. It is significant inquiry, if only to add a word to the discussion of the ponderous legal quandaries of physicians who care for terminal patients. The problem is also of wider significance for the theory of tort and criminal liability. The area of liability for omissions bristles with moral, analytic, and institutional puzzles. In the course of this inquiry, we shall confront some of these problems and others we shall catalogue in passing.

I

The question is posed: is the physician's discontinuing aid to a terminal patient an act or omission? To be sure, the choice of legal track does not yield radically different results. For some omissions, physicians are liable in much the same way as they are for unpermitted operations and negligent treatment. One need only consider the following turn of events. Doctor Brown is the family doctor of the Smith family and has been for several years. Tim Smith falls ill with pneumonia. Brown sees him once or twice at the family home and administers the necessary therapy. One evening, upon receiving a telephone call from the Smith family that Tim is in a critical condition, Dr. Brown decides that he should prefer to remain at his bridge game than to visit the sick child. Brown fails to render aid to the child; it is clear that Brown would be liable criminally and civilly if death should ensue.[1] That he has merely omitted to act, rather than asserted himself intentionally to end life, is immaterial in assessing his criminal and civil liability. Of course, the doctor would not be under an obligation to respond to the call of a stranger who said that he needed help. But there is a difference between a stranger and someone who has placed himself in the care of a physician. The factor of reliance and reasonable expectation that the doctor will render aid means that the doctor is legally obligated to do so. His failure to do so is then tantamount to an intentional infliction of harm. As his motive, be it for good or ill, is irrelevant in analyzing his liability for assertive killing, his motive is also irrelevant in analyzing his liability for omitting to render aid when he is obligated to do so.

Thus, it makes no difference whether a doctor omits to render aid because he prefers to continue playing bridge or if he does so in the hope that the patient's misery will come quickly to a natural end. A doctor may be criminally and civilly liable either for intentionally taking life or for omitting to

[1] The Queen v. Instan, [1893] 1 Q.B. 450.

act and thus permitting death to occur. However, the sources of these two legal proscriptions are different. And this difference in the source of the law may provide the key for the analysis of the doctor's liability in failing to prolong life in the case discussed at the outset of this article. That a doctor may not actively kill is an application of the general principle that no man may actively kill a fellow human being. In contrast, the principle that a doctor may not omit to render aid to a patient justifiably relying upon him is a function of the special relationship that exists between doctor and patient. Thus, in analyzing the doctor's legal duty to his patient, one must take into consideration whether the question involved is an act or an omission. If it is an act, the relationship between the doctor and patient is irrelevant. If it is an omission, the relationship is all-controlling.

With these points in mind, we may turn to an analysis of specific aspects of the medical decision not to prolong life. The first problem is to isolate the relevant medical activity. The recurrent pattern includes: stopping cardiac resuscitation, turning off a respirator, a pacemaker, or a kidney machine, and removing the tubes and devices used with these life-sustaining machines. The initial decision of classification determines the subsequent legal analysis of the case. If turning off the respirator is an "act" under the law, then it is unequivocally forbidden: it is on a par with injecting air into the patient's veins. If, on the other hand, it is classified as an "omission," the analysis proceeds more flexibly. Whether it would be forbidden as an omission would depend on the demands imposed by the relationship between doctor and patient.

There are gaps in the law; and we are confronted with one of them. There is simply no way to focus the legal authorities to determine whether the process of turning off the respirator is an act or an omission. That turning off the respirator takes physical movement need not be controlling. There might be "acts" without physical movement, as, for example, if one should sit motionless in the driver's seat as one's car heads toward an intended victim. Surely that would be an act causing death; it would be first-degree murder regardless of the relationship between the victim and his assassin. Similarly, there might be cases of omissions involving physical exertion, perhaps even the effort required to turn off the respirator. The problem is not whether there is or there is not physical movement; there must be another test.

That other test, I should propose, is whether on all the facts we should be inclined to speak of the activity as one that causes harm or one merely tnat permits harm to occur. The usage of the verbs "causing" and "permitting" corresponds to the distinction in the clear cases between acts and omissions. If a doctor injects air into the veins of a suffering patient, he causes harm. On the other hand, if the doctor fails to stop on the highway to aid a stranger injured in an automobile accident, he surely permits harm to occur, and he might be morally blameworthy for that; but as the verb "cause" is ordinarily used, his failing to stop is not the cause of the harm.

As native speakers of English, we are equipped with linguistic sensitivity for the distinction between causing harm and permitting harm to occur. That sensitivity reflects a commonsense perception of reality; and we should employ it in classifying the hard cases arising in discussions of the prolongation of life. Is turning off the respirator an instance of causing death or permitting death to occur? If the patient is beyond recovery and on the verge of death, one balks at saying that the activity causes death. It is far more natural to speak of the case as one of permitting death to occur. It is significant that we are inclined to refer to the respirator as a means of prolonging life; we would not speak of insulin shots for a diabetic in the same way. The use of the term "prolongation of life" builds on the same perception of reality that prompts us to say that turning off the respirator is an activity permitting death to occur, rather than causing death. And that basic perception is that using the respirator interferes artificially in the pattern of events. Of course, the perception of the natural and of the artificial is a function of time and culture. What may seem artificial today, may be a matter of course in ten years. Nonetheless, one *does* perceive many uses of the respirator today as artificial prolongations of life. And that perception of artificiality should be enough to determine the legal classification of the case. Because we are prompted to refer to the activity of turning off the respirator as activity permitting death to occur, rather than causing death, we may classify the case as an omission, rather than as an act.

To clarify our approach, we might consider this scenario. A pedestrian D notices that a nearby car, parked with apparently inadequate brakes, is about to roll down hill. P's house is parked directly in its path. D rushes to the front of the car and with effort he is able to arrest its movement for a few minutes. Though he feels able to hold back the car for several more minutes (time enough perhaps to give warning of the danger), he decides that he has had enough; and he steps to one side, knowing full well that his quarry will roll squarely into P's front yard. That is precisely what it does. What are P's rights against D? Again, the problem is whether the defendant's behavior should be treated as an act or as an omission. If it is an act, he is liable for trespass against P's property. If it is an omission, the law of trespass is inapplicable; and the problem devolves into a search for a relationship between P and D that would impose on D the duty to prevent this form of damage to P's property. Initially, one is inclined to regard D's behavior as an act bringing on harm. Like the physician's turning off a respirator, his stepping aside represents physical exertion. Yet as in the physician's case, we are led to the opposite result by asking whether under the circumstances D caused the harm or merely permitted it to occur. Surely, a newspaper account would employ the latter description; D let the car go, he permitted it to roll on, but he is no more a causal factor than if he had not initially intervened to halt its forward motion. We deny D's causal contribution for reasons akin to those in the physician's case. In both instances, other factors are sufficient in themselves to bring on the harmful result. As the car's brakes were inadequate to hold it on the hill, so the patient's hopeless condition brought on his death. With sufficient causal factors present, we can imagine the harm's occurring without the physician's or the pedestrian's contribution. And thus we are inclined to think of the behavior of each as something less than a causal force.

One might agree that as a matter of common sense, we can distinguish between causing harm and permitting harm to occur and yet balk at referring to the way people ordinarily describe phenomena in order to solve hard problems of legal policy. After all, what if people happen to describe things differently? Would that mean that we would have to devise different answers to the same legal problems? To vindicate a resort to common sense notions and linguistic usage as a touchstone for separating acts from omissions, we must clarify the interlacing of these three planes of the problem: (1) the distinction between acts and omissions, (2) the ordinary usage of the terms "causing" and "permitting" and (3) resorting in cases of omissions, but not in cases of acts, to the relationship between the agent and his victim in setting the scope of the agent's duties. The question uniting the second and third variables is this: is there good reason for being guided by the relationship between the parties in cases where the agent has permitted harm to occur, but not in cases where the agent has intentionally and directly caused harm to a stranger? To answer this question, we need to turn in some detail to the function of causal judgments in analyzing liability, whereupon we may clarify the link between the first and second variables of the analysis, namely, between the category of omissions and the process of permitting harm to occur.

Ascribing liability for tortious and criminal harm may be looked upon as a two-stage process. The first stage is the isolation of a candidate for liability. In virtually all dimensions of the law of crimes and torts, we rely upon the concept of causation to separate from the mass of society those individuals who might prove to be liable for the proscribed harm. Upon reducing the number of potentially liable parties to those that have caused the harm, the final stage of analysis demands an evaluation of the facts under the apt rules of liability, e.g., those prescribing negligence and proximate cause as conditions for liability.

The one area of the law where one has difficulty isolating candidates for liability is the area of omissions. When others have stood by and permitted harm to occur, we either have too many candidates for liability or we have none at all. A helpless old woman succumbs to starvation. Many people knew of her condition and did nothing; the postman, her hired nurse, her daughter, the bill collector, the telephone operator—each of them allowed her to die. Could we say, on analogy to causing death, that permitting the death to occur should serve as the criterion for selecting these people as candidates for liability? If we say that all of them are candidates for liability, then the burden falls to the criteria of fault to decide which of them, if any, should be liable for wrongful death and criminal homicide. The problem is whether the criteria of fault are sufficiently sensitive to resolve the question of liability. What kinds of questions should we ask in assessing fault? Did each voluntarily omit to render aid? Did any one of them face a particular hazard in doing so? Were any of them in a particularly favorable position to avert the risk of death? If these are the questions we must ask in assessing fault and affixing liability, we are at a loss to discriminate among the candidates for liability. Each acted voluntarily with knowledge of the peril; none faced personal hazard in offering assistance; and their capacities to avert the risk were equal. Thus, we may use the concept of permitting as we do the notion of causation to narrow the field to those who should be judged on criteria of fault. But if we do, the criteria of fault are useless (at least in the type of case sketched here) for discriminating among the candidates.

One wonders why this is so. In the arena of caused harms, one may have a large number of candidates for liability. The conventional test of causing harm sweeps wide in encompassing all those but for whose contribution the harm would not have occurred. Yet the criteria of liability—reasonableness of risk, ambit of risk, proximate cause—are effective in further reducing the field to those we might fairly hold liable. The reason is that each causal agent is chargeable with a different risk that loss of the given kind would occur. The risks differ in quantum and scope. Some bear a remote relationship to the harm; others seem reasonable in light of other circumstances. These differences in the posture of each causal agent toward the risk of harm enable us to assess their individual fault with some sensitivity.

In contrast, those who permit harm to occur do not bear individualized responsibility for the risk of harm. Their status derives not from the creation of the risk, but merely from knowledge that the risk exists and from the opportunity to do something about it. One could speak of the likelihood that each could avert the harm. And in some cases, this approach might be useful; a doctor's failing to render aid to a man lying in the street is more egregious than a layman's turning the other way. Yet in the general run of case—the starvation of the old woman discussed above, the Kitty Genovese incident—the risks assignable to passive bystanders are of the same murky order: each could have done something but did not.

Even if a man might be charged with a specific risk for having failed to avert harm, it is often difficult to assess the reasonableness of his permitting that likelihood of harm. Causal agents take risks that are evaluated by reference to the agent's reasons for acting. A motorist risks the death of others by embarking on an automotive trip, yet the risk is reasonable in light of his conventionally acceptable purpose of traveling by car. One cannot so readily evaluate the risks ascribable to those who fail to avert harm. Men generally do not further their goals by letting events turn as they may. Is it reasonable or unreasonable for a father to let his 16-year-old son participate in drag races on the city streets? He promotes no end of his own by failing to intervene. His reasons are those of indifference and fear of involvement—the same reasons that prompted 38 people in New York City to witness the murder of Kitty Genovese. Reasons of this kind do not lend themselves to a calculus of reasonableness: how does one weigh a man's fear of involvement against the occurrence of harm? And without a calculus of reasonableness, one may hardly expect to discern differences in the personal fault of those who permit harm to occur.

Affixing liability fairly in cases of omission requires a more sensitive filtering mechanism prior to the application of the traditional criteria of personal fault. The concept of permitting harm sweeps too wide; and the criteria of personal fault tend to be of little avail in narrowing the field. Thus one can understand the role of the relationship between the parties as a touchstone of liability. Legal systems, both common law and continental, have resorted to the relationship between the parties as a device for narrowing the field to those individuals whose liability may be left to depend on personal fault. According to the conventional rules, the old woman's nurse and daughter are candidates potentially liable for permitting death to occur. Liability would rest on personal fault, primarily on the voluntariness of each in omitting to render aid. Thus the conventional rules as to when one has a duty to render aid fulfill the same function as the causal inquiry in its domain: these rules, like the predication of causation, isolate individuals whose behavior is then scrutinized for the marks of negligent and intentional wrongdoing.

By demonstrating the parallel between the causal concept in cases of acts and the relationship between the parties in cases of omissions, we have come a long way in support of our thesis. We have shown that in cases of permitting harm to occur, one is required to resort to the relationship between the parties in order fairly to select those parties whose liability should turn on criteria of personal fault. In the absence of a causal judgment, with its attendant assignment of differentiated responsibility for the risk of harm, one can proceed only by asking: is this the kind of relationship, e.g., parent-child, doctor-patient, in which one person ought to help another? And on grounds ranging from common decency to contract, one derives individual duties to render aid when needed.

One step of the argument remains: the conclusion that cases of permitting harm are instances of omissions, not of acts. This is a step that turns not so much on policy and analysis, as on acceptance of the received premises of the law of homicide. One of these premises is that acting intentionally to cause death is unconditionally prohibited: the relationship between the defendant and his victim is irrelevant. One may resort to the relationship between the parties only in cases of omissions indirectly resulting in harm.[2] With these two choices and no others, the logic of classification is ineluctable. Cases of permitting harm, where one must have recourse to the rela-

[2] Rex v. Smith, 2 Car. & P. 448, 172 E.R. 203 (Gloucester Assizes 1826).

tionship between the parties, cannot be classified as cases of acts: to do so would preclude excusing the harm on the ground that the relationship between the parties did not require its avoidance. Thus, to permit recourse to relationship of the parties, one must treat cases of permitting harm as cases of omissions.

To complete our inquiry, we need attend to an asymmetry in the analysis of causing and permitting. As Professors Hart and Honore have shown in *Causation in the Law* (1957), some omissions may be the causes of harm. And thus, the category of causing harm includes some cases of omitting as well as all cases of acting to bring on harm. Suppose, for example, that an epileptic regularly takes pills to avert a seizure. Yet on one occasion he omits to take the pills in the hope that he is no longer required to. He has a seizure. The cause of his seizure is clear: he omitted to take the prescribed pill. In the same way, a physician failing to give a diabetic patient a routine shot of insulin would be the cause of harm that might ensue. The taking of the pill and the giving of the shot are the expected state of affairs. They represent normality, and their omission, abnormality. Because we anticipate the opposite, the omission explains what went wrong, why our expectations were not realized. In contrast, if pills to avert epileptic seizures had just been devised, we would not say, as to someone who had never taken the pills, that his failure to do so had brought on his attack. In that case, our expectations would be different, the omission to take pills would not represent an abnormality, and the anticipated omission would not be a satisfying causal explanation of the attack.

A doctor's failure to give his diabetic patient an insulin shot is a case warranting some attention. By contemporary standards, insulin shots, unlike mechanical respirators, do not interfere artifically in the course of nature; because the use of insulin is standard medical practice, we would not describe its effect as one of prolonging life. We would not say that withholding the shot permits death; it is a case of an omission causing harm. With the prohibition against causing death, one should not have to refer to the doctor-patient relationship to determine the criminality of the doctor's omission. Yet in fact, common-law courts would ground a conviction for omitting to give the shot on the doctor's duty to render aid to his patient—a duty derived from the doctor-patient relationship. Thus we encounter an apparent inconsistency: a case of causing in which one resorts to the relationship of the parties to determine criminality. We can reconcile the case with our thesis by noting that cases of omissions causing harm possess the criteria—regularity of performance and reliance—that give rise to duties of care. The doctor is clearly under a duty to provide his patient with an insulin shot if the situation demands it. And the duty is so clear precisely because one expects an average doctor in the 1960s to use insulin when necessary; this is the same expectation that prompts us to say that his failure to give the shot would be the cause of his patient's death.

That an omission can on occasion be the cause of harm prompts us slightly to reformulate our thesis. We cannot say that causing harm may serve as the criterion for an act as opposed to an omission because some instances of causation are omissions. But we may claim with undiminished force that permitting harm to occur should be sufficient for classification as an omission. Upon analysis, we find that our thesis for distinguishing acts from omissions survives only in part; it works for some omissions, but not for all. Yet, so far as the stimulus of this investigation is concerned, the problem of physicians permitting death to come to their terminal patients, the thesis continues to hold: permitting a patient to die is a case in which one appropriately refers to the relationship of the parties to set the scope of the physician's legal duty to his patient; in this sense it functions as an omission in legal analysis.

II

By permitting recourse to the doctor-patient relationship in fixing the scope of the doctor's duties to his patient, we have at least fashioned the concepts of the common law to respond more sensitively to the problems of the time. We have circumvented the extravagant legal conclusion that a physician's turning off a kidney machine or a respirator is tantamount to murder. Yet one critical inquiry remains. How does shunting the analysis into the track of legal omissions actually affect the physician's flexibility in the operating room? We say that his duties are determined by his relationship with his patient; specifically, it is the consensual aspect of the relationship that is supposed to control the leeway of the physician. Yet there is some question as to where the control actually resides.

To take a clear case, let us suppose that prior to the onset of a terminal illness, the patient demands that his physician do everything to keep him alive and breathing as long as possible. And the physician responds, "Even if you have a flat EEG reading and there is no chance of recovery?" "Yes," the patient replies. If the doctor agrees to this bizarre demand, he becomes obligated to keep the respirator going indefinitely. Happily, cases of this type do not occur in day-to-day medical practice. In the average case, the patient has not given a thought to the problem; and his physician is not likely to alert him to it. The problem then is whether there is an implicit understanding between physician and patient as to how the physician should proceed in the last stages of a terminal illness. But would there be an implicit understanding about what the physician should do if the patient is in a coma and dependent on a mechanical respirator? This is not the kind of thing as to which the average man has expectations. And if he did, they would be expectations that would be based on the customary practices of the time. If he had heard about a number of cases in which patients had been sustained for long periods of time on respirators, he might (at least prior to going into the coma) expect that he would be similarly sustained.

Thus, the analysis leads us along the following path. The doctor's duty to prolong life is a function of his relationship with his patient; and, in the typical case, that relationship devolves into the patient's expectations of the treatment he will receive. Those expectations, in turn, are a function of the practices prevailing in the community at the time, and practices in the use of respirators to prolong life are no more and no less than what doctors actually do in the time and place. Thus, we have come full circle. We began the inquiry by asking: is it legally permissible for doctors to turn off respirators used to prolong the life of doomed patients? And the answer after our tortuous journey is simply: it all depends on what doctors customarily do. The law is sometimes no more precise than that.

The conclusion of our circular journey is that doctors are in a position to fashion their own law to deal with cases of prolongation of life. By establishing customary standards, they may determine the expectations of their patients and thus regulate the understanding and the relationship between doctor and patient. And by regulating that relationship, they may control their legal obligations to render aid to doomed patients.

Thus the medical profession confronts the challenge of developing humane and sensitive customary standards for guiding decisions to prolong the lives of terminal patients. This is not a challenge that the profession may shirk. For the doctor's legal duties to render aid derive from his relationship with the patient. That relationship, along with the expectations implicit in it, is the responsibility of the individual doctor and the individual patient. With respect to problems not commonly discussed by the doctor with his patient, particularly the problems of prolonging life, the responsibility for the patient's expectations lies with the medical profession as a whole.

17

A Patient's Decision to Decline Lifesaving Medical Treatment: Bodily Integrity versus the Preservation of Life

〜〜〜〜〜〜〜

Norman L. Cantor

THE scene is a local community hospital. The patient is a 25-year-old man or woman suffering from a perforated ulcer, potentially fatal but curable by a simple operation. The patient is unmarried, childless, and fully coherent. With the threat of death looming, physicians request that the patient consent to surgery and an accompanying blood transfusion. The patient refuses because: (a) religious convictions forbid either the surgery or the blood transfusion (e.g., Jehovah's Witnesses believe that blood transfusions violate biblical injunctions against "eating blood"); (b) the patient wants to die because of shame and anxiety over recent financial or romantic setbacks; (c) the patient wants to die because he or she is also the victim of a terminal illness which will inevitably entail considerable pain and gradual bodily degeneration; or (d) the patient is refusing treatment as a symbolic protest against a governmental policy, such as Vietnam, and will only submit to surgery when that policy is officially changed. The hospital administrator, acting on

Reprinted from the *Rutgers Law Review* 26 (Winter 1973): 228–64, with the permission of the publisher. Copyright 1973 by Rutgers University (The State University of New Jersey). Some footnotes omitted.

the principle that a hospital's paramount mission is to preserve life, seeks a judicial order appointing himself temporary guardian for purposes of consenting to the necessary lifesaving medical treatment.

Can or should a judge grant the relief requested? Does refusal to intervene entail acceptance of a "right to die" in the context of suicide and euthanasia? Does it matter whether the patient is motivated by reasons of conscience or simply by the will to die? Does it matter that the patient has dependents who will be disadvantaged by his or her death? The strong temptation is to respond positively to the opportunity to preserve life. Judges have been anguished by the knowledge that failure to order treatment would likely mean the patient's death, particularly where the patient did not really wish to die but was only following religious dictates. Religious freedom, bodily integrity, or individual self-determination appear as evanescent or ephemeral principles in the face of an immediate threat to life. Yet, both religious freedom and control of one's body are cherished values in our society, and both are of constitutional dimension when threatened by governmental invasion.

The above questions should not be resolved by visceral reaction. Careful analysis of legal protections for bodily integrity, constitutional standards, and governmental interests asserted as justifications for judicial intervention is necessary. While the reported cases are relatively few, there has been no dearth of legal commentary on judicial compulsion of lifesaving medical treatment. Previous treatments of this topic, however, have largely failed to examine all the potential interests, or to assess the degree of harm posed to these interests by refusal of medical care. This article is intended to avert that weakness. Hopefully, it will contribute to resolution of a public-policy issue—judicially compelled lifesaving treatment—which undoubtedly arises with considerably more frequency than the number of reported cases would indicate. Additionally, fixing the delicate constitutional balance between bodily integrity and the preservation of life in this context may have significant ramifications for such issues as abortion, contraception, sterilization, and population control.

I. Background—Cases and Commentators

Judicial intervention to secure lifesaving medical treatment most commonly involves minors whose parents voice religious objections to blood transfusions or operations. In these situations, the cases have uniformly upheld state interference with parents' control in order to safeguard the children. Religious objections have been overridden by resort to the state's traditional parens patriae authority—its right and duty to protect the disabled, meaning those unable to care for themselves. Normally, this parens patriae doctrine is embodied in "neglect" statutes authorizing state intervention for parental failure to provide necessary medical care. But there have been indications that such intervention would be forthcoming even in the absence of specific legislation. In short, protection of child welfare has been viewed as a paramount state interest and courts have consistently ordered lifesaving medical treatment for minors.

No similar "neglect" statutes authorize judicial interference when competent adults fail to secure necessary medical treatment, nor does the common-law parens patriae doctrine extend beyond protection of the disabled. Moreover adults' cases have usually entailed religious or other principled objections to treatment raised by the patient whose own bodily integrity is threatened. The cases involving adults' refusal of treatment are, therefore, considerably more complex than those involving minors and the judicial results have varied accordingly.

Where the patient declining care was a parent of a minor child, the courts have been prone to appoint a guardian to authorize treatment. The most famous example is *Application of the President and Directors of Georgetown College.*[1] There, a 25-year-old female Jehovah's Witness had refused a blood transfusion despite mortal danger posed by a ruptured ulcer. The patient was the mother of a seven-month-old child but both the patient and her husband refused to authorize the transfusion. After a United States district court judge had rejected the hospital's request for judicial intervention, Circuit Judge J. Skelly Wright authorized the transfusion, citing a number of considerations to support his decision. Primarily, he viewed the case as embodying an extension of the traditional parens patriae doctrine. Since the state could generally guard a child's well-being, and prevent the child's abandonment, it could also act to prevent this "ultimate abandonment" of a child by its parent. He failed, however, to clearly indicate whether the state's precise interest lay in avoiding a fiscal burden or in preserving the emotional well-being of a minor. Presumably, the latter was the predominant factor, since a

[1] 331 F.2d 1000 (D.C. Cir.), *cert. denied*, 377 U.S. 978 (1964).

spouse remained to provide economic security for the surviving child. Judge Wright also noted the interests of the hospital and physicians who had assumed responsibility for treatment and cure and wanted to pursue their professional skills. To let the patient die without a transfusion would run counter to their professional judgments and might expose them to civil or criminal liability. This dilemma could be obviated by judicial authorization of treatment. Judge Wright also contended that court authorization would entail only minor infringement upon the patient's religious beliefs. According to the court, the religious prohibition attached to consenting to a blood transfusion; thus, submission to a court-ordered transfusion would not contravene the patient's religious scruples. Finally, in an effort to glean further support for judicial intervention, Judge Wright analogized a refusal of medical treatment to suicide and pointed toward criminal penalties for attempted suicide as proof of legitimate legislative opposition to suicide. He could not rely heavily on the suicide analogy only because the legal status of attempted suicide in his jurisdiction was unclear.

The District of Columbia Circuit Court en banc refused to address the merits of the *Georgetown College* case, so it cannot be considered strong precedent in that jurisdiction. Nonetheless, the case has had a considerable persuasive impact. It has been followed where minor dependents were involved, where only a spouse would have survived the patient, and where no dependents were present.

The recent decision of the New Jersey Supreme Court in *John F. Kennedy Memorial Hospital* v. *Heston* represents a major appellate call for judicial intervention even in the absence of minor children.[2] The case dealt with a 22-year-old, unmarried woman who had been severely injured in an automobile accident. Although there was considerable dispute over the woman's competency at the time of hospital admission, it was clear that she had been for some time a Jehovah's Witness opposed to blood transfusions, and her mother, also a Jehovah's Witness, refused to authorize a necessary blood transfusion. Upon petition of the hospital, a lower court judge appointed a temporary guardian and the transfusion was given. On appeal, New Jersey's highest court unanimously upheld the judicial action. The opinion by Chief Justice Weintraub cited two interests sufficient to justify judicial intervention—the state's interest in preserving life and the hospital's

[2] 58 N.J. 576, 279 A.2d 670 (1970).

interest in pursuing its functions without the threat of liability. The interest in "life" was recited without much elaboration as to the precise governmental concerns involved, whether economic, political, or simply paternalistic. As evidence of the state's legitimate concern with sustaining life, the opinion pointed to the legislative proscription of attempted suicide. Chief Justice Weintraub observed that through the police, the state commonly intervenes to prevent suicide. He concluded that whatever interests justify such intervention also support the overriding of an individual's refusal of lifesaving attention. According to the court, "if the State may interrupt one mode of self-destruction, it may with equal authority interfere with the other."

The court next considered the position of the hospital and staff in the controversy. Not to pursue lifesaving treatment would violate professional creeds. Moreover, civil liability might flow from failure to render treatment, unless a valid release was available. The court preferred to authorize treatment over the patient's objections rather than subject the professional staff to the task of assessing the patient's competency or a release's validity.

The preceding discussion notwithstanding, judicial sentiment is by no means unanimous in favor of court-ordered treatment. The most articulate statement for the position opposing interference with a patient's decision is *In re Brooks' Estate*.[3] There, the patient, a female Jehovah's Witness, refused a transfusion necessary to the treatment of a peptic ulcer. The patient had a spouse and adult children, but they did not oppose her refusal. In a unanimous decision, the Supreme Court of Illinois upheld the patient's right to determine her own fate. Although the hospital's representative asserted an overriding societal interest in protecting the lives of citizens, the court perceived no immediate threat to the public health, safety, or welfare sufficient to outweigh the patient's interest in religious freedom. The court commented: "Even though we may consider [Mrs. Brooks'] beliefs unwise, foolish, or ridiculous, in the absence of an overriding danger to society we may not permit interference therewith . . . for the sole purpose of compelling her to accept medical treatment forbidden by her religious principles, and previously refused by her with full knowledge of the probable consequences." In dictum, the opinion conceded that the result might be different if Mrs. Brooks had minor children, since the state would then have

[3] 32 Ill. 2d 361, 205 N.E.2d 435 (1965).

an interest in preventing the children from becoming wards of the state.

Judicial refusal to override a patient's rejection of medical treatment has been reached in several other cases. In *Erickson* v. *Dilgard*, the court supported the patient's refusal of a blood transfusion despite a "very great chance" that the consequence would be death from internal bleeding.[4] No reasons for the refusal, religious or otherwise, was articulated in the opinion. The court nonetheless ruled in favor of individual self-determination, commenting: "It is the individual who is the subject of a medical decision who has the final say and . . . this must necessarily be so in a system of government which gives the greatest possible protection to the individual in the furtherance of his own desires."

In an unreported 1972 case, a Milwaukee judge declined to appoint a temporary guardian for a 77-year-old woman who had refused to permit amputation of a gangrenous leg.[5] Although the patient was physically weak, the court noted her clear determination to avoid the surgical procedure and ruled that competent adults have the prerogative of making life-and-death medical decisions about their own bodies. The court's opinion observed: "I believe we should leave [the patient] depart in God's own peace." The patient died several weeks after the decision.

Commentators upon patients' refusal of lifesaving treatment have expressed views almost as varied as those of the courts. There is widespread support for judicial intervention where the patient has a minor child, grounded on the public interest both in avoiding an economic burden and in protecting the emotional well-being of a youngster. Beyond this point, attitudes toward compelled treatment diverge. Some sources (Cawley 1969) regard the state's interest in preserving life as too chimerical to justify interference with an adult's private decision on how to control his body. They perceive no real threat to public safety or welfare, or to the welfare of any third parties from a patient's refusal of treatment, and, therefore, find no basis to override an individual's convictions. They note that although the law generally compels adults to care for their dependents, it does not compel self-care. Other sources (Sharpe and Hargest 1968) concede governmental power to intercede and render lifesaving treatment but counsel against exercise of such authority. According to this view, preservation of life promotes a healthy and thriving population and therefore constitutes an important so-

---

[4] 44 Misc. 2d 27, 252 N.Y.S. 2d 705 (Sup. Ct. 1962).

[5] *In re* Raasch, No. 455–996 (Prob. Div., Wilwaukee County Ct. Jan. 21, 1972).

cietal interest. However, respect for individual self-determination and recognition that refusals of lifesaving treatment do not pose a substantial threat to societal well-being dictate against judicial intervention.

There is some sentiment that judicial compulsion of lifesaving treatment is not only permissible, but desirable (Hegland 1965). According to this view, the state's interest in preserving life—even by overriding individual choice—is real and compelling. Not only is society preserved and strengthened by the sustenance of the patient, but general respect for the sanctity of life is reinforced. The traditional negative attitude of the law toward suicide and euthanasia is cited as support for interference with individual decisions consenting to death. These sources consider compelled treatment to be only a minor infringement upon religious liberty since the individual may follow all his religious dictates except in the life-and-death situation. Submission to court-ordered treatment would not violate the patient's religious convictions.

These divergent viewpoints, both judicial and scholarly, reflect the complexity of the issues involved in refusal of lifesaving medical assistance. Before attempting resolution of these delicate issues, however, it is important to consider the legal framework in which judges contemplating intervention must operate.

II. Constitutional and Common-law Standards

The "right" of an individual to determine when bodily invasions will occur is by no means a novel jurisprudential concept. Bodily integrity has often been recognized by the judiciary as an important value and has enjoyed protection under both the common law and the Constitution. In an 1891 decision repudiating attempts to compel a personal injury plaintiff to undergo pretrial medical examination, the United States Supreme Court commented: "No right is held more sacred, or is more carefully guarded, by the common law, than the right of every individual to the possession and control of his own person, free from all restraint or interference by others, unless by clear and unquestionable authority of law."[6]

More recently, the medical patient's right to bodily control has been emodied in the tort doctrine of informed consent. Under this doctrine, no medical procedure may be performed without a patient's consent, obtained

[6] Union Pacific Ry. v. Botsford, 141 U.S. 250, 251 (1891).

after explanation of the nature of the treatment, substnatial risks, and alternative therapies. The theory is variously expressed as assault, battery, negligence, malpractice, or even trespass, but the underlying concept of protection of bodily integrity remains the crux of informed consent. The doctrine recognizes that the consequence of a physician's explanation and consultation may be a patient's refusal of treatment and assumption of the risk of harm. Indeed, it has been acknowledged that the exercise of self-determination by the patient may mean the spurning of lifesaving assistance. As expressed by one court:

> Anglo-American law starts with the premise of thorough-going self-determination. It follows that each man is considered to be master of his own body, and he may, if he be of sound mind, expressly prohibit the performance of lifesaving surgery, or other medical treatment. A doctor might well believe that an operation or form of treatment is desirable or necessary, but the law does not permit him to substitute his own judgment for that of the patient by any form of artifice or deception.[7]

There is an exception to the informed consent requirement in "emergency" situations, grounded not on the imminence of death, but on the patient's incapacity and the presumption that the patient would, if physically able, authorize medical treatment. The emergency exception does not, therefore, affect the case of a competent adult or that of an adult whose convictions are asserted by a valid representative.

It is not suggested that the doctrine of informed consent precludes judicial intervention to compel lifesaving treatment. The doctrine is a judicial construct which can either be narrowly interpreted to bar only non-judicially authorized treatment or can be modified. Moreover, the threat of civil liability for lifesaving treatment cannot be a very effective deterrent for physicians since the value of the benefit conferred—preservation of life—must be set off against any damages from the technical trespass. But the doctrine of informed consent does demonstrate profound legal concern for bodily integrity and individual self-determination. These latter interests are directly at stake in resolving the issue of compelled lifesaving treatment.

The Constitution also bears directly upon resolution of the issue. Many, if not most, of the reported cases involve religiously motivated rejection of treatment, usually a Jehovah's Witness's refusal of a blood transfusion. In

[7] Natanson v. Kline, 186 Kan. 393, 406–07, 350 P.2d 1093, 1104 (1960).

such instances, the free exercise clause of the First Amendment (as applied to the states through the Fourteenth Amendment) is inevitably raised as the guarantor of individual choice. Since religious liberty is not absolute, the issue is how to appraise compelled treatment in light of the First Amendment. The applicable constitutional standard has been articulated as requiring a finding of "grave abuses" endangering "paramount state interests" to justify infringement of religious liberty.[8] The search for a paramount state interest is, therefore, an integral part of any free exercise case. The basic approach, however, requires balancing the state interests involved against the constitutional liberties at stake, keeping in mind that society, as well as the individual, benefits from the maintenance of basic liberties.

Last term, in *Wisconsin v. Yoder*, the Supreme Court made eminently clear that balancing is the appropriate approach in a free exercise case.[9] The Court addressed a Wisconsin statute requiring school attendance until age 16. The law was alleged to infringe upon free exercise of the Amish religion, which demanded devotion to nature and the soil and avoidance of worldly influence. The Amish contended that continued exposure to secular education beyond age 14 would undermine their youngsters' beliefs and eventually destroy the religion. In a six-to-one decision the Court upheld the Amish claim, finding that the threats to the Amish religion posed by the compulsory attendance law outweighed state interests in promoting an effective political system (educated electorate) and a self-reliant population. Chief Justice Burger's majority opinion clearly articulated a balancing test.

Yoder also demonstrates that use of a balancing test entails much more than the abstract weighing of "state interests" and "individual freedom." Assessment of the extent of harm threatened by enforcement or nonenforcement of the disputed statute or policy is required. For example, the *Yoder* opinion considered the magnitude of harm posed to the Amish religion by two additional years of education and the societal benefits derived from the two years. The Court could not perceive significant benefits to the quality of citizenship or to the self-reliance of the population stemming from two more years of education. In short, the Court looked to the actual impact of the law upon both the state interests and religious freedoms invoked.

This intricate balancing technique has important implications for the issue of court-ordered medical treatment. It suggests that abstract weighing

[8] Sherbert v. Verner, 374 U.S. 398, 406 (1963).   [9] 406 U.S. 205 (1972).

of bodily integrity against the preservation of life is too simplistic. The underlying state interests must be determined and the harm to those interests from allowing patients to die must be assessed. For example, if the social harm lies in a diminished populace, the number of people likely to reject lifesaving medical treatment must be appraised. Similarly, the degree of interference with religious or philosophical tenets must be gauged. This type of analysis will be applied in succeeding pages.

Of course, the free exercise clause does not provide the only constitutional bulwark for bodily integrity. The emerging concept of privacy undoubtedly gives constitutional dimension to the individual's asserted right to control his body. A "right to be let alone" (Griswold 1960) has long been discussed in the context of the Fourth Amendment. In *Schmerber* v. *California*, concerning a police-ordered blood test to procure proof of drunken driving, the Supreme Court applied Fourth-Amendment limitations to a bodily invasion to obtain evidence of crime.[10] While upholding the governmental intrusion in the context of that case, the Court acknowledged that "the integrity of an individual's person is a cherished value in our society," and that the human dignity and privacy at stake are "fundamental human interests." Moreover, it is clear that personal privacy is protected by constitutional provisions other than the Fourth Amendment. *Griswold* v. *Connecticut* indicated that the constitutional source of personal privacy lies in the First, Fourth, Fifth, Ninth, and Fourteenth Amendments.[11] While *Griswold* only dealt with marital privacy, there can be little doubt that the right to personal privacy extends well beyond a married couple's use of contraceptives. Last term, in *Eisenstadt* v. *Baird*, a case involving the regulation of contraceptive dissemination, four Justices observed: "If the right of privacy means anything, it is the right of the *individual*, married or single, to be free from unwarranted governmental intrusion into matters so fundamentally affecting a person as the decision whether to bear or beget a child."[12]

Nor can the concept of personal privacy be limited to matters of sexual privacy. In the context of challenges to abortion laws, several federal courts have spoken broadly of a woman's right to control her own body. Indeed, this broad approach is necessary, for if only the decision of whether to beget children is constitutionally protected, it could be argued in abortion cases that the availability of contraceptives satisfies that interest. *Stanley* v.

[10] 384 U.S. 757 (1966).   [11] 381 U.S. 479 (1965).   [12] 405 U.S. 438 (1972).

Georgia also reinforces the notion that personal privacy extends well beyond matters of procreation.[13] In ruling that a person could not be punished for private possession of obscene material, the Court acknowledged the "fundamental . . . right to be free, except in very limited circumstances, from unwarranted governmental intrusions into one's privacy." These cases, taken together, indicate that basic physical privacy is entitled to constitutional protection from governmental invasion.

It would not be accurate to talk about an undifferentiated "right to privacy." There are many different facets of personal privacy including personal appearance, sexual conduct, confidentiality of personal information, a physical zone of privacy, privacy of belief and thought, and freedom from bodily intrusion. Not all of these interests may be regarded as fundamental. Moreover, different constitutional provisions may protect different aspects of privacy. For example, governmental intrusions to obtain evidence of crime are governed by the Fourth Amendment, while personal belief is guarded by the First Amendment and nonevidentiary bodily invasions are protected by a penumbral right of personal privacy. The point remains, however, that no more basic aspect of personal privacy can be found than bodily integrity, and this interest is entitled to concomitant constitutional protection.

In many instances, including refusal of medical treatment, a matter relating to bodily control also entails significant ramifications for a person's future life-style or condition. Refusal of treatment determines not just whether a bodily invasion will take place, but whether the patient will live. Abortion determines not just whether an operation takes place or a birth proceeds, but whether the mother will have an offspring to nurture, support, and raise. Because of such long-range implications, I have referred to the refusal of lifesaving treatment as involving a right to self-determination, meaning liberty to choose a life-style or course of conduct. This interest has a constitutional dimension and is covered by the Fourteenth-Amendment guarantee of liberty, that is, substantive due process. However, bodily control or integrity involves not just liberty to act, but preservation of a domain of personal privacy. Protection of the immediate person and surroundings of an individual is explicitly provided in the First, Fourth, and Fifth amendments, and by a broader right of privacy deriving from these explicit provisions. My thesis is that this broader right of privacy will be viewed as a fundamental

[13] 394 U.S. 557 (1969).

aspect of personal liberty, a prerequisite or predicate to the exercise of all other liberties. A strict scrutiny approach, including a search for a compelling state interest, should, therefore, be employed where governmental invasions of bodily privacy occur. Although refusal of treatment involves both self-determination (liberty) and bodily control, it must be judged according to the stricter protections surrounding personal privacy.

This constitutional protection has import for consideration of compelled treatment. The person who declines medical assistance for philosophical or personal reasons, as opposed to religious commands, can also invoke the Constitution. Of course, bodily control is no more an absolute prerogative than religious freedom, but the constitutional standard used to test the validity of judicially compelled treatment will remain substantially the same whether the patient relies upon the free exercise clause or penumbral guarantees of privacy. That is, to justify an invasion of bodily integrity the state will have to demonstrate that a compelling state interest exists, and that it outweighs countervailing interests in individual rights. As previously noted, this entails careful assessment of the asserted state interests and the extent of harm posed to them by upholding the individual's privacy and self-determination. With this standard in mind, consideration of the specific interests at stake in the issue of lifesaving treatment can be undertaken.

III. Analysis of Interests

A variety of public interests have been arrayed both by courts and commentators in support of judicial intervention to order lifesaving medical treatment for a reluctant patient. These interests run the gamut from a noble reference to the sanctity of life to a banal concern for the economic burden left by a patient who dies after refusing treatment. Most of these interests have been described briefly in the prior discussion of case law on point. A few have not. All deserve careful scrutiny.

Preservation of Society

One writer (Hegland 1965) has argued that the "importance of the individual's life to the welfare of society" precludes allowing a patient to spurn lifesaving treatment. This is an appealing notion, but it cannot withstand critical examination. Certainly, a society and its duly constituted institutions have a strong and legitimate interest in their own preservation. Any significant diminution in population might be a matter of real concern, but no one has ever suggested that the volume of persons declining medical treatment constitutes a threat to the maintenance of population levels. Nor is the refusal of treatment an act likely to be widely imitated or duplicated if openly allowed; it is unlike narcotics addiction in that respect. In short, society's existence is by no means threatened by patients' refusals of treatment.

The state also has a legitimate interest in promoting a thriving and productive population. Compulsory education laws are one manifestation of such an interest, yielding both economic and political benefits to society as a whole. In this context, the state might assert an interest in the productivity of an individual—talents, skills, taxpaying potential, military service potential—justifying compelled treatment to keep the individual alive. It is submitted, however, that this concern with productivity cannot override the competing interests in bodily integrity or religious liberty. In the first place, the marginal social utility involved is generally outweighed by the direct and immediate invasion of the patient's personal privacy both because of the small numbers involved and the attenuated impact on the economy. Secondly, in each instance of refusal, the societal interest would vary according to the individual patient's attributes. In terms of productivity, for example, an industrialist or nuclear physicist has more "social worth" than a vagrant. The problem here is obvious. It is both unseemly and unrealistic to measure the social worth of each patient who declines medical treatment. One solution would be to assume the high value of every patient. But this approach exalts the interest of government, the state, or society over individual self-determination. It is also a fictive approach since in reality the vast majority of us do not contribute so much to the social fabric as to enable the state to claim a paramount interest in our preservation.

Sanctity of Life

The state has an indisputable interest in the preservation of life. The criminal law and police power are focused on the protection of public safety. But this use of governmental authority is grounded on the assumption that citizens invariably want to enjoy bodily safety and uninterrupted life. Where a competent individual chooses to decline lifesaving treatment, the normal congruity of interest between individual welfare and state protection against death is disrupted. Entirely new interests, self-determination and privacy from state intrusions, are asserted. The assumption that the citizen demands self-preservation can no longer be operative.

Some writers have nonetheless argued that preservation of a resisting patient's life is relevant to the lives and safety of the general public. The theory is that by denying the patient an opportunity to choose death, a court promotes general respect for life. If a court acquiesced in a patient's rejection of treatment and consequent death, the value of life would be degraded since "any exception to the sanctity of life cannot but cheapen it" (Hegland).

This argument cannot be taken lightly. Sanctity of life is not just a vague theological precept. It is the foundation of a free society. Indeed, libertarians recently campaigned against capital punishment on a similar theory that destruction of life (even the life of a convicted malefactor) degrades the value of life and undermines a society's regard for its sanctity. The countervailing consideration, of course, is the dignity tied up with bodily control and self-determination: "Control by men over their circumstances of action is, along with knowledge of their circumstances, an indispensable part of their personal integrity. Knowledge and control are what make the difference between puppets and people" (Fletcher 1954).

It is true that noninterference in an individual's decision to refuse treatment may mean that the patient dies for a reason which may appear silly or inconsequential to most observers. But the rejection of lifesaving medical treatment normally represents a principled invocation of personal or religious convictions, not a deprecation of life. Restraint by courts would be impelled by profound respect for the individual's bodily integrity and religious freedom, not by disregard or disdain for the sanctity of life. Human dignity is enhanced by permitting the individual to determine for himself what beliefs are worth dying for. Through the ages, a multitude of noble causes, religious and secular, have been regarded as worthy of self-sacrifice. Certainly, most governments and societies, our own included, do not consider the sanctity of life to be the supreme value. Nations still insist on the prerogative to engage in mass killing for furtherance of the "national interest," "wars of liberation," or the "defense of democracy." Bodily control, self-determination, and religious freedom are beneficial both to the individual and to the society whose atmosphere and tone are determined by the human values which it respects.

Public Morals

As the debate over so-called victimless crimes (e.g., homosexuality, prostitution, drug abuse) illustrates, the use of law to reinforce a dominant morality without tangible benefit to public health, safety, and welfare is fraught with difficulties. This is particularly true where the moral underpinnings of laws no longer enjoy a wide community consensus. Many laws aimed primarily at morality nonetheless have been enacted and we must acknowledge that all law is infused with some moral view.

These factors are relevant here because the rejection of lifesaving treatment is a form of suicide—in that it is a voluntary act undertaken with knowledge that death will likely result. Suicide, in turn, has traditionally been anathema in a Judeo-Christian culture. In the religious sphere, the revulsion toward suicide is grounded primarily on the Sixth Commandment and the belief that only a divinity can control the withdrawal of life (St. John-Stevas 1964). Antipathy toward suicide, however, extends well beyond the theological realm and public attitudes have sometimes mirrored religious ones. The English common law attached both criminal and civil penalties to suicide or attempted suicide (Williams 1957). Suicide was viewed as an offense against nature, violating instincts of self-preservation, as well as an offense against God, the society, and the King. The common revulsion of Western culture toward self-imposed death has, then, an ethical or moral base as well as a religious one. Self-destruction is considered to be contrary to man's natural inclinations, a deprivation of a person's productive capacity, an evil example to others, and even a rude expression of contempt for society. "Public morals," specifically the "immorality" of self-destruction, cannot provide a legitimate basis for intervention in the patient's decision, however. Contemporary condemnation of suicide as "immoral" is largely clerical in nature and public attitudes toward suicide have markedly changed. While embarrassment about the subject persists, the individual is no longer generally regarded as a sinner or crazed demon. Changes in law have accompanied changes in public opinion. In the vast majority of states, attempted suicide is no longer covered by the criminal law. To the extent that antisuicide laws remain on the books, they are directed toward authorizing officials to take temporary custody of the individual to prevent the immediate infliction of harm and to render psychological assistance (Curran and Shapiro 1970). Suicide is no longer considered, either legally or popularly, as inherently immoral. A morality grounded on an individual's service to the state would be threatened by a patient's conduct in refusing treatment. However, that moral scheme is not widely accepted within a democratic society which stresses maximum individual liberty compatible with the comfort and welfare of others.

Protection of the Individual against Himself

Normally, the state's police power is exercised for the general public's health, safety, or welfare. This is so even in the case of certain ostensibly individual invasions, such as compulsory immunizations or blood tests. There are a few areas of law, however, where the state apparently undertakes to protect the individual against his own imprudence.

The "snake cases," involving statutory prohibition of the public handling of snakes, provided one commonly cited example of government paternalism. A number of courts have sustained the validity of such statutes against claims by fundamentalist religious sects that the prohibitions interfere with their expression of religious faith. These cases do not, however, stand for the proposition that government can readily interfere with an individual's course of conduct in order to prevent the individual from harming himself. For these statutes undoubtedly protect observers and peripheral participants, as well as the snake handlers themselves. No court has addressed the issue of whether a legislature could protect the handler alone.

The motorcycle helmet cases are more apposite. Scores of state cases have considered challenges to statutes requiring motorcyclists to wear protective helmets. Motorcyclists claim that their individual liberty and privacy are infringed without a corresponding protection of legitimate public interests. The majority of courts have avoided the basic issue of whether state concern for the welfare of the cyclist can justify such requirements; they have made strained findings that all highway travelers are protected because cyclists struck by stones or limbs might lose control of their vehicles and injure others. Thus, the public health, safety, and welfare is being promoted. A number of courts have proceeded beyond this fictive argument to address whether the state may protect an individual from himself. The results are inconclusive. Several cases have urged that the police power encompasses authority to protect individuals despite their reluctance to be safeguarded. A few cases have ruled that the helmet statutes constitute unconstitutional infringements of liberty, since they have only a tenuous relation to public safety or welfare. It is submitted that without a clearer judicial consensus, and without Supreme Court guidance, the motorcycle helmet cases provide no resolution of whether the state can generally protect individuals against themselves. Certainly, they do not determine the outcome where a patient resists compelled treatment and invokes religious freedom or a right to bodily integrity as his protection. Indeed, constitutional standards may differ where liberty (substantive due process) is invoked as opposed to religious freedom or bodily privacy.

There is, however, an area of paternalistic state conduct which has universally been upheld despite its ostensible interference with individual freedom of choice. A plethora of pure food and drug laws, licensure schemes, and regulations controlling noxious substances exists which incidentally prevents consumers from injuring themselves. Even where the restrictions apply to sellers or distributors, the objective is to prevent the buyer from subjecting himself to risks which the government deems unadvisable. Some observers have articulated concern about the legal implications of this interference with individual self-determination, but these protective health measures nonetheless proliferate. They are generally salutary and seldom challenged. Yet they may occasionally prevent consumer access to an enjoyable food (for example, swordfish, cyclamate-containing beverages) or to an experimental drug which might be highly beneficial. The individual is effectively precluded from selecting his own risks. Because such protective laws remain judicially inviolate, the question arises whether they provide an effective precedent for governmental prevention of individual risk taking which might be extended to the lifesaving medical treatment problem.

Most protective legislation is clearly warranted because it guards against abuses which individual consumers are generally helpless to detect or control. For example, most consumers cannot determine the minimum competency of a physician, the iodine content of a food, or the spoilage of meat without regulatory controls. Furthermore, consumers alone may be impotent to eliminate the dangerous products of an entire industry (for example, flammable fabrics or unsafe cars). The regulated items also have such wide potential distribution that the public safety and welfare is actually promoted by the protective legislation. These observations about regulatory schemes, however, in no way apply to refusal of medical treatment, since judicial intervention to compel treatment is a very different matter than common regulatory controls. Although both forms of governmental action interfere with individual choice, the regulatory schemes are generally impelled by conditions which preclude real individual choice. The elimination of dangerous products also constitutes, in most instances, a lesser deprivation than interference with religious liberty or bodily integrity. Thus, while precedents may be cited for governmental efforts to preclude individual risk taking, none sanctions judicial intervention to protect a patient against his own decision to decline treatment. Clearly, there are limitations on attempts to guarantee the individual's safety, for otherwise an individual's personal habits, including eating and sleeping, would be potentially subject to governmental dictates. The rights to freedom of religion and personal privacy circumscribe paternalistic impulses in the context of compelled medical treatment.

Protection of Third Parties

The patient's important interests in religious freedom or bodily integrity could be overridden if refusal of medical treatment were shown to inflict legally cognizable harm on persons other than the patient. Various third party injuries have been suggested by courts and commentators discussing compelled treatment. They all warrant consideration.

Surviving Adults. The death of a relative or close friend may provoke grief, despair, or other emotional harm in the surviving person. This phenomenon will undoubtedly be present in cases of compelled treatment, and may be urged as a ground for judicial intervention. It is submitted, however, that this factor cannot justify a court in overriding a patient's determination. A variety of conduct by an individual may inflict emotional harm upon his loved ones. The dissolution of a marriage by separation or divorce, or simply abusive conduct toward loved ones can cause emotional wounds, yet no court would contemplate a judicial order to force an adult to be considerate or kind to adult relatives. A similar independence of conduct must be accorded to the patient who may be asserting religious or personal principles in his refusal of treatment. The emotional consequences to survivors will likely be temporary, should be tempered by respect for the patient's principled decision, and, in any event, do not outweigh the patient's interests at stake.

Fellow Patients. One source (Hegland) has argued that a patient's rejection of lifesaving treatment will distract physicians, provoke turmoil in the hospital staff, and generally disrupt hospital procedure to the detriment of other patients. This argument is speculative and seems rather farfetched. If the patient's choice is honored, precisely the converse of the predicted result should follow. That is, by declining treatment, medical care may well be reduced to the administration of analgesics, freeing staff to attend to other functions. Once a policy of judicial nonintervention is established and publicized, the hospital staff will not expend futile effort in seeking court orders. Although there may be occasions when the rejection of therapy engenders medical complications which necessitate diverting staff to the patient, this situation is more likely to be the exception than the rule and cannot operate as a general justification for judicial interference with patients' decisions.

Physicians. Several courts have noted the interests of physicians in compelling lifesaving treatment. One concern is that the physician, if required to respect the patient's choice to decline treatment, must act against his best professional judgment. It is difficult for a physician, trained and dedicated to preservation of life, to allow a salvageable patient to die. In addition, by withholding therapy, the physician may theoretically risk subsequent civil or criminal liability, particularly if the physician were found to have honored an incompetent patient's choice.

While a physician's interest in proper practice of medicine is both valid and legally cognizable, the above concerns do not justify judicial intervention to compel lifesaving treatment. Unfettered exercise of medical judgment has never been a sacrosanct value. The doctrine of informed consent is grounded on the premise that a physician's judgment is subservient to the patient's right to self-determination. Further, other situations exist where a physician's professional judgment is legally restricted or precluded. Laws governing contraception, narcotics, experimental drugs, and compulsory reporting (e.g., of child abuse and venereal disease) demonstrate that professional judgment is not always a paramount consideration. The assertion of constitutional interests in bodily integrity and free exercise of religion in the context of refusal of care deserve no less deference, even in derogation of a physician's best judgment. While it may be harrowing for a physician to determine whether a patient is voluntarily and competently declining lifesaving treatment, difficult medical decisions must inevitably be made. This is so, for example, whenever a patient is certified as mentally ill for purposes of civil commitment or when a patient ostensibly consents to medical operations which entail substantial risks.

Surviving Minors. As previously noted, both courts and commentators have supported judicial intervention to compel medical treatment where the patient is the parent of a minor child, based on an extension of the parens patriae doctrine. Since the state can generally act to safeguard a child's welfare, it can act to prevent "ultimate abandonment" of a child by the parent's self-destruction. By keeping the parent alive, the child presumably benefits emotionally, by continued love and reassurance from the parent, and economically, by continued financial support.

The argument that a court should act to preserve the emotional well-being of children is an appealing one. The legitimacy of the state's interest can be sustained on either of two grounds: there may be altruistic concern with providing each child with a healthful environment, or, development of stable children may be viewed as promoting the political and social well-being of the country. Of course, the loss of a parent will not always produce emotional harm in a child. Not all parents are loving and supportive of their children. It is conceivable that in some instances the surviving child would benefit emotionally from a court's acquiescence in the parent's decision to decline lifesaving treatment. But judicial inquiry, on a case-by-case basis, into the complex emotional relationships among parents and children might well be too time-consuming and unpleasant to be undertaken. Assuming that the death of a parent will likely provoke some emotional harm to a surviving child, the question becomes whether that harm justifies exercise of the state's parens patriae authority to compel a patient to undergo unwanted treatment.

There are numerous situations where a child may be left alone by a parent with consequent emotional upheaval in the child. Death of a parent from natural causes, service in the armed forces, divorce, or even extended travel might cause some emotional wounds. Yet these unintended inflictions of emotional harm are never the source of state intervention; to suggest such intervention would undoubtedly provoke indignant cries of interference with personal liberty. Indeed, an infinite variety of parental conduct could be regulated if prevention of the infliction of emotional harm upon children were accepted as an unlimited basis for interference with parental conduct not intended to harm the child. The state could, under such a theory, compel medical checkups or dictate diets in order to preserve the health of parents.

Some interference with parental conduct is not only justified, but necessary, as the existence of "neglect" statutes demonstrates. Nevertheless, the loss of one of two parents because of the parent's adherence to religious or personal convictions in declining treatment is, arguably, too remote from the state's interest in a child's emotional well-being to support judicial intervention. Perhaps a legislature could make a contrary judgment and dictate intervention, but a court operating without such authorization must hesitate to intervene on the basis of protecting children's psychic well-being.

A second, less speculative basis exists for judicial intervention to preserve parents' lives—the economic interest of the state in avoiding the burden of supporting surviving children. In many contexts, protection of the public fisc has served as a justification for state conduct or regulations which otherwise would be considered to infringe upon fundamental personal rights. This has been the case with compulsory sterilization laws, motorcycle helmet laws, and certain welfare regulations having an indirect impact on parents' behavior. In *Wisconsin* v. *Yoder*, the Supreme Court treated avoidance of "public wards" as a legitimate state interest to be balanced against competing individual rights. It must be conceded, then, that some judicial concern with the financial plight of a patient's survivors is both understandable and proper.

The economic issue is placed in even sharper perspective if the refusal of medical treatment threatens permanent disability but not death; for example, where rejection of a blood transfusion results in insufficient oxygen to the brain and consequent neurological damage. The ensuing permanent disability could result in the patient, as well as the surviving family, becoming public economic burdens. In such an instance, the economic impact would be direct and probably substantial. Judicial intervention to avoid that impact would likely be sustained even in the face of constitutional challenges bottomed on privacy and religious freedom. Similar considerations would probably support judicial intervention where the patient by declining treatment would die and leave an impecunious family to be sustained by the public.

Despite this concession, an important caveat should be considered before a court intervenes to compel treatment on an "avoidance of public wards" theory. The economic factors justifying intervention are not present in every case of a parent's refusal of treatment. The surviving spouse, accumulated savings, or other sources may be available to avoid penury even if the patient dies. Thus, the problem would have to be approached on a case-by-case basis and the economic circumstances sifted in each instance. This type of judicial inquiry is neither difficult nor unseemly; courts commonly examine financial status with regard to support payments, bankruptcy, and enforcement of judgments, to cite a few examples. However, tying the question of judicial intervention to financial circumstances of the patient may prove distasteful to the judiciary. The effect is to tell the patient that his convictions will not be respected because he does not have enough money. It is at least arguable that this de facto wealth discrimination would violate the equal protection clause. In any event, it appears rather mercenary to hinge exercise of rights of privacy and free exercise upon wealth. Perhaps the public should be expected to absorb the economic burden when the refusal of medical treatment leaves indigent survivors. Courts might well take this approach. In light of the relatively small number of people who can be expected to spurn medical treatment when they know their family will be left impecunious, the overall economic burden shifted to the public can be expected to be slight. Judges who rely on the public ward theory to compel lifesaving medical treatment will likely be impelled not by real concern for the public coffers, but by their personal distaste for the patient's decision.

IV. Implications for Other Areas of Law

Suicide

I have argued that a patient should normally have the prerogative of declining lifesaving medical treatment, both because of the constitutional principles involved and the lack of a sufficiently strong basis for judicial intervention. This raises important questions with regard to the legal status of suicide. Does a right to decline treatment imply a broader right to die? Or can judicial acquiescence in refusal of treatment be reconciled with traditional efforts of the legal system to prevent suicide? What of the patient whose rejection of treatment is tantamount to suicide because the patient wishes to die?

Several sources (e.g., Hegland) have contended that there is a close analogy between refusal of treatment and suicide, even where the refusal is not accompanied by a wish to die. They argue that if an individual has a right to dictate his own death, the form—nonfeasance in refusal of treatment as opposed to misfeasance in suicide—should not matter. They point to the apparent legitimacy of governmental efforts to preclude suicide, and assert that the same interests which justify such efforts also justify intervention to preclude refusal of treatment. According to this view, it would be anomalous to permit refusal of treatment but to prevent suicide since the person who wishes to die is then obstructed but the person who wishes to live is permitted to die.

The meaning of "suicide," as contained in criminal statutes, may well exclude the case of a principled decision to refuse lifesaving medical treatment because such criminal enactments probably require a finding of specific intent to die, a factor lacking in the religiously or philosophically motivated rejection of treatment. Although an actor is ordinarily presumed to intend the natural consequences of his act, this presumption would probably not be applied in this context; to do so would label the person who jumps in front of a car to save another a suicide. Similarly, refusal of treatment should not be considered to fall within the term "suicide" as contained in the criminal law. It is also true that attempted suicide has been eliminated from criminal codes in the vast majority of states. Legislatures have recognized that deterrence is not accomplished by criminal sanctions of attempted suicide, and that intervention to secure treatment or assistance for the victim can be accomplished without need of the criminal law. Yet, neither of these factors—narrowness of the technical definition of suicide or elimination of attempted suicide from the criminal law—negates the arguments of those who assert that the same interests supporting governmental intervention to block suicide also support judicial intervention to compel medical treatment. The issues of whether refusal of treatment is legally tantamount to suicide, or whether attempted suicide is a criminal offense, are therefore not determinative of whether a state can validly compel a reluctant patient to undergo treatment. If government efforts to prevent suicide are valid, and if the same interests supporting such efforts are applicable to the refusal of treatment, then the proponents of compelled treatment would appear to have a strong case. Their first premise, that efforts to prevent suicide by direct state intervention are valid, seems correct. One case raising a constitutional challenge to an attempted-suicide statute was dismissed for want of a substantial federal question.[14] The question remains, however, whether the interests involved in suicide and refusal of treatment are sufficiently distinct to justify divergent legal treatment of the two phenomena.

The principal objective of governmental intervention in the area of suicide is to secure assistance for the individual. Such assistance is appropriate

[14] Penney v. Municipal Ct., 312 F. Supp. 938 (D.N.J. 1970).

because many suicide attempts are the product of rash, unbalanced, or confused judgments. Admittedly, there is no simple explanation for the phenomenon of suicide. "A profound ambiguity of motives" (Alvarez 1970) characterizes both suicide in general and the actions of any particular individual. For this reason, it is impossible to accurately categorize or quantify types of suicide. However, there seems to be a consensus that many suicide attempts are the products of mental disorder. Some attempts are also acknowledged to be either conscious or subconscious cries for help, rather than determined efforts to die (Farberow and Shneidman 1961). No criticism can be directed toward governmental efforts to reach and assist persons who do not wish to die or whose action is the product of a temporary derangement. While it is true that the laws of practices aimed at preventing suicide do not differentiate according to the individual victim's motives, it is equally true that those factors cannot readily be determined without some initial intervention. "The natural and human thing to do with a person who is suddenly discovered attempting suicide is to interpose to prevent it" (Williams 1957). Moreover, if the individual has made a deliberate choice to die, the state's intervention constitutes more a temporary postponement than a permanent proscription. A determined individual can likely find alternative times, places, and means to consummate his intended act. In the interim, intervention will only have ensured that the self-destruction is the product of a fixed and unalterable desire.

Other elements differentiate the problem of suicide from refusal of medical treatment. The sheer magnitude of the suicide phenomenon makes it a cause of societal alarm. Over 20,000 people per year successfully commit suicide in the United States. This accounts for 1 percent of annual deaths and places suicide among the 12 leading causes of death. Even these figures do not expose the true magnitude of the problem; suicide is grossly underreported and many attempts at suicide are unsuccessful. In addition, there is some evidence that suicide produces an imitative effect, sometimes causing "epidemics" of self-destruction. Even without this last speculative factor, the magnitude of the suicide phenomenon warrants serious governmental concern.

In sum, both the magnitude of the problem and certain attributes of the suicide phenomenon provide a solid basis for government intervention to prevent suicide. These factors are not, for the most part, present in refusal of lifesaving medical treatment. The volume of such refusals must be miniscule in comparison to attempted suicide. Most instances of refusal represent careful decisions to abide by religious or philosophical principles, and not rash attempts at self-destruction. There is normally an opportunity to test the sincerity, firmness, and rationality of a patient's decision to decline treatment without mooting the issue by medical intervention. By insisting on his position, the patient directly invokes important constitutional principles of either religious freedom or personal privacy. Thus, there is ample basis for espousing governmental intervention in suicide cases while eschewing similar intervention to compel lifesaving medical treatment.

This leaves the problem of the patient who rejects medical treatment with the intent and wish to die, the patient who really is committing suicide by refusing treatment. This may be a small percentage of refusals of treatment; virtually every case which has come to my attention has involved a religiously motivated decision. But the suicidal refusal, particularly when the patient is suffering from serious illness and is threatened with loss of faculties, is not entirely implausible. At the outset of this article I hypothesized several situations where the patient refusing treatment might be seeking death—the despondent patient who has lost the will to live, the terminally ill patient who wishes to avoid a painful deterioration and loss of dignity, and the protesting patient who hopes to become a political martyr. Even though these patients might not be making "principled" decisions in the sense of open reliance upon religious or philosophical scruples, serious considerations of bodily integrity and self-determination are still involved.

The important state interest in preventing rash or unbalanced self-destruction must be honored in this situation. Medical inquiry (or judicial inquiry if a court has been petitioned for intervention) into the patient's state of mind is appropriate. The patient must be competent and his decision to reject treatment must be deliberate and firm. Otherwise, temporary intervention to provide psychological assistance (and medical treatment if the patient would die in the interim) is warranted, even if the patient's suicide wish is temporarily frustrated. If there is a genuine emergency, with no opportunity to assess the patient's state of mind, medical intervention should proceed. If the patient demonstrates the requisite state of mind, however, and persists in refusal of treatment, that decision should be respected though tantamount to suicide. The distinction between principled and unprincipled action is not strong enough to warrant a different approach toward the suicide patient than that taken toward the religiously motivated patient when both in reality are asserting rights to bodily integrity, personal privacy, and self-determination. This position, that the patient wishing to die should be permitted to decline treatment, has distinct implications for legal approaches to suicide generally. In effect, it means that the "serious suicide," the person whose decision to die is clearly competent, deliberate, and firm, should be permitted to die. The form of self-destruction, refusal of treatment versus slashing of wrists or whatever, should not matter.

Euthanasia

Euthanasia, or mercy killing, is generally defined as the deliberate killing by a physician or other party of a person suffering from a painful and terminal illness. Although an affirmative act by the physician (e.g., an injection) is normally thought to be a component of euthanasia, the withholding of medical treatment or therapy may be considered to be a form of euthanasia. I have argued that withholding of medical treatment at the request of a competent adult patient is not only legally defensible, but that a court cannot constitutionally intervene to authorize treatment. This raises several issues. Does my position conflict with established legal postures toward euthanasia? Does my position mean that euthanasia in the form of affirmative killing must also be countenanced?

It is well established in criminal law that an affirmative act of euthanasia constitutes homicide (Curran and Shapiro 1970). A person is not legally permitted to consent to the infliction of death upon himself by another. While judges and juries appear to show extreme solicitude toward persons accused of euthanasia, the act is clearly illegal under contemporary doctrine. The legal status of the physician who merely withholds treatment at the request of the patient is in great dispute. Most commentators merely state that the legality of such an act of omission is uncertain. The precise issue is whether the special physician-patient relationship imposes upon the physician an automatic duty to take every step to preserve the patient's life. Glanville Williams (1956) asserts that a physician's inaction at the patient's behest is probably lawful. Yale Kamisar (1958) argues that the physician who withholds life-preserving treatment "commits criminal homicide by omission." All sources agree that no physician has ever been indicted or convicted for any such crime.

The legal relationship between the physician and the dying patient is murky. Physicians commonly administer analgesics which shorten a patient's life. No one apparently regards this as illegal. Even though death may be accelerated, the countervailing necessity to relieve suffering prevails. Also, a point is inevitably reached in the demise of a terminally ill patient when medical treatment no longer preserves life, but rather prolongs the act of dying. It seems inconceivable that the patient's competent exercise of a right to decline further treatment could be denied at that point. Some authorities meet this last situation by acknowledging that "extraordinary" medical techniques need not be employed to keep a patient alive. Presumably, this would permit disconnecting extraordinary equipment. Yet no one has defined the term "extraordinary" with precision; blood transfusions and intravenous feeding are probably considered "ordinary," while heart-lung machines and artificial respirators are not.

In light of this general confusion regarding the physician's responsibility toward the dying patient, I have little difficulty extending my basic position—that a physician must legally respect a patient's decision to reject treatment—to the terminally ill patient. The same considerations of bodily integrity and self-determination apply. They assume added importance where the patient faces a loss of faculties and dignity before inevitably succumbing. I stop short, however, of espousing euthanasia in the form of affirmative physicians' acts to kill a patient.

The arguments in favor of affirmative acts of euthanasia are appealing; indeed, they rely on some of the same values which support the patient's refusal of treatment. The basic contention is that voluntary euthanasia supports human dignity. The suffering patient in the throes of terminal illness is relieved of the indignity of a life endured without faculties or self-control. A host of objections have, however, been raised against legalization. Some of them are spurious, but others are substantial. For example, Professor Kamisar discusses at length the problem of assessing the "voluntariness" of a consent by a patient who, by definition, is a victim of terminal illness and is either experiencing considerable pain or is drugged. Several sources (e.g., St. John-Stevas) also contend that legal acceptance of an act of killing where a life is "not worth living" would undermine respect for life and lay a foundation for acceptance of involuntary euthanasia. Proponents of euthanasia have advanced a variety of protective procedural schemes to forestall some of these criticisms. Mandatory time intervals to allow a patient to contemplate or reconsider and intervention of neutral third parties or referees to confirm the diagnosis and verify the patient's consent have been proposed.

The most serious argument against voluntary euthanasia—that it would eventually lead to involuntary euthanasia—is not convincing. So long as careful attention is paid to the capacity of a person to request euthanasia, there is a large gap between voluntary euthanasia and involuntary elimination of societal misfits. One does not necessarily flow from the other. I am bothered, however, by authorizing an affirmative act which would destroy another human being. A patient's request to terminate further therapy should be honored, but affirmative acts (injections, etc.) to terminate patients' lives should not be condoned. If affirmative medical conduct to end the patient's life is prohibited, the patient is allowed maximum opportunity to change his mind and demand treatment. The patient declining treatment normally remains alive for a period and thereby receives some opportunity to articulate or demonstrate any change of mind or to eliminate any mistake on the physician's part in comprehending the patient's wishes. Authorization of affirmative acts of mercy killing would necessitate changes in state criminal law which might arguably constitute official recognition of the "worthlessness" of some life. A physician's deference to a patient's decision to refuse medical treatment is not currently criminal, and no statutory changes are needed to sustain refusals of treatment. The physician who respects the patient's choice, as required by the doctrine of informed consent, is not concurring in the dying patient's possible evaluation of his life as "worthless," as might be the case if the physician voluntarily administered fatal drugs.

The line between withholding treatment at the patient's request and active administration of death may be difficult to draw and may seem somewhat arbitrary. This is particularly so where the "affirmative acts" are the disconnection of life-sustaining equipment or placement of a poison capsule within reach of the patient. Both acts fall somewhere in the spectrum between passive withholding of treatment and active administration of a fatal injection. While a determination can eventually be made as to whether disconnection of life-sustaining equipment is an "affirmative act," that determination will probably be based on a subjective characterization of the physician's action. More importantly, it is not clear that active administration of death at the patient's request is morally very different from withholding treatment. Nonetheless, the considerations mentioned in the preceding paragraph lead me to the position that affirmative acts of euthanasia should continue to be proscribed while the patient's decision to decline lifesaving treatment must be respected. In any event, it is clear that acceptance of a right to decline treatment does not compel broad acceptance of euthanasia in all forms. . . .

V. Conclusion

As to an independent adult who genuinely objects to treatment, the patient's decision to refuse lifesaving treatment must be respected by the judiciary no matter what the reason for refusal. Respect for bodily integrity, as dictated by constitutional rights of personal privacy, mandates this result in light of the inadequacy or inapplicability of asserted governmental interests in compelling treatment. Even where familial circumstances would constitutionally permit judicial intervention, a judge should normally respect the patient's decision. Intervention to protect survivors' emotional or economic interests, with concomitant government avoidance of fiscal burdens, would too often reflect judicial distaste for a decision to accept death rather than recognition of compelling state interests sufficient to override a patient's decision.

Acceptance of a patient's right to decline lifesaving treatment will mean emotional strain for both physicians and judges. On occasion, it will even be difficult to determine whether the patient's decision is the product of a sound mind. Yet deference to the patient's refusal of treatment reflects sensitivity toward personal interests in bodily integrity and self-determination, not callousness toward life.

References

Alvarez, A. *The Savage God: A Study of Suicide.* New York: Random House, 1972.
Cawley, C. C. *The Right to Live.* South Brunswick, N.J.: A. S. Barnes, 1969.
Curran, William J., and E. Donald Shapiro. *Law, Medicine, and Forensic Science.* Boston: Little, Brown, 1970.
Farberow, Norman L., and Edwin Shneidman, eds. *The Cry for Help.* New York: McGraw-Hill, 1961.
Fletcher, Joseph. *Morals and Medicine.* Princeton, N.J.: Princeton University Press, 1954.
Griswold, Erwin N. "The Right to Be Let Alone." *Northwestern University Law Review* 55 (May-June 1960): 216–26.
Hegland, Kennedy F. "Unauthorized Rendition of Lifesaving Medicial Treatment." *California Law Review* 53 (August 1965): 860–77.

Kamisar, Yale. "Some Non-Religious Views against Proposed Mercy Killing Legislation." *Minnesota Law Review* 42 (May 1958): 969–1042

St. John-Stevas, Norman. *Life, Death, and the Law.* Cleveland: World Publishing Company, 1964.

Sharpe, David J., and Robert F. Hargest. "Lifesaving Treatment for Unwilling Patients." *Fordham Law Review* 36 (May 1968): 695–706.

Williams, Glanville. *The Sanctity of Life and the Criminal Law.* New York: Knopf, 1957.

18

In the Matter of KAREN QUINLAN, An Alleged Incompetent

SUPERIOR COURT OF NEW JERSEY
CHANCERY DIVISION MORRIS COUNTY

Opinion

THE case presented is:

Given the facts that Karen Quinlan is now an incompetent in a persistent vegetive state, that at the outset of her unconsciousness her parents placed her under the care and treatment of Dr. Morse, and through him Dr. Javed and St. Clare's Hospital, urging everything be done to keep her alive, that the doctors and hospital introduced life-sustaining techniques, does this Court have the power and right, under the mantle of either its equity jurisdiction, the constitutional rights of free exercise of religion, right of privacy or privilege against cruel and unusual punishment, to authorize the withdrawing of the life-sustaining techniques? . . .

The judicial conscience and morality involved in considering whether the Court should authorize Karen Quinlan's removal from the respirator are inextricably involved with the nature of medical science and the role of the physician in our society and his duty to his patient.

When a doctor takes a case, there is imposed upon him the duty "to exercise in the treatment of his patient the degree of care, knowledge, and skill ordinarily possessed and exercised in similar situations by the average member of the profession practicing in his field."[1] If he is a specialist he

---

[1] Schueler v. Strelinger, 43 N.J. 330, 344 (1964).

"must employ not merely the skill of a general practitioner,but also that special degree of skill normally possessed by the average physician who devotes special study and attention to the particular organ or disease or injury involved, having regard to the present state of scientific knowledge."[2] This is the duty that establishes his legal obligations to his patients.

There is a higher standard, a higher duty, that encompasses the uniqueness of human life, the integrity of the medical profession, and the attitude of society toward the physician and therefore the morals of society. A patient is placed, or places himself, in the care of a physician with the expectation that he (the physician) will do everything in his power, everything that is known to modern medicine, to protect the patient's life. He will do all within his human power to favor life against death.

The attitudes of society have over the years developed a significant respect for the medical profession. Society has come to request and expect this higher duty.

But the doctor is dealing in a science which lacks exactitude, a science that has seen significant changes in recent years, a science that will undoubtedly have prodigious advancements in the future but a science which still does not know the cause of some afflictions and which does not know all the interrelationships of the body functions. . . .

Doctors, therefore, to treat a patient, must deal with medical tradition and past case histories. They must be guided by what they do know. The extent of their training, their experience, consultations with other physicians, must guide their decision-making processes in providing care to their patient. The nature, extent, and duration of care by societal standards is the responsibility of a physician. The morality and conscience of our society places this responsibility in the hands of the physician. What justification is there to remove it from the control of the medical profession and place it in the hands of the courts? Aside from the constitutional arguments, plaintiff suggests because medical science holds no hope for her recovery, because if Karen was conscious she would elect to turn off the respirator, and finally because there is no duty to keep her alive.

None of the doctors testified there was *no* hope. The hope for recovery is remote but no doctor talks in the absolute. Certainly he cannot and be cred-

[2] Clark v. Wichman, 72 N.J. Super. 486, 493 (App. Div. 1962).

ible in light of the advancements medical science has known and the inexactitudes of medical science.

There *is* a duty to continue the life-assisting apparatus, if within the treating physician's opinion, it should be done. Here Dr. Morse has refused to concur in the removal of Karen from the respirator. It is his considered position that medical tradition does not justify that act. There is no mention in the doctor's refusal of concern over criminal liability and the Court concludes that such is not the basis for his determination. It is significant that Dr. Morse, a man who demonstrated strong empathy and compassion, a man who has directed care that impressed all the experts, is unwilling to direct Karen's removal from the respirator. . . .

The breadth of the power to act and protect Karen's interests is, I conclude, controlled by a judicial conscience and morality that dictate the determination whether or not Karen Ann Quinlan be removed from the respirator is to be left to the treating physician. It is a medical decision, not a judicial one. I am satisfied that it may be concurred in by the parents but not governed by them. This is so because there is always the dilemma of whether it is the conscious being's relief or the unconscious being's welfare that governs the parental motivation.

It is also noted the concept of the Court's power over a person suffering under a disability is to *protect* and aid the best interests. As pointed out, the *Hart* and *Strunk* cases deal with protection as it relates to the future life of the infants or incompetent. Here the authorization sought, if granted, would result in Karen's death. The natural processes of her body are not shown to be sufficiently strong to sustain her by themselves. The authorization, therefore, would be to permit Karen Quinlan to die. This is not protection. It is not something in her best interests, in a temporal sense, and it is in a temporal sense that I must operate whether I believe in life after death or not. The single most important temporal quality Karen Ann Quinlan has is life. This Court will not authorize that life to be taken from her. . . .

Robert Muir, Jr.
Judge of the Superior Court
November 10, 1975

In the Matter of KAREN QUINLAN, An Alleged Incompetent

SUPREME COURT OF NEW JERSEY

IT is the issue of the constitutional right of privacy that has given us most concern, in the exceptional circumstances of this case. Here a loving parent, *qua* parent and raising the rights of his incompetent and profoundly damaged daughter, probably irreversibly doomed to no more than a biologically vegetative remnant of life, is before the court. He seeks authorization to abandon specialized technological procedures which can only maintain for a time a body having no potential for resumption or continuance of other than a "vegetative" existence. . . .

The claimed interests of the State in this case are essentially the preservation and sanctity of human life and defense of the right of the physician to administer medical treatment according to his best judgment. In this case the doctors say that removing Karen from the respirator will conflict with their professional judgment. The plaintiff answers that Karen's present treatment serves only a maintenance function; that the respirator cannot cure or improve her condition but at best can only prolong her inevitable slow deterioration and death; and that the interests of the patient, as seen by her surrogate, the guardian, must be evaluated by the court as predominant, even in the face of an opinion *contra* by the present attending physicians. Plaintiff's distinction is significant. The nature of Karen's care and the realistic chances of her recovery are quite unlike those of the patients discussed in many of the cases where treatments were ordered. In many of those cases the medical procedure required (usually a transfusion) constituted a minimal bodily invasion and the chances of recovery and return to functioning life were very good. We think that the State's interest *contra* weakens and the individual's right to privacy grows as the degree of bodily invasion increases and the prognosis dims. Ultimately there comes a point at which the individual's rights overcome the State interest. It is for that reason that we believe Karen's choice, if she were competent to make it, would be vindicated by the law. Her prognosis is extremely poor,—she will never resume cognitive life. And the bodily invasion is very great,—she requires 24-hour intensive nursing care, antibiotics, the assistance of a respirator, a catheter and feeding tube.

Our affirmation of Karen's independent right of choice, however, would ordinarily be based upon her competency to assert it. The sad truth, however, is that she is grossly incompetent and we cannot discern her supposed choice based on the testimony of her previous conversations with friends, where such testimony is without sufficient probative weight.[1] Nevertheless we have concluded that Karen's right of privacy may be asserted on her behalf by her guardian under the peculiar circumstances here present. . . .

We glean from the record here that physicians distinguish between curing the ill and comforting and easing the dying; that they refuse to treat the curable as if they were dying or ought to die, and that they have sometimes refused to treat the hopeless and dying as if they were curable. In this sense, as we were reminded by the testimony of Drs. Korein and Diamond, many of them have refused to inflict an undesired prolongation of the process of dying on a patient in irreversible condition when it is clear that such "therapy" offers neither human or humane benefit. We think these attitudes represent a balanced implementation of a profoundly realistic perspective on the meaning of life and death and that they respect the whole Judeo-Christian tradition of regard for human life. No less would they seem consistent with the moral matrix of medicine, "to heal," very much in the sense of the endless mission of the law, "to do justice."

Yet this balance, we feel, is particularly difficult to perceive and apply in the context of the development by advanced technology of sophisticated and artificial life-sustaining devices. For those possibly curable, such devices are

[1] 137 N.J. Super. at 260.

of great value, and, as ordinary medical procedures, are essential. Consequently, as pointed out by Dr. Diamond, they are necessary because of the ethic of medical practice. But in light of the situation in the present case (while the record here is somewhat hazy in distinguishing between "ordinary" and "extraordinary" measures), one would have to think that the use of the same respirator or like support could be considered "ordinary" in the context of the possibly curable patient but "extraordinary" in the context of the forced sustaining by cardio-respiratory processes of an irreversibly doomed patient. And this dilemma is sharpened in the face of the malpractice and criminal action threat which we have mentioned. . . .

Having concluded that there is a right of privacy that might permit termination of treatment in the circumstances of this case, we turn to consider the relationship of the exercise of that right to the criminal law. We are aware that such termination of treatment would accelerate Karen's death. The County Prosecutor and the Attorney General stoutly maintain that there would be criminal liability for such acceleration. Under the statutes of this State, the unlawful killing of another human being is criminal homicide.[2] We conclude that there would be no criminal homicide in the circumstances of this case. We believe, first, that the ensuing death would not be homicide but rather expiration from existing natural causes. Secondly, even if it were to be regarded as homicide, it would not be unlawful.

These conclusions rest upon definitional and constitutional bases. The termination of treatment pursuant to the right of privacy is, within the limitations of this case, *ipso facto* lawful. Thus, a death resulting from such an act would not come within the scope of the homicide statutes proscribing only the unlawful killing of another. There is a real and in this case determinative distinction between the unlawful taking of the life of another and the ending of artificial life-support systems as a matter of self-determination. . . .

We thus arrive at the formulation of the declaratory relief which we have concluded is appropriate to this case. . . . Upon the concurrence of the guardian and family of Karen, should the responsible attending physicians conclude that there is no reasonable possibility of Karen's ever emerging from her present comatose condition to a cognitive, sapient state and that the life-support apparatus now being administered to Karen should be dis-

[2] N.J.S.A. 2A:113–1, 2, 5.

continued, they shall consult with the hospital "Ethics Committee" or like body of the institution in which Karen is then hospitalized. If that consultative body agrees that there is no reasonable possibility of Karen's ever emerging from her present comatose condition to a cognitive, sapient state, the present life-support system may be withdrawn and said action shall be without any civil or criminal liability therefor on the part of any participant, whether guardian, physician, hospital or others. We herewith specifically so hold. . . .

March 3, 1976

FOUR
Euthanasia

19

An Alternative to the Ethic
of Euthanasia

Arthur J. Dyck

CONTEMPORARY society and modern medicine face difficult policy decisions. This is illustrated most recently in the Voluntary Euthanasia Act of 1969, submitted for consideration in the British Parliament. The purpose of that act is to provide for "the adminstration of euthanasia to persons who request it and who are suffering from an irremediable condition" (Downing 1971) and to enable such persons to make such a request in advance. For the purposes of that act, euthanasia means "the painless inducement of death" to be administered by a physician (i.e., "a registered medical practitioner").

The declaration that one signs under this act, should one become incurably ill and wish to have euthanasia administered, reads as follows:

If I should at any time suffer from a serious physical illness or impairment reasonably thought in my case to be incurable and expected to cause me severe distress or render me incapable of rational existence, I request the administration of euthanasia at a time or in circumstances to be indicated or specified by me or, if it is apparent that I have become incapable of giving directions, at the discretion of the physician in charge of my case. In the event of my suffering from any of the conditions specified above, I

Reprinted from Robert H. Williams, ed., *To Live or To Die*, pp. 98–112, with the permission of Springer-Verlag, Inc. Copyright © 1973 by Springer-Verlag, Inc.

request that no active steps should be taken . . . to prolong my life or restore me to consciousness.
This declaration is to remain in force unless I revoke it, which I may do
at any time. . . . I wish it to be understood that I have confidence in the
good faith of my relatives and physicians, and fear degeneration and indignity far more than I fear premature death.

The ethic by which one justifies making such a declaration has been
eloquently expressed by Joseph Fletcher. He speaks of "the right of spiritual
beings to use intelligent control over physical nature rather than to submit
beastlike to its blind workings." For Fletcher, "Death control, like birth control, is a matter of human dignity. Without it persons become puppets. To
perceive this is to grasp the error lurking in the notion—widespread in medical circles—that life as such is the highest good."

Within our society today there are those who agree with the ethic of
Joseph Fletcher. They agree also that an ethic that places a supreme value
upon life is dominant in the medical profession. In a candid editorial ("New
Ethic for Medicine" 1970), the traditional Western ethic with its affirmation
of "the intrinsic worth and equal value of every human life regardless of its
stage or condition" and with its roots in the Judaic and Christian heritage, is
declared to be the basis for most of our laws and much of our social policy.
What is more, the editorial says, "the reverence for each and every human
life" is "a keystone of Western medicine and is the ethic which has caused
physicians to try to preserve, protect, repair, prolong, and enhance every
human life which comes under their surveillance." Although this medical
editor sees this traditional ethic as still clearly dominant, he is convinced
that it is being eroded and that it is being replaced by a new ethic that he
believes medicine should accept and applaud. This editor sees the beginning
of the new ethic in the increasing acceptance of abortion, the general practice of which is in direct defiance of an ethic that affirms the "intrinsic and
equal value for every human life regardless of its stage, condition, or status."
For, in the opinion of this editor, human life begins at conception, and
abortion is killing. Such killing is to be condoned and embraced by the new
ethic.

In the above editorial a case is made for what is called "the quality of
life." To increase the quality of life, it is assumed that the traditional Western ethic will necessarily have to be revised or even totally replaced. This, it
is argued, is because it "will become necessary and acceptable to place rela-

tive rather than absolute values on such things as human lives, the use of scarce resources, and the various elements which are to make up the quality of life or of living which is to be sought." On such a view, the new ethic aids medicine in improving the quality of life; the ethic designated as the old ethic, rooted in Judaism and Christianity, is treated as an impediment to medicine's efforts to improve the quality of life. What kind of ethic should guide contemporary decisions regarding sterilization, abortion, and euthanasia—decisions as to who shall live and who shall die? Given the limits of this article, we shall discuss and assess the ethic (moral policy) of those who favor a policy of voluntary euthanasia and the ethic (moral policy) of those who oppose it. The term "euthanasia" is used here, exactly as in the Voluntary Euthanasia Act of 1969, to mean "the painless inducement of death."

The Ethic of Euthanasia

What then is the ethic that guides those who support legislation like the Voluntary Euthanasia Act of 1969 and its Declaration? The arguments for euthanasia focus upon two humane and significant concerns: compassion for those who are painfully and terminally ill; and concern for the human dignity associated with freedom of choice. Compassion and freedom are values that sustain and enhance the common good. The question here, however, is how these values affect our behavior toward the dying.

The argument for compassion usually occurs in the form of attacking the inhumanity of keeping dying people alive when they are in great pain or when they have lost almost all of their usual functions, particularly when they have lost the ability or will to communicate with others. Thus, someone like Joseph Fletcher cites examples of people who are kept alive in a hopelessly debilitated state by means of the latest medical techniques, whether these be respirators, intravenous feeding, or the like. Often when Fletcher and others are arguing for the legalization of decisions not to intervene in these ways, the point is made that physicians already make decisions to turn off respirators or in other ways fail to use every means to prolong life. It is this allegedly compassionate behavior that the law would seek to condone and encourage.

The argument for compassion is supplemented by an argument for greater freedom for a patient to choose how and when he or she will die. For one thing, the patient should not be subjected to medical treatment to which that patient does not consent. Those who argue for voluntary euthanasia extend this notion by arguing that the choice to withhold techniques that would prolong life is a choice to shorten life. Hence, if one can choose to shorten one's life, why cannot one ask a physician by a simple and direct act of intervention to put an end to one's life? Here it is often argued that physicians already curtail life by means of pain-killing drugs, which in the doses administered, will hasten death. Why should not the law recognize and sanction a simple and direct hastening of death, should the patient wish it?

How do the proponents of euthanasia view the general prohibition against killing? First of all, they maintain that we are dealing here with people who will surely die regardless of the intervention of medicine. They advocate the termination of suffering and the lawful foreshortening of the dying process. Secondly, although the patient is committing suicide, and the physician is an accomplice in such a suicide, both acts are morally justifiable to cut short the suffering of one who is dying.

It is important to be very clear about the precise moral reasoning by which advocates of voluntary euthanasia justify suicide and assisting a suicide. They make no moral distinction between those instances when a patient or a physician chooses to have life shortened by failing to accept or use life-prolonging techniques and those instances when a patient or a physician shorten life by employing a death-dealing chemical or instrument. They make no moral distinction between a drug given to kill pain, which also shortens life, and a substance given precisely to shorten life and for no other reason. Presumably these distinctions are not honored, because regardless of the stratagem employed—regardless of whether one is permitting to die or killing directly—the result is the same, the patient's life is shortened. Hence, it is maintained that, if you can justify one kind of act that shortens the life of the dying, you can justify any act that shortens the life of the dying when this act is seen to be willed by the one who is dying. Moral reasoning of this sort is strictly utilitarian; it focuses solely on the consequences of acts, not on their intent.

Even though the reasoning on the issue of compassion is so strictly utilitarian, one is puzzled about the failure to raise certain kinds of questions. A strict utilitarian might inquire about the effect of the medical practice of promoting or even encouraging direct acts on the part of physicians to shorten the lives of their patients. And, in the same vein, a utilitarian might also be very concerned about whether the loosening of constraints on physicians may not loosen the constraints on killing generally. There are two reasons these questions are either not raised or are dealt with rather summarily. First, it is alleged that there is no evidence that untoward consequences would result. And second, the value of freedom is invoked, so that the question of killing becomes a question of suicide and assistance in a suicide.

The appeal to freedom is not strictly a utilitarian argument, at least not for some proponents of voluntary euthanasia. Joseph Fletcher, for example, complains about the foolishness of nature in bringing about situations in which dying is a prolonged process of suffering. He feels strongly that the failure to permit or encourage euthanasia demeans the dignity of persons. Fletcher has two themes here: On the one hand, the more people are able to control the process of nature, the more dignity and freedom they have; on the other hand, people have dignity only insofar as they are able to choose when, how, and why they are to live or to die. For physicians this means also choices as to who is to die, because presumably one cannot assist in the suicide of just any patient who claims to be suffering, or who thinks he or she is dying.

The ethic that defends suicide as a matter of individual conscience and as an expression of human dignity is a very old ethic. Both the Stoics and the Epicureans considered the choice of one's own death as the ultimate expression of human freedom and as an essential component of the dignity that attaches to rational personhood. This willingness to take one's life is an aspect of Stoic courage (Tillich 1952). A true Stoic could not be manipulated by those who threatened death. When death seemed inevitable, they chose it before someone could inflict it upon them. Human freedom for the Stoics was not complete unless one could also choose death and not compromise oneself for fear of it. All the "heroes" in literature exhibit this kind of Stoic courage in the face of death.

A euthanasia ethic, as exemplified already in ancient Stoicism, contains the following essential presuppositions or beliefs:

1. that an individual's life belongs to that individual to dispose of entirely as he or she wishes;
2. that the dignity that attaches to personhood by reason of the freedom to make moral choices demands also the freedom to take one's own life;

3. that there is such a thing as a life not worth living, whether by reason of distress, illness, physical or mental handicaps, or even sheer despair for whatever reason;
4. that what is sacred or supreme in value is the "human dignity" that resides in man's own rational capacity to choose and control life and death.

This commitment to the free exercise of the human capacity to control life and death takes on a distinct religious aura. Speaking of the death control that amniocentesis makes possible, Robert S. Morison declares that "the birth of babies with gross physical and mental handicaps will no longer be left entirely to God, to chance, or to the forces of nature."

An Ethic of Benemortasia

From our account of the ethic of euthanasia, those who oppose voluntary euthanasia would seem to lack compassion for the dying and the courage to affirm human freedom. They appear incompassionate because they oppose what has come to be regarded as synonymous with a good death—namely, a painless and deliberately foreshortened process of dying. The term "euthanasia" originally meant a painless and happy death with no reference to whether such a death was induced. Although this definition still appears in modern dictionaries, a second meaning of the term has come to prevail: euthanasia now generally means "an act or method of causing death painlessly so as to end suffering" (*Webster's New World Dictionary*, 1962). In short, it would appear that the advocates of euthanasia (i.e., of *causing* death) are the advocates of a good death, and the advocates of voluntary euthanasia seek for all of us the freedom to have a good death.

Because of this loss of a merely descriptive term for a happy death, it is necessary to invent a term for a happy or good death—namely, benemortasia. The familiar derivatives for this new term are *bene* (good) and *mors* (death). The meaning of "bene" in "benemortasia" is deliberately unspecified so that it does not necessarily imply that a death must be painless and/or induced in order to be good. What constitutes a good or happy death is a disputable matter of moral policy. How then should one view the arguments for voluntary euthanasia? And, if an ethic of euthanasia is unacceptable, what is an acceptable ethic of benemortasia?

An ethic of benemortasia does not stand in opposition to the values of compassion and human freedom. It differs, however, from the ethic of euthanasia in its understanding of how these values are best realized. In particular, certain constraints upon human freedom are recognized and emphasized as enabling human beings to increase compassion and freedom rather than diminish them. For the purposes of this essay, we trace the roots of our ethic of benemortasia to Jewish and Christian sources. This does not mean that such an ethic is confined to those traditions or to persons influenced by them any more than an ethic of euthanasia is confined to its Stoic origins or adherents.

The moral life of Jews and Christians alike is and has been guided by the Decalogue, or Ten Commandments. "Thou shalt not kill" is one of the clear constraints upon human decisions and actions expressed in the Decalogue. It is precisely the nature of this constraint that is at stake in decision regarding euthanasia.

Modern biblical scholarship has discovered that the Decalogue, or Mosaic Covenant, is in the form of a treaty between a Suzerain and his people. The point of such a treaty is to specify the relationship between a ruler and his people, and to set out the conditions necessary to form and sustain community with that ruler. One of the most significant purposes of such a treaty is to specify constraints that members of a community must observe if the community is to be viable at all. Fundamentally, the Decalogue articulates the indispensable prerequisites of the common life.

Viewed in this way the injunction not to kill is part of a total effort to prevent the destruction of the human community. It is an absolute prohibition in the sense that no society can be indifferent about the taking of human life. Any act, insofar as it is an act of taking a human life, is wrong, that is to say, taking a human life is a wrong-making characteristic of actions.

To say, however, that killing is prima facie wrong does not mean that an act of killing may never be justified (Ross 1930). For example, a person's effort to prevent someone's death may lead to the death of the attacker. However, we can morally justify that act of intervention only because it is an act of saving a life, not because it is an act of taking a life. If it were simply an act of taking a life, it would be wrong.

A further constraint upon human freedom within the Jewish and Christian traditions is articulated in a myth concerning the loss of paradise. The loss of Eden comes at the point where man and woman succumb to the temptation to know good and evil, and to know it in the perfect and ultimate sense in which a perfect and ultimate being would know it. To know who should live and who should die, one would have to know everything about people, including their ultimate destiny. Only God could have such knowledge. Trying to decide who shall live and who shall die is "playing god." It is tragic to "play god" because one does it with such limited and uncertain knowledge of what is good and evil.

This constraint upon freedom has a liberating effect in the practice of medicine. Nothing in Jewish and Christian tradition presumes that a physician has a clear mandate to impose his or her wishes and skills upon patients for the sake of prolonging the length of their dying where those patients are diagnosed as terminally ill and do not wish the interventions of the physician. Thus the freedom of the patient to accept his or her dying and to decide whether he or she is to have any particular kind of medical care is surely enhanced. A patient who has every reason to believe that he or she is dying would lose the last vestige of freedom were he or she denied the right to choose the circumstances under which the terminal illness would take its course. Presumably that patient is someone who has not chosen to die, but who does have some choices left as to how the last hours and days will be spent. Interventions, in the form of drugs, drainage tubes, or feeding by injection or whatever, may or may not be what the patient wishes or would find beneficial for these last hours or days. People who are dying have as much freedom as other living persons to accept or to refuse medical treatment when that treatment provides no cure for their ailment. There is nothing in the Jewish or Christian tradition that provides an exact blueprint as to what is the most compassionate thing to do for someone who is dying. Presumably the most compassionate act is to be a neighbor to such a person and to minister to such a person's needs. Depending upon the circumstances, this may or may not include intervention to prolong the process of dying.

Our ethic of benemortasia acknowledges the freedom of patients who are incurably ill to refuse interventions that prolong dying and the freedom of physicians to honor such wishes. However, these actions are not acts of suicide and assisting in suicide. In our ethic of benemortasia, suicide and assisting in suicide are unjustifiable acts of killing. Unlike the ethic of those who would legalize voluntary euthanasia, our ethic makes a moral distinction between acts that *permit* death and acts that *cause* death. As George P.

Fletcher notes, one can make a sharp distinction, one that will stand up in law, between "permitting to die" and "causing death." Jewish and Christian tradition, particularly Roman Catholic thought, have maintained this clear distinction between the failure to use extraordinary measures (permitting to die) and direct intervention to bring about death (causing death). A distinction is also drawn between a drug administered to cause death and a drug administered to ease pain which has the added effect of shortening life (see, for example, Smith 1970).

Why are these distinctions important in instances where permitting to die or causing death both have the effect of shortening life? In both instances there is a failure to try to prolong the life of one who is dying. It is at this point that one must see why consequential reasoning is in itself too narrow, and why it is important also not to limit the discussion of benemortasia to the immediate relationship between a patient and his or her physician.

Where a person is dying of a terminal illness, it is fair to say that no one, including the dying person and his or her physician, has wittingly chosen this affliction and this manner or time of death. The choices that are left to a dying patient, an attendant physician, others who know the patient, and society concern how the last days of the dying person are to be spent.

From the point of view of the dying person, when could his or her decisions be called a deliberate act to end life, the act we usually designate as suicide? Only, it seems to me, when the dying person commits an act that has the immediate intent of ending life and has no other purpose. That act may be to use, or ask the physician to use, a chemical or an instrument that has no other immediate effect than to end the dying person's life. If, for the sake of relieving pain, a dying person chooses drugs administered in potent doses, the intent of this act is not to shorten life, even though it has that effect. It is a choice as to how to live while dying. Similarly, if a patient chooses to forgo medical interventions that would have the effect of prolonging his or her life without in any way promising release from death, this also is a choice as to what is the most meaningful way to spend the remainder of life, however short that may be. The choice to use drugs to relieve pain and the choice not to use medical measures that cannot promise a cure for one's dying are no different in principle from the choices we make throughout our lives as to how much we will rest, how hard we will work, how little and how much medical intervention we will seek or tolerate, and the like. For society or physicians to map out life-styles for individuals with respect to such decisions is surely beyond anything that we find in Stoic, Jewish, or Christian ethics. Such intervention in the liberty of individuals is far beyond what is required in any society whose rules are intended to constrain people against harming others.

But human freedom should not be extended to include the taking of one's own life. Causing one's own death cannot generally be justified, even when one is dying. To see why this is so, we have to consider how causing one's death does violence to one's self and harms others.

The person who causes his or her own death repudiates the meaningfulness and worth of his or her own life. To decide to initiate an act that has as its primary purpose to end one's life is to decide that that life has no worth to anyone, especially to oneself. It is an act that ends all choices regarding what one's life and whatever is left of it is to symbolize.

Suicide is the ultimately effective way of shutting out all other people from one's life. Psychologists have observed how hostility for others can be expressed through taking one's own life. People who might want access to the dying one to make restitution, offer reparation, bestow last kindnesses, or clarify misunderstandings are cut off by such an act. Every kind of potentially and actually meaningful contact and relation among persons is irrevocably severed except by means of memories and whatever life beyond death may offer. Certainly for those who are left behind by death, there can remain many years of suffering occasioned by that death. The sequence of dying an inevitable death can be much better accepted than the decision on the part of a dying one that he or she has no worth to anyone. An act that presupposes that final declaration leaves tragic overtones for anyone who participated in even the smallest way in that person's dying.

But the problem is even greater. If in principle a person can take his or her own life whenever he or she no longer finds it meaningful, there is nothing in principle that prevents anyone from taking his or her life, no matter what the circumstances. For if the decision hinges on whether one regards his or her own life as meaningful, anyone can regard his or her own life as meaningless even under circumstances that would appear to be most fortunate and opportune for an abundant life.

What about those who would commit suicide or request euthanasia in order to cease being a "burden" on those who are providing care for them? If it is a choice to accept death by refusing noncurative care that prolongs dying, the freedom to embrace death or give one's life in this way is honored by our ethic of benemortasis. What is rejected is the freedom to cause death whether by suicide or by assisting in one.

How a person dies has a definite meaning for those to whom that person is related. In the first year of bereavement, the rate of death among bereaved relatives of those who die in hospitals is twice that of bereaved relatives of those who die at home; sudden deaths away from hospital and home increase the death rate of the bereaved even more (Lasagna 1970).

The courage to be, as expressed in Christian and Jewish thought, is more than the overcoming of the fear of death, although it includes that Stoic dimension. It is the courage to accept one's own life as having worth no matter what life may bring, including the threat of death, because that life remains meaningful and is regarded as worthy by God, regardless of what that life may be like.

An ethic of benemortasia stresses what Tillich has called the "courage to be as a part"—namely, the courage to affirm not only oneself, but also one's participation as a self in a universal community of beings. The courage to be as a part recognizes that one is not merely one's own, that one's life is a gift bestowed and protected by the human community and by the ultimate forces that make up the cycle of birth and death. In the cycle of birth and death, there may be suffering, as there is joy, but suffering does not render a life meaningless or worthless. Suffering people need the support of others; suffering people should not be encouraged to commit suicide by their community, or that community ceases to be a community.

This consideration brings us to a further difficulty with voluntary euthanasia and its legalization. Not only does euthanasia involve suicide, but also, if legalized, it sanctions assistance in a suicide by physicians. Legislation like the Voluntary Euthanasia Act of 1969 makes it a duty of the medical profession to take someone else's life for him. Here the principle not to kill is even further eroded and violated by giving the physician the power and the encouragement to decide that someone else's life is no longer worth living. The whole notion that a physician can engage in euthanasia implies acceptance of the principle that another person's life is no longer meaningful enough to sustain, a principle that does not afford protection for the lives of any of the most defenseless, voiceless, or otherwise dependent members of a community. Everyone in a community is potentially a victim of such a principle, particularly among members of racial minorities, the very young, and the very old.

Those who would argue that these consequences of a policy of voluntary euthanasia cannot be predicted fail to see two things: that we have already had an opportunity to observe what happens when the principle that sanctions euthanasia is accepted by a society; and that regardless of what the consequences may be of such acts, the acts themselves are wrong in principle.

With respect to the first point, Leo Alexander's (1949) very careful analysis of medical practices and attitudes of German physicians before and during the reign of Nazism in Germany should serve as a definite warning against the consequences of making euthanasia a public policy. He notes that the outlook of German physicians that led to their cooperation in what became a policy of mass murders,

> started with the acceptance of that attitude, basic in the euthanasia movement, that there is such a thing as life not worthy to be lived. This attitude in its early stages concerned itself merely with the severely and chronically sick. Gradually the sphere of those to be included in this category was enlarged to include the socially unproductive, the racially unwanted, and finally all non-Germans. But it is important to realize that the infinitely small wedged-in lever from which this entire trend of mind received its impetus was the attitude toward the nonrehabilitable sick.

Those who reject out of hand any comparison of what happened in Nazi Germany with what we can expect here in the United States should consider current examples of medical practice in this nation. The treatment of mongoloids is a case in point. Now that the notion is gaining acceptance that a fetus diagnosed in the womb as mongoloid can, at the discretion of a couple or the pregnant woman, be justifiably aborted, instances of infanticide in hospitals are being reported. At Johns Hopkins Hospital, for example, an allegedly mongoloid infant whose parents would not permit an operation that is generally successful in securing normal physical health and development, was ordered to have "nothing by mouth," condemning that infant to a death that took 15 days. By any of our existing laws, this was a case of murder, justified on the ground that this particular life was somehow not worth saving. (If one argues that the infant was killed because the parents did not want it, we have in this kind of case an even more radical erosion of our restraints upon killing.)

Someone may argue that the mongoloid was permitted to die, not killed. But this is faulty reasoning. In the case of an infant whose future life and happiness could be reasonably assured through surgery, we are not dealing with someone who is dying and with intervention that has no curative effect. The fact that some physicians refer to this as a case of permitting to die is an ominous portent of the dangers inherent in accepting the principle that a physician or another party can decide for a patient that his or her life is not worth living. Equally ominous is the assumption that this principle, once accepted, can easily be limited to cases of patients for whom no curative intervention is known to exist.

With all the risks that attend changing the physician's role from one who sustains life to one who induces death, one may well ask why physicians should be called upon to assist a suicide?

M. R. Barrington, an advocate of suicide and of voluntary euthanasia, is aware of the difficulty of making this request of physicians and of the necessity for justifying legalization of such requests. She suggests that the role of the physician in assisting suicide is essential, "especially as human frailty requires that it should be open to a patient to ask the doctor to choose a time for the giving of euthanasia that is not known to the patient" (Barrington 1971). This appeal to "human frailty" is very telling. The hesitation to commit suicide and the ambivalence of the dying about their worth should give one pause before one signs a declaration that empowers a physician to decide that at some point one can no longer be trusted as competent to judge whether or not one wants to die. Physicians are also frail humans, and mistaken diagnoses, research interests, and sometimes errors of judgment that stem from a desire for organs, are part of the practice of medicine.

Comatose patients pose special problems for an ethic of benemortasia as they do for the advocates of voluntary euthanasia. Where patients are judged to be irreversibly comatose and where sustained efforts have been made to restore such persons to consciousness, no clear case can be made for permitting to die, even though it seems merciful to do so. It seems that the best we can do is to develop some rough social and medical consensus about a reasonable length of time for keeping "alive" a person's organ systems after "brain death" has been decided (Ramsey 1970). Because of the pressures to do research and to transplant organs, it may also be necessary to employ special patient advocates who are not physicians and nurses. These patient advocates, trained in medical ethics, would function as ombudsmen.

In summary, even if the practice of euthanasia were to be confined to those who voluntarily request an end to their lives, no physician could in good conscience participate in such an act. To decide directly to cause the death of a patient is to abandon a cardinal principle of medical practice—namely, to do no harm to one's patient. The relief of suffering, which is surely a time-honored role for the physician, does not extend to an act that presupposes that the life of a patient who is suffering is not worthy to be lived. As we have argued, not even the patient who is dying can justifiably and unilaterally universalize the principle by which a dying life would be declared to be worthless.

Some readers may remain unconvinced that euthanasia is morally wrong as a general policy. Perhaps what still divides us is what distinguishes a Stoic from a Jewish and Christian way of life. The Stoic heritage declares that my life and my selfhood are my own to dispose of as I see fit and when I see fit. The Jewish and Christian heritage declares that my life and my selfhood are not my own, and are not mine to dispose of as I see fit. In the words of H. Richard Niebuhr (1963),

> I live but do not have the power to live. And further, I may die at any moment but I am powerless to die. It was not in my power, nor in my parents' power, to elect my *self* into existence. Though they willed a child or consented to it they did not will *me*—this I, thus and so. And so also I now, though I *will* to be no more, cannot elect myself out of existence, if the inscrutable power by which I am, elects otherwise. Though I wish to be mortal, if the power that threw me into being in this mortal destructible body elects me into being again there is nothing I can do about that. I can destroy the life of my body. Can I destroy myself? This remains the haunting question of the literature of suicide and of all the lonely debates of men to whom existence is a burden. Whether they shall wake up again, either here in this life or there in some other mode of being, is beyond their control. We can choose among many alternatives; but the power to choose self-existence or self-extinction is not ours. Men can practice birth-control, not self-creation; they can commit *bio*cide; whether they can commit suicide, self-destruction, remains a question.

Although one has the power to commit biocide, this does not give one the right to do so. Niebuhr views our lives as shaped by our responses to others and their responses to us. All of us are in responsible relations to others. The claim that an act of suicide (biocide) would harm no one else is unrealistic. To try to make that a reality would require an incredibly lonely existence cut off from all ties of friendship, cooperation, and mutual dependence. And in so doing, we would repudiate the value and benefits of altruism.

The other points at which the proponents of euthanasia and the advocates of benemortasia part company concern the perception of the context in which all moral decisions are made. Here again the division has religious overtones. Those who decide for euthanasia seem to accept an ethic which ultimately privatizes and subjectivizes the injunction not to kill. Those who oppose euthanasia see the decision not to kill as one that is in harmony with what is good for everyone, and indeed is an expression of what is required of everyone if goodness is to be pervasive and powerful on earth. Once again, H. Richard Niebuhr has eloquently expressed this latter position:

> All my specific and relative evaluations expressed in my interpretations and responses are shaped, guided, and formed by the understanding of good and evil I have *upon the whole*. In distrust of the radical action by which I am, by which my society is, by which this world is, I must find my center of valuation in myself, or in my nation, or in my church, or in my science, or in humanity, or in life. Good and evil in this view mean what is good for me and bad for me; or good and evil for my nation, or good and evil for one of these finite causes, such as mankind, or life or reason. But should it happen that confidence is given to me in the power by which all things are and by which I am; should I learn in the depths of my existence to praise the creative source, . . . all my relative evaluations will be subjected to the continuing and great correction. They will be made to fit into a total process producing good—not what is good for me (though my confidence accepts that as included), nor what is good for man (though that is also included), nor what is good for the development of life (though that also belongs in the picture), but what is good for being, for universal being, or for God, center and source of all existence.

Our ethic of benemortasia has argued for the following beliefs and values:

1. that an individual person's life is not solely at the disposal of that person; every human life is part of the human community that bestows and protects the lives of its members; the possibility of community itself depends upon constraints against taking life;
2. that the dignity that attaches to personhood by reason of the freedom to make moral choices includes the freedom of dying people to refuse non-curative, life-prolonging interventions when one is dying, but does not extend to taking one's life or causing death for someone who is dying;
3. that every life has some worth; there is no such thing as a life not worth living;
4. that the supreme value is goodness itself to which the dying and those who care for the dying are responsible. Religiously expressed the supreme value is God. Less than perfectly good beings, human beings, require

constraints upon their decisions regarding those who are dying. No human being or human community can presume to know who deserves to live or to die.

At the same time, we have implied throughout that religion and the Jewish and Christian expressions of it are not obstacles to modern medicine and a better life; rather they help foster humanity's quest to preserve and enhance human life on this earth.

References

Alexander, Leo. "Medical Science under Dictatorship." *New England Journal of Medicine* 241 (July 14, 1949): 39–47.

Barrington, Mary Rose. "Apologia for Suicide." In *Euthanasia and the Right to Death*, edited by A. B. Downing. Los Angeles: Nash Publishing, 1969.

Downing, A. B., ed. *Euthanasia and the Right to Death*. Los Angeles: Nash Publishing, 1969.

Dyck, Arthur J. "Population Policies and Ethical Acceptability." In *Rapid Population Growth: Consequences and Policy Implications*, edited by Roger Revelle et al. Baltimore: Johns Hopkins University Press, 1971.

Fletcher, George P. "Prolonging Life: Some Legal Considerations." In *Euthanasia and the Right to Death*, edited by A. B. Downing. Los Angeles: Nash Publishing, 1969.

Fletcher, Joseph. "The Patient's Right to Die." In *Euthanasia and the Right to Death*, edited by A. B. Downing. Los Angeles: Nash Publishing, 1969.

Jakobovits, Immanuel. *Jewish Medical Ethics*. New York: Bloch Publishing Company, 1959.

Kamisar, Yale. "Euthanasia Legislation: Some Non-Religious Objections." In *Euthanasia and the Right to Death*, edited by A. B. Downing. Los Angeles: Nash Publishing, 1969.

Lasagna, Louis. "The Prognosis of Death." In *The Dying Patient*, edited by Orville Brim et al. New York: Russell Sage Foundation, 1970.

Morison, Robert S. "Chairman's Introduction." In *Early Diagnosis of Human Genetic Defects*, edited by M. Harris. Washington, D.C.: Department of Health, Education, and Welfare, 1971.

"A New Ethic for Medicine and Society." *California Medicine* 113 (September 1970): 67–68.

Niebuhr, H. Richard. *The Responsible Self.* New York: Harper & Row, 1963.

Ramsey, Paul. *The Patient as Person.* New Haven: Yale University Press, 1970.

Ross, W. D. *The Right and the Good.* Clarendon: Oxford University Press, 1930.

Smith, Harmon L. *Ethics and the New Medicine.* New York: Abingdon Press, 1970.

Tillich, Paul. *The Courage to Be.* New Haven: Yale University Press, 1952.

20

Should There Be a Legal Right
to Die?

ROBERT F. DRINAN

IN the escalating controversies over abortion and the law some of the opponents of abortion suggest that the legalization of feticide may and/or will lead to infanticide and to euthanasia. Such assertions may be exaggerated rhetoric but they do suggest nonetheless that a fundamental struggle over the very meaning of the taking of a human life is developing in America and in the Western world.

Without entering into the truth or falsity of the assertion that allowing a parent to abort a fetus may lead to other invasions of the sanctity of life, it seems appropriate to analyze and evaluate those currents of thought which would legalize suicide or which, to put it another way, would establish a "legal right to die."

The proponents of this idea do not always seem to appreciate the fact that Anglo-American law has for centuries placed the severest sanctions on the taking of life. The only exception to the grave prohibition of the law's interdiction of the extinguishing of life has been the death penalty for murderers and certain other criminals. We witness in our day, by a strange twisting of logic, a vehement assertion by many groups that the state has no right to execute murderers and an equally vehement affirmation by the same groups

Reprinted from the *American Ecclesiastical Review* 159 (1968): 277–86, with the permission of the author and the Catholic University of America Press.

that it has the right and even the duty to authorize the death of unborn children and of persons who are incurably sick or aged.

The opponents of capital punishment who simultaneously advocate abortion and euthanasia may insist that they are not being illogical but the central question is—who has the right to extinguish the life of a human being?

The Preciousness of Life

It has been cardinal in Anglo-American law that a human life is more precious than any other conceivable object. The right to hold property or even to possess liberty has been subordinated in our law to the values attributed to human life. It is probably true to state that the preciousness of human life has been more rather than less realized in our statutory and decisional law within the past two generations. For example, a trend in the law will now allow recovery by a child for prenatal injuries sustained by the negligence of a third party. This new tendency to expand the rights of even unborn children is rooted in the ever expanding concept of the value of every life.

Until recently it had been assumed in our law that human life was precious because it was a gift of God. Today this idea has been eroded so that life, however precious, is now considered to be the possession of man himself. Consequently, it follows that man may surrender that life by suicide if he finds it intolerable and society may demand the life of an unborn child if the birth of such child will cause physical or psychological harm to its mother.

Every argument in favor of "mercy killing" or euthanasia must presuppose that man has a right to commit suicide. Such a presupposition necessarily is rooted in a man-centered idea of human destiny.

It is amazing and distressing to see the sweeping assumptions of the ever increasing numbers in our society who are campaigning to abolish all of our laws which by the severest penalties make it a crime to commit suicide or "mercy murder."

Theoretically any discussion of the position of those who would allow the extinguishing of life by human hands should center on the nature of the right and duty to preserve a human life. Such a discussion can hardly be fruitful, however, if a law of divine origin common to all men cannot be assumed. In this regard one is reminded of the opinion expressed by Reinhold

Niebuhr that the natural law, regarded hopefully by Catholics as a "bridge" between Catholics and non-Catholics, is in Niebuhr's view the great obstacle to effective communication between Catholics and Protestants.

It is well, therefore, to approach the question of the right and duty to preserve life from a practical, factual point of view. We will consequently treat of (1) the history and present status of the euthanasia movement, (2) the limitations and practical difficulties latent in the arguments advanced for legalizing "mercy murder" and (3) the approach which Catholics should have with regard to militant attempts to effect radical changes in our legal-moral institutions.

History of the Euthanasia Idea

The boldest yet the most scholarly and respected plea to legalize euthanasia that has been published in recent times is without doubt contained in the volume *The Sanctity of Life and the Criminal Law*, by Sir Glanville Williams (1967). In this expanded version of the Carpentier lectures given in 1956 at the Columbia University Law School, Mr. Williams makes a forthright presentation of his case that suicide and voluntary euthanasia should be legalized. He also advocates the legalization of human sterilization, artificial insemination, abortion and, of course, birth control. Mr. Williams' position is therefore that of the consistent, logical advocate of the elimination of all religious and even moral concepts from the civil law. Professor Williams, a distinguished English legal scholar, argues openly and forthrightly that a "prohibition imposed by a religious belief should not be applied by law to those who do not share the belief."

Professor Williams chronicles a good deal of information about the rise and contemporary frustration of the British Voluntary Euthanasia Legalization Society. Since this group is the parent of the Euthanasia Society of America, it will be profitable to review its efforts to create a "legal right to die."

In 1936 sensational headlines in England and America reported the debate in the House of Lords over a bill designed to legalize voluntary euthanasia. This bill was the result of the work of an organization under the presidency of Lord Moynihan, President of the Royal College of Surgeons. Endorsement of the euthanasia bill came from many famous names which included Julian Huxley, H. G. Wells, G. B. Shaw, Sir James Jeans, Dean

Inge, and several others. Some clergymen of every church except the Roman Catholic endorsed the bill although the proposal by no means could claim the support of the majority of non-Catholic clerics.

The bill debated by the House of Lords in 1936 was restricted to persons (1) over 21 years of age, (2) suffering from an incurable and fatal disease, (3) accompanied by severe pain, and (4) who, in the presence of two witnesses, sign a statutory form requesting euthanasia. The public debate on this proposal (contained in *Parliamentary Debates*, December 1, 1936) reveals the basic instincts of doctors, clergymen, and almost all others which explain why the bill was defeated by a vote of 35 to 14 and why indeed no nation of the world has yet legalized euthanasia. The late Lord Lang, Archbishop of Canterbury, spoke against the bill and urged that doctors be allowed to continue to exercise their best judgment—aware always of the difference between prolonging life and prolonging the act of dying. A somewhat unclear assumption involved in the House of Lords debate was that physicians may and do, consciously or subconsciously, treat patients where, in the words of the Archbishop of Canterbury, "some means of shortening life may be justified."

Professor Williams finds the outcome of the debate "indefensible." In his view there is no legal protection for the conscientious physician who, following his own best judgment and the wishes of his patient, terminates the life of an incurably sick person.

Americans and "The Right To Die"

In January 1938, the Euthanasia Society of America (ESA) was incorporated. Charles Francis Potter, its founder, said in 1938: "We have been for years active in the birth-control movement, and since that fight is largely won, we feel free to transfer some of our efforts to the euthanasia enterprise." According to a newspaper story on February 4, 1936, the same Rev. Dr. Potter had advocated the lethal chamber for incurable imbeciles.

The Euthanasia Society of America has not yet found a legislator to introduce a bill along the English pattern, although attempts have been made in New York State, Nebraska, and elsewhere. The support which ESA has attracted is, however, surprising. Clergymen who have signed ESA's ethical statement professing that they see no contradiction between euthanasia and the principles of Christianity include Dr. Harry Emerson Fosdick and Dr. Ralph W. Sockman.

Among the more well-known Americans who have allowed their endorsement of legalized "mercy murder" to be publicized are Robert Frost, Eugene O'Neill, Max Eastman, Rex Stout, Arthur Garfield Hays, Fannie Hurst, and Dr. Walter C. Alvarez.

Although some physicians have conceded the desirability of enacting a "legal right to die," no medical society in America has ever endorsed the legalization of euthanasia. It is difficult to see how a doctor or a medical group could advocate such a measure in view of the statement in the Hippocratic Oath where a new doctor affirms that ". . . neither will I administer a poison to anyone when asked to do so, nor will I suggest such a course."

Public opinion concerning euthanasia probably parallels attitudes among physicians—who have never been adequately polled on the matter. There does exist, however, a widespread sympathy for the idea of what someone has named "assisted suicide." Many persons in good faith feel that an "easy way out" should be available for the aged and the incurably sick. The ever deepening problems surrounding the prolongation of life by new medical techniques of both the aged and the hopelessly afflicted suggest as one solution a less rigid application of the moral and legal prohibition of suicide.

A Nonphilosophical Case against Euthanasia

It is distressing to those who have certainty concerning some basic truths knowable by the light of the natural law to be confronted with serious and conscientious critics of society who urge that civil law should allow and even encourage human beings to go against man's primary instinct—the instinct of self-preservation.

In confrontation therefore with the rejection of the very basic philosophical first principles one can hardly hope to conduct a "dialogue" grounded in mutually accepted premises derived from a moral consensus. There are, however, a few relative absolutes left among the opponents of the traditional natural-law morality. One of these semiabsolutes affirms that life should not be taken away unless the person whose life is in question has given full and free consent. A second principle asserts that all human beings should avoid doing those acts which will produce in their lives an unreasonable guilt or anxiety. Popularized law and oversimplified psychology seem to have left at least these two principles in the minds of those who advocate euthanasia. Building on this admittedly frail foundation, what *practical* difficulties can be anticipated in connection with these two principles if the state should ever allow a sick person to "consent" to have another assist him to extinguish his own life?

Let us explore some of the situations which might well occur if the law ever allowed a "legal right to die."

Is Free Consent Possible For One in Pain?

The necessity of *severe* pain was included in the British proposal to legalize euthanasia. The English bill in effect sought to remove the criminal stigma of suicide from those who, incurably sick and suffering severe pain, gave free consent in writing to two physicians. Aside from the moral question of suicide would it ever really be possible to obtain the *free* consent of a person with *severe* pain? Pain does different things to different people. Drugs to alleviate pain have similarly different reactions. When is *free* consent to be obtained—when the patient is in agonizing pain or when he is enjoying a mild euphoria after the administration of drugs? It seems clear that consent obtained at either of these times might well be deemed not to be *free*.

Could a fixed period be established during which the patient could rescind his own freely invoked "right to die"? Even with this provision great difficulties would often present themselves concerning the question of the "freedom" of the conset. For example, what if the patient became unconscious after he gave his "free" consent and had not returned to consciousness at the end of the statutory period allowed for revocation of consent? Does the consent perdure? Must the next of kin be consulted since the patient is now legally incompetent?

An analogy concerning the legal and moral sacredness and inviolability of one's "freedom" of consent can be seen in the legal safeguards surrounding the surrender of a child by its mother. If a mother consents for good reason to allow her own child to be adopted by someone else, the full freedom of the natural mother's consent is essential to the validity of the child's transfer. The law affirms that when a mother gives up something as precious as her own child her consent *must* be free and, if it is not, she has the right to rescind it.

Consent to give up one's life—one's most precious possession—must similarly be protected not merely on behalf of the individual concerned but for the peace of society. If it were generally thought that something less than full and free consent to die was accepted by hospital authorities, great fear and apprehension might result in the souls of those possibly eligible to exercise their "right to die."

An article in a recent issue of the *Journal of the American Medical Association* [see Oken article] suggests a further practical problem never confronted by the advocates of a legal "right to die." In a survey of 193 members of the staff of a Chicago hospital, 88 percent of these physicians said that not telling a cancer patient that he has cancer was "their usual policy." Only 12 percent stated that it was their usual policy to tell the cancer victim of his disease. Ninety of the 193 doctors said that they "very rarely" tell their cancer patients the full story and 18 of the 193 said they "never" tell.

This sampling of doctors was reported to be representative of high-quality medical practitioners. The results reflect previous surveys showing similar tendencies on the question of how much information to give the cancer patient.

It is reported in the same article in the AMA *Journal*, however, that doctors are virtually unanimous on two points—(1) that some member of the family of the cancer patient be told if the patient is not and that (2) a physician, whatever his policy on telling the patient, should have a "resolute and determined purpose . . . to sustain and bolster the patient's hope."

It can be seen therefore that the family of most cancer patients will inevitably be deeply involved if any question of a "right to die" should arise. This fact is well to bear in mind when we discuss later the guilt which may affect the soul of those who cooperate in "assisted suicide."

Enormous problems therefore surround the implementation of the proposal of the euthanasiasts that a person may secure his right to die only if he gives his *free consent*. A consideration of these problems leads us to an even more difficult problem—is man *ever* capable of giving *free* consent to surrendering his right to life?

Is Free Consent Ever Possible?

It is a common conviction today that any person who attempts suicide is afflicted with a serious mental illness. Psychiatry has been able to identify, classify, and control to some extent certain suicidal tendencies which arise in disturbed lives. Although the Catholic tradition places the severest sanctions on suicide, the Church nonetheless is most sympathetic to the idea that those who attempt suicide are sick rather than sinful.

If an incurably sick person desires to extinguish his life it is not easy to distinguish such a desire from the ordinary suicidal impulse which overwhelms certain individuals because of a severe disappointment or a deep mental depression. No one could say that these latter individuals have "freely" consented to die, although their subjective despair may be greater and their desire to die more "free" than persons incurably sick who desire euthanasia.

In a certain sense, therefore, it is impossible for any observer of another individual, who is either hopelessly sick or mentally depressed, to judge the quality of "freedom" which has gone into his decision to seek death. Who can distinguish in would-be suicides the calm Stoic from the irrational exhibitionist? Yet someone must do so and be responsible to society for the "freedom" of the choice of those who seek death. Otherwise the law would simply allow physicians or other officials to cooperate with and practically sponsor the suicide of those in their care who have expressed even once a desire to be free from their sufferings forever.

If it is impossible then to obtain a consent to die which one can know objectively is "free," is it ever feasible to have a law allowing "mercy deaths" yet insisting that the patient give "free" consent? Switzerland, the only nation in the world to allow even "semi-euthanasia," authorizes a physician to place a deadly dose of medicine within the reach of any incurably sick patient who has requested it. The law would seem to assume, however, that the doctor must make a judgment that the request to "drink the hemlock" results from a decision communicated to and participated in by the patient's family and is on the whole a wise one. Any doctor in Switzerland and elsewhere would ponder deeply whether he would be ethically able to cooperate with what has become a part of Swiss law.

Anxiety and Guilt

If *free* consent to die is difficult or impossible to obtain from anyone and especially from those with severe pain, it follows that in any case where a consent to exercise one's "right to die" could be obtained under a euthanasia statute other individuals beside the patient would be deeply involved in the formation and acceptance of the consent required to die. It follows that the survivors of a person who exercised a legal "right to die" would be confronted with countless opportunities to regret the influences which they inevitably would have exercised over the decisions of their relative or friend now departed.

The wisest voices in modern society recognize that every man must live with his past and with himself. Everywhere we see that bitter regrets about past conduct produce feelings of guilt which may result in permanent anxiety, neuroses, or even psychoses. To the Christian all of this is explainable in the truths of original sin and the tenderness of Christ in establishing the tribunal of penance. But the secular humanist must create a formula by which guilt concerning the past—an unavoidable feeling with most people—can be so moderated that peace in the present is possible.

Nothing can be imagined more likely to arouse guilt, even in the most firm disbeliever in the notion of sin, than cooperation in an "assisted suicide" with a loved one. It is not the actual death that would produce guilt and anxiety in the survivor but the uncertainty of the evidence on which one acted.

In any case where an incurably sick person has requested the exercise of his "right to die," his family can oppose, support, or acquiesce in his decision. If a family firmly opposes the patient's decision and does whatever is possible to prevent the "mercy murder," they would have no cause for subsequent regret. If, however, the family supported or even acquiesced in the decision there could arise countless possible eventualities after the patient's death which would cause the gravest disturbances in the souls of the survivors. Consider the following circumstances and cases:

1. Much research today indicates that cancer is a viral disease. We are told that it may soon be possible to have a dramatic breakthrough on cancer as spectacular as the Salk vaccine. What if this should occur a short time after a family has acquiesced in the exercise of the "right to die" of one of their members?

2. Pain-killing medicines are continuously improving. It may be that there will be discovered within the near future a drug which can eliminate virtually all pain associated with certain incurable diseases while another drug could supply an energizing force to offset the weakening effects of a debilitating illness. What if this medical advance came about shortly after

the death of a patient by legalized suicide with the consent of the patient's family? What feelings of remorse will the family have if they realize that their decision deprived their loved one of several months of pain-free, almost normal living?

3. What would be the reaction of a family who acquiesced in the "mercy death" of a loved one if they discovered subsequently that the deceased person had experienced irrational suicidal tendencies all through his life?

One can see therefore that any weakening of the present prohibition on suicide, even for the most humanitarian reasons—will bring about moral crises and problems of conscience for those who participate even to a small degree in the decision of one who decides to determine on his own the moment of his death.

Such are but a very few of the many considerations of a practical nature which would be involved in the legalization of euthanasia. Clearly the whole thrust of the spirit and letter of Christianity is opposed to "mercy murder." But arguments from this source will hardly have any effect upon the advocates of euthanasia who in their official bulletin announce that "we no longer believe that physical suffering is the will of God, to be accepted with resignation."

From the background of the euthanasia movement in England and America one can see that there is a gathering storm which claims that the right to life is not divinely controlled but that it can be in certain circumstances humanly manipulated.

How strong and threatening is the movement to legalize euthanasia? How strong, in other words, is the emotional and man-centered reasoning which can so overturn traditional moral concepts that it can grant to man or the state the right to take an innocent life?

The attempt to legalize euthanasia shows no signs of abating although there is some encouragement in the fact that, as the *Encyclopedia of Religion and Ethics* states, euthanasia has never been institutionalized in the history of mankind.

What attitudes and what principles should the Church adopt in the face of a severe assault upon the right to life now protected by our civil law as one of man's most sacred possessions?

A Three-sided Attitude toward New Assaults
on the Right to Life

It seems clear that Catholics will confront in the near future an unprecedented attempt by an alliance of many non-Catholic and secular forces to weaken or abolish the protection now given to human life in Anglo-American civil law. Although the proper Catholic attitude in any case that may arise will differ according to various circumstances, the following three suggestions are made as guidelines for the conduct of Catholics and all others grounded in a natural-law tradition.

1. It is never profitable to question the good faith of those who advocate the repeal of certain laws which to Catholics are so fundamental that their repeal is unthinkable. The advocates of euthanasia operate from a code of moral ultimates which is entirely different from that assumed by the traditionalists who assert that the life of an innocent human being cannot under any circumstances be taken by human hands.

2. It should always be remembered that civil law is never expected to enforce *all* the morality of the society which it governs. Many directives of the moral law—as, for example, the disclosing without adequate reason of the true but immoral acts of others—are clearly immoral but have never been illegal.

It may be therefore that certain unenforceable statutes which are now legally binding could be repealed without great harm or possibly with profit.

3. Pluralism as a theory of society in America seems to include the idea that different groups allow the morality of other groups to exist even though it is contrary to the wishes and even the consciences of a majority or of several minority groups. In other words, pluralism means that our public morality is not retained or made by the use of the political power of any minority or even a majority.

Catholics will have many opportunities to ponder the implications of these principles in the immediate future. In the interim Catholics and all believers in the sanctity of human life should deepen and radiate their profoundest convictions about the inviolability of the life of every human being.

21

Justifying the Final Solution

HELGE HILDING MANSSON

THE taking of human life has been a part of man's history and evolution.
The social control of killing, therefore, has been of great concern to social
thinkers and has received increased popular attention since World War II
and the Nuremberg trials. But social control, sometimes bolstered by statutory and moral law, appears to be more successful in determining who the
victims will be rather than in reducing their number. The act of killing has
its roots in biological, psychological, and social determinants of such a
complex nature that understanding through traditional individual psychology alone or any other particular branch of science is unlikely to be accomplished. This, however, does not mean that psychology has nothing to
offer. Just as we can study the relationship of attitudes to behaviors, so can
we study some of the conditions leading to the acceptance of ideas and attitudes which provide individuals with a variety of justifications for their endorsement of force, violence, and even killing.

Milgram (1963), in his very provocative study on obedience, has pointed
out that "obedience is as basic an element in the structure of social life as
one can point to." He cites the figure of 45 million people who were systematically slaughtered on command between 1933 and 1945. He demonstrated
in his study the link that obedience represents between individual action and

Reprinted from *Omega* 3 (May 1972): 79–87, with the permission of the publisher. Copyright
© 1972 by the Baywood Publishing Company, Inc.

political purposes. Without in any way wishing to detract from Milgram's most ingenious and important study, this investigator believes that obedience is not, in and of itself, sufficient as an explanatory concept for the behaviors that we associate with willingness to tolerate harm to others, even killing and genocide.

The acceptance and tolerance of aggression and the use of force are part of our cultural values which, in turn, affect our attitudes toward aggressors and victims alike. To many people, the establishment of personal justifications that sanction killing seems to be of greater importance than is the "evilness" or "goodness" of killing per se. Jean-Paul Sartre in his recent article (1968) on genocide calls attention to a 23-year-old student who had "interrogated" prisoners for ten months and who could scarcely live with his memories. This 23-year-old said, "I'm a middle-class American, I look like any other student, yet somehow I am criminal." And Sartre points out that he (the soldier) was right when he added, "Anyone in my place would have acted as I did." It is a moot question whether this soldier's method of "interrogating" prisoners was because of blind obedience to command or because the element of genocide exists within all of us.

The infamous case of Kitty Genovese, who was murdered in New York in 1964, gained national attention because, of the 38 people who were known to have observed the assault and her killing, not one person had come to her aid or had alerted the police. This case inspired a number of studies (Lerner and Simons 1966; Walster 1966; Lerner and Mathews 1967; Latane and Darley 1968) concerned with the so-called "Innocent Bystander Phenomenon." In these studies, obedience to authority did not seem to be crucial. Instead, a mixture of fear, hostility, anonymity, and a variety of self-justifications are offered as explanations for why men not only remain uninvolved but even increase their dislike of, and hostility toward, victims. The central idea that emerged from these studies is that this is "a just and orderly world where good behavior is rewarded and bad behavior brings pain." Stated differently: if you are fit, you survive—if unfit, you perish.

The present study investigated some of the conditions that affect people's attitudes toward killing. It was hypothesized that social distance (i.e., the degree of identification with and the degree of perceived threat by persons judged to be "unfit") would increase the respondents' willingness to endorse their killing as a final solution—as long as the final solution was carried out objectively, i.e., scientifically.

Method

The subjects (Ss) were 570 male and female full and part-time University of Hawaii students, ranging from age 17 to 48 years, who were tested in four separate studies. From 20 to 30 subjects were present in each session conducted in a normal classroom.

General Justification for Scientific Application

In the first study 70 Ss were presented with the following statement:

In recent times, a growing concern with the increasing menace of population explosion has taken place. Of particular concern is the fact that the unfit, i.e., the mentally and emotionally unfit, are increasing the population much faster than the emotionally fit and intelligent humans. Unless something drastic is done about this, the day will come when the fit and the intelligent part of the population will find itself in danger. Education and birth-control devices are not succeeding in controlling this population explosion, and unfortunately it has now become necessary to devise new methods of coping with this problem—and new measures are being considered by several of the major powers in the world including our own. One of these devices is euthanasia, which means mercy killing. Such killing is considered by most experts as not only being beneficial to the unfit because it puts them out of their misery or lives, but more importantly it will be beneficial to the healthy, fit, and more educated segment of the population. It is therefore a "final solution" to a grave problem. This should not be a surprising thought since we already practice it in many countries—including our own. We do decide when a human is unfit to live as in the case of capital punishment. What is not clear, however, is which method of killing should be applied, which method is least painful, and who should do the killing and/or decide when killing should be resorted to. For these reasons further research is required and our research project is concerned with this problem. We need to relate intelligent and educated people's decisions to such problems and we are therefore asking for you to help us out. The findings of our studies will be applied to humans once the system has been perfected. At the moment, we need to try this out with animals first and only when the necessary data has been obtained will it be applied to human beings in this and other countries.

It is important that this be studied and applied scientifically. After the experimenter had presented this statement (in a manner denoting the utmost seriousness), the Ss were asked whether they approved of such research provided it was done scientifically.

Present versus Future Threat

In the second study, 120 Ss were presented the same statement with the following additions and changes. Sixty Ss were told that the fit and intelligent population "such as ourselves will be in danger within the next 15 to 20 years." The other 60 Ss were told that the danger to the fit and intelligent population "such as ourselves will come to pass in about another 70 to 100 years."

The Use of Warfare versus Application of Scientific Methods

In the third study, 110 Ss were tested. Fifty-five Ss were also told that "only intelligent and selective warfare" would be helpful in reducing the population of the unfit. The other 55 Ss were read the standard statement, i.e., scientific application.

Degrees of Identification

In the fourth and final study, 270 Ss were tested in three groups of 90 Ss each. Again the basic statement was presented to them with the following variations. Group I was told that "the unfit population was increasing in the U.S.A." Group II was told only that "minority groups were increasing too fast," and group III was told "the Asian population explosion was getting out of hand."

After all the Ss in each of the studies had anonymously indicated whether or not they approved of the respective solutions, they were asked to respond to seven additional questions, most of which were concerned with practical aspects of "systematic" killing.

When all the data had been obtained, the experimenter carefully explained the true purpose of the study and invited further discussion and comments. It was clear that the respondents had taken the basic statement very seriously, as indicated by the emotional statements and rationalizations that many of the respondents expressed.

Results

It will be recalled that the responses obtained from 570 Ss were distributed over four different studies. Each of these presented a different set of justifications endorsing the need to kill people and, in so doing, providing for a final solution to the danger of population increase of unfits, minority groups, and Asians. Table 21.1 shows the number of people in each of the four studies who endorsed the idea of killing as a final solution, as well as the number of people who did not endorse it.

In the first study, 70 Ss were told that the population explosion was

Table 21.1 Distribution of Subjects Approving or Disapproving of a "Final Solution"

		Approve	Disapprove	N	P
Study I.	Do you approve or disapprove of scientific research and application of the final solution to the emotionally and mentally unfit?	47	23	70	<.01
Study II.	. . . the fit and intelligent population such as ourselves will be in danger within the next				
	15–20 years	41	19	60	
	70–100 years	26	34	60	
		67	53	120	<.05
Study III.	Do you approve or disapprove of application of the final solution through				
	warfare	16	39	55	
	science	35	20	55	
		51	59	110	<.01
Study IV.	Do you approve or disapprove of the application of the scientific research to achieve a final solution? The unfit population was defined as				
	in U.S.A.	57	33	90	
	minority groups	61	29	90	
	Asian populations	43	47	90	
		161	109	270	<.05
Total for all conditions		326	244	570	<.05

greater among "the emotionally and mentally unfit." Of the 70 Ss, 47 of them endorsed such scientific and objective research. The remaining 23 Ss said that it would not be a good idea. In other words, almost two-thirds of the Ss endorsed the idea of the final solution, provided it was done "scientifically."

In the second study, which involved 120 Ss, 60 Ss were told that the population explosion of these emotionally and mentally unfit would present a danger to the healthy and fit like ourselves within the next 15 to 20 years (i.e., within our own lifetime). The other 60 Ss were told the same except that the dangers presented by the population explosion of the emotionally and otherwise unfit would not materialize for another 70 to 100 years, e.g., the implication being that they would be a future threat but not a threat within the lifetime of the subject. Of the 60 Ss who believed that the population explosion would present a danger within their own lifetime, 41 Ss (about two-thirds) approved of the scientific study and application of the final solution. Only 19 Ss (about one-third) did not express their endorsement. Among the other 60 Ss who believed that the danger would not materialize in their own lifetime, only 26 Ss expressed their endorsement. The remaining 34 Ss did not endorse such research. This, too, is significant ($p < .05$). Hence the dimension of time (i.e., the perception of present versus future threat) seems to be important.

The third study involved 110 Ss, of whom 55 Ss were given the standard story. The other 55 Ss were told a modified story. Instead of involving scientific application, the experimenter explained that experts have concluded that only intelligent and selective application of modern warfare can achieve the necessary elimination of the "unfit" segments in the world population. Consistent with our earlier findings, 35 Ss endorsed and 20 Ss did not endorse the scientific approach to the final solution. Of the other 55 Ss, however, only 16 endorsed the final solution through warfare, whereas 39 Ss rejected warfare as a desirable ($p < .01$). Whether this is to be interpreted as a general disapproval or fear of warfare, or of its application to the final solution, is unclear. Warfare implies danger to everyone in spite of official claims to the contrary. Science is seen as systematic, controlled, and true. In view of the other findings, it is not likely that most of these subjects were opposed to a final solution per se.

The last study was conducted with 270 Ss, who were randomly assigned to each of three groups of 90 Ss each. The first group was given the same basic story with the exception that the problem population was defined as "the unfits in U.S.A." The second group was told that the population was the "minority groups." The third group had the "Asian populations" defined as the source of danger. Table 21.1 shows the distribution of the 270 Ss endorsing or not endorsing the final solution. Of the 90 Ss, 57 indicated their endorsement of the final solution for the "unfit populations in U.S.A.," whereas 61 Ss did, and 29 Ss did not, endorse the killing of the "minority groups." By contrast, only 43 Ss endorsed the final solution for the Asian population, whereas 47 Ss disapproved (p < .05). It is noteworthy that the proportion of Ss indicating their endorsement of a final solution for the Asian populations was much smaller than for either of the other two. The fact that approximately 230 of the subjects were Americans of Oriental ancestry may, of course, account for this finding.

The data presented do not clearly support our expectation that Ss' willingness to give their endorsement was related to social distance or identification with the victims. It is reasonable to assume that identification with others is an important variable, but that it was not tested adequately in this study. The expectation that perception of present-versus-future threat would affect the Ss endorsement of a "final solution" was supported. The overall finding that a large majority of the Ss was willing to endorse the application of the final solution to others shows how readily that justifications for killing are accepted.

Table 21.2 shows the responses to a set of seven questions asked verbally of each of the 570 Ss regardless of whether they had favored or not favored scientific control of population explosion (by scientific killing). The Ss were told:

> Regardless of whether you endorse or do not endorse the systematic application of science or other means to the elimination of people presenting a threat to the welfare of the fit population, please answer each of the following questions as conscientiously as you can.

It is clear that a surprisingly large number of the Ss took these questions seriously, and that psychological or other constraints are not very evident. All that is evident is the uncritical acceptance of a final solution—legitimized through accepted justifications. It is of interest to note that the largest number of "no" responses are to Question 2 which asked whether "persons who make the decision should also carry out the act of killing." From

Table 21.2 Distribution of Subjects Responding to Each of Seven Verbally Asked Questions

		N
1.	Do you agree that there will always be people who are more fit in terms of survival than not?	
	(a) yes	516
	(b) no	54
2.	If such killing is judged necessary, should the person or persons who make the decisions also carry out the act of killing?	
	(a) yes	325
	(b) no	245
3.	Would it work better if one person was responsible for the killing and another person carried out the act?	
	(a) yes	451
	(b) no	119
4.	Would it be better if several people pressed a button but only one button would cause death? This way anonymity would be preserved and no one would know who actually did the killing.	
	(a) yes	367
	(b) no	203
5.	What would you judge to be the best and most efficient method of induced death?	
	(a) electrocution	10
	(b) painless poison	53
	(c) painless drugs	517
6.	If you were required by law to assist would you prefer to be:	
	(a) the one who assists in the decision?	483
	(b) the one who assists in the killing?	46
	(c) the one who assists with both the decision and the killing?	8
	(d) no answer	33
7.	Most people agree that in matters of life and death, extreme caution is required. Most people also agree that under extreme circumstances, it is entirely just to eliminate those judged dangerous to the general welfare. Do you agree?	
	(a) yes	517
	(b) no	27
	(c) undecided	26

the responses to the other questions one can interpret this as a reluctance to be directly involved in killing but not as a reluctance to assist otherwise with the process. The distribution of responses to Question 6 is consistent with such interpretation.

Discussion

The overall data demonstrate that the values ordinarily associated with a commitment to, and a belief in, the sacredness or worthwhileness of human life are not unqualifiedly shared by everyone. Many explanations have been offered to questions about genocide, mass killing, and violence of any sort (e.g., wicked leadership, concepts of duty, man's destructive instincts, and psychological variables such as obedience). These reasons, however, do not clearly explain why people sanction such actions and develop the required attitudes and rationalizations to support them. While Milgram pointed out that "the crux of the study of obedience is to systematically vary the factors believed to alter the degree of obedience to the experimental command," he also recognized that *many* aspects can be varied, such as the source of command, the content and form of command, the instrumentalities for its execution, the target object, the general social setting, etc. These aspects were in varying degrees present in this study. Hence a few comments are in order.

1. To the subjects, the experimenter was perceived as an authority (i.e., a professor of social psychology). This made the experimenter trustworthy and his statement legitimate. The social setting, therefore, was such that the respondents could express their belief without being coerced. It should be remembered that the subjects responded in private and anonymously.

2. The perception by the subjects that the "final solution" was serving a worthy purpose (putting the unfit out of their misery and at the same time removing the danger to the fit like themselves) no doubt influenced their responses.

3. While the subjects had not voluntarily committed themselves to helping out the experimenter, the fact that they were asked for their assistance was flattering. The tendency to agree with the experimenter is thus made stronger—especially in combination with their perception of him as an authority, and of the proposal as serving a real need.

4. To state their approval makes the subjects not only agree with the experimenter's position that further research is needed, but is also consistent

with their wish to do what they can to reduce any potential danger to themselves. Under such circumstances, the psychological identification with the potential victims remains weak or nonexistent.

5. As in Milgram's study, the experiment gave the subjects little time for reflection before they responded. The responses were raw, immediate, and unthinking, and thus likely to reflect some basic attitudes.

6. The conflict was perceived in terms of who should survive, the "fit" or the "unfit." It was not a conflict in Milgram's sense of a disposition not to harm others and a disposition to obey or agree with authority. To be unwilling to approve harm to others increases the likelihood that harm will come to ourselves. It is either them or us. Either they are eliminated, or we may all perish.

This study indicates that the attitudes existing among the general population, the way individuals perceive their relationship to others, and the extent to which such relationships carry different degrees of trust and feelings of personal security, all play a significant role in determining the acceptance or rejection of violence and killing. In any case, the attitudinal disposition not to harm others seems to be weak, and especially so when others are perceived to represent some threat to one's own security. The experimental reasons provided the subjects were agreed to and eagerly adopted as justification for eliminating the unfit—in the absence, it must be stressed, of any obedience to command.

It is possible to argue that such genocidal attitudes directed toward the helpless and the unfit are ordinarily not particularly salient to the average person. Once, however, threat is perceived, such attitudes do become salient, and the justifications offered by the experimenter are readily endorsed. They did believe that the final solution was justified, but they needed to have the justification articulated.

During the postexperimental session when the subjects were informed that the original statement was not to be taken seriously and that no such scientific research was planned, the subjects became exceedingly defensive; not so much because they had been deceived by the experimenter, but due to their discovery that they did harbor attitudes that under normal circumstances they would have denied. Once they had committed themselves to the "just" idea of the final solution, they began to defend themselves. A typical defense was that "self-preservation is the first law of life." Some pointed out that some clergy had said that it was okay to shoot anyone trying to enter their bunker during nuclear attacks. It is not necessary to go into all the rationalizations offered—all variants of Social Darwinism. Suffice it to say that most subjects worked hard to justify their original endorsement: "War has always existed and killing is part of man and therefore must serve a purpose." The strength and intensity with which the subjects stuck to their justifications were real. And so were their beliefs that mass killings can be justified.

Social critics have pointed out that America has a history of violence associated with the conquering of a new continent and the racial groups in the population. Conflicts and tensions are built into the American system and may well account for the ease with which justifications are offered and accepted by so many of the subjects. It is possible that racism, claimed by some (Sartre 1968; Presidential Commission on Civil Disorder 1968) to be a basic American attitude, such as antiblack, anti-Asiatic, anti-Mexican, etc., and which has deep historical roots, is associated with the readiness with which our respondents endorsed the idea of scientific research and application of the final solution.

It is proper to conclude by quoting from a poem by Merton entitled, "Chant to be used in processions around a site with furnaces." It is a monologue by a commander of a Nazi extermination camp who is to be hanged for genocide and was cited by Jerome Frank (1966). Merton concluded his poem with the lines:

> You smile at my career, but would do as I did if you know yourself and dared. In my day we worked hard. We say what we did. Our self-sacrifice was conscientious and complete. Our work was faultless and detailed. Do not think yourself better because you burn up friends and enemies with long-range missiles without ever seeing what you have done.

To this poem it may be added: Do not think we are better as long as so many of us seem unthinkingly to endorse programs which in their spirit are genocidal, even though we may believe we have legitimate justification such as self-preservation, or merely because such programs are advocated in the respectable name of science.

References

Frank, J. "Group Psychology and the Elimination of War." In *Peace Is Possible*, edited by Elizabeth Hollins. New York: Grossman, 1966.

Latane, B., and J. Darley. "When Will People Help in a Crisis?" *Psychology Today*, December 1968.

Lerner, Melvin J., and Gail Matthews. "Reactions to Suffering of Others under Conditions of Indirect Responsibility." *Journal of Personality and Social Psychology* 5 (1967): 319–25.

Lerner, Melvin J., and Carolyn H. Simmons. "Observers' Reaction to the 'Innocent Victim'—Compassion or Rejection?" *Journal of Personality and Social Psychology* 4 (1966): 203–10.

Milgram, Stanley. "Behavioral Study of Obedience." *Journal of Abnormal and Social Psychology* 67 (1963): 371–78.

Sartre, Jean-Paul. "On Genocide." *Ramparts*, February 1968.

Walster, Elaine. "Assignment of Responsibility for an Accident." *Journal of Personality and Social Pscyhology* 4 (1966): 73–79.

22

Deciding for Yourself:
The Objections

DANIEL MAGUIRE

IT is fair to say that if you do not know the objections to your position, you do not know your position. This was a firm conviction in the great medieval universities, where the position of the adversaries was given unique prominence. The *Summa* of Thomas Aquinas, for example, leads off each article with the objections to his position, and quite regularly he makes the principal points of his case not in exposition but rather in response to the objections. There is a wisdom in this medieval tactic (I refuse to accept the term *medieval* as pejorative) that we could well reappraise and reappropriate. In modern terms, it recognized the dialectical nature of our approach to truth, or, more simply, it recognized that the delicate reality of truth is grasped by our minds only in the tension of point and counterpoint, position and counterposition. "We know in part," said Paul the Apostle with masterful epistemological insight. And only by staying in contact with the parts that others are on to can we move our knowledge from more imperfect to less imperfect. That said, let us look at the main objections to the idea of choosing to end your own life by positive means.

Reprinted from *Death By Choice,* pp. 131–40, 141–55, and 156–64, with the permission of the author and Doubleday & Company, Inc. Copyright 1973, 1974 by Daniel Maguire. Some footnotes omitted.

The Domino Theory

Writing in the *Indiana Law Journal*, Luis Kutner (1968) observes matter-of-factly that efforts to legalize "voluntary euthanasia" have been persistently rejected because they "appear to be an entering wedge which opens the door to possible mass euthanasia and genocide." What Kutner says is a commonplace in the literature that treats of death by choice. He is evoking, of course, the ghost of Nazi Germany, where some 275,000 people are thought to have perished in "euthanasia centers." There is no precedent that is more regularly brought forward than this one, and well it should be, for what happened in Germany did not happen in an ancient tribe centuries ago, but in a modern state with which we have not a few bonds of cultural kinship.

Analogies, of course, are our way of knowing. We meet something new and immediately a number of similar or analogous realities come to mind. We come to know the unknown by relating it to the related known. That is all well and good. But analogies are also tricky, and the mind can indulge in false analogues. By this I mean that we can compare a present situation to a past one and be so impressed by the possible similarities that we miss the differences.

It is argued that German euthanasia in the Nazi period began at a more moderate level. It was to involve only the severely and hopelessly sick. Originally, it was not to be allowed for Jews since it was seen as a privilege for "true" Germans. But once begun it grew and spread preposterously, until hundreds of thousands of socially unproductive, defective, and, eventually, racially "tainted" persons were liquidated. "Useless eaters," Hitler called them. And it all started, as Leo Alexander (1949) writes, "from small beginnings." The conclusion drawn from this is that if we allow any exceptions, any "small beginnings," we too shall fall into the excesses of the Nazis. For this reason positive acts to end the lives of consenting persons, or life-ending actions taken by those persons themselves, are to be seen as absolutely unconscionable.

Let me begin to confront this Nazi analogy by the technique which past logicians called *retorqueo argumentum* . . . turning the example back on the one who uses it. This technique does not disprove the argument offered, but it does conduct exploratory surgery on its presuppositions.

Therefore, let it be similarly argued that the Nazi war machine began from "small beginnings." It began when the first humans began to kill one another to settle differences. Through the process of military evolution, this grew to the preposterous point of *Blitzkrieg* and the Nazi military atrocities of World War II. Therefore, relying on the Nazi experience and relying on many other ghastly historical examples of the abuse of military kill-power (which can make this case stronger than that against euthanasia) we can conclude that all forms of killing, even in self-defense, should be morally banned. We should, in a word, become absolute pacifists, and not allow the "small beginnings," which have throughout history generated bloodbath after bloodbath. If the Nazi analogy forbids euthanasia, then it should also, and indeed *a fortiori*, given the history of military carnage, forbid war.

We could make a similar *retorqueo* argument regarding sterilization. The Nazi practice of eugenic sterilization might be argued as the basis for an absolutist stance against all sterilization. Add to the Nazi experience here the excesses revealed in the United States, where children were sterilized apparently without consent (*Time*, July 23, 1973). Given these facts of abuse, should not the possibility of abuse be precluded by an absolute moral ban on sterilization?

Similarly, and finally, could not a case be constructed against the morality of developing and retaining nuclear weapons by citing the Hiroshima and Nagasaki atrocities? Such attacks could happen again. Development and deployment are not even "small beginnings." Therefore, if the thrust of the Nazi analogy used against death by choice is valid, all these should be considered, again *a fortiori*, as beyond the moral pale.

The answer that would be given to my *retorqueo* arguments here would be that I am overworking analogies and not noting the differences between past and present situations. I would make the same response to the analogy regarding death by choice.

There are many differences between our setting and that of Nazi Germany, however many alarming similarities can be found. I shall note four of them. First, the euthanasia program of the Nazis was an explicit repudiation of the individualistic philosophy that animates this country. Mercy killing for the benefit of the patient was not the point in Germany, and was rejected. People were killed because their life was deemed to be of no value to German society. The uselessness of the patient to the community was decisive. Though this idea was resisted heroically by many Germans, and though the mass destruction of mental patients even had to be revoked by the Nazis due to public outcry, still the German context was all too susceptible to this collectivist form of ethic. The motif of individual rights simply was not as ingrained in the society of Nazi Germany as it is today in our society. Indeed, in our society, it tends to be exaggerated. This makes for a major difference to which the Nazi analogists should advert.

A second weakness in the Nazi analogy is that our society is not nearly so homogeneous as German society. American society, we are discovering as we emerge from illusions of oneness, is made up of "unmeltable ethnics" and conflicting cultures. This does not mean that the whole country cannot get jelled into oneness when civil religion gets activated by some national crisis, though even that is getting more difficult to do. But it does suggest that on matters of individual morality, our pluralism is incorrigible. This would seem to augur well for the possibilities of critical debate on any issue such as death by choice. Again, it is a difference worth noting before we concede that the Nazi "parade of horrors" will be our portion if we admit the possibility of some exceptions in the area of voluntary imposition of death.

A third reason to limit the Nazi analogy is the Nazi experience itself. We now have that grotesque episode emblazoned on our cultural memory. The stark experiences of Nazism have become important symbols in our collective consciousness. This does not mean that knowledge is virtue, but it does suggest that deeply ingrained knowledge of human wickedness can help to deter. The wickedness has a harder time now slipping in unbeknownst. Our *when* is different from their *when*, and that is a difference. Their experience gives us a vantage point that makes our situation to that degree advantageously dissimilar.

Fourthly and finally, the opening of the question of voluntary dying is now arising in an atmosphere where death is being reevaluated as a potential good, not in an atmosphere where the utilitarian value of certain lives is the issue. How a question arises is important for the conclusions that may follow. The question currently is not whether life is worth living, but whether death, in its own good time, is worth dying. This cultural reevaluation of death is another major and influential difference.

In conclusion then, on the Nazi analogy, it is illuminating. It gives us an example of the iniquity of men that in our earlier naïveté we might have thought implausible. It must never be allowed to leak out of our memories, for of such chastening memories is moral progress made. We must face the painful fact that the Nazis were, like us, members of the species that calls itself *sapiens*, but is nevertheless capable of staggering malice. One can grant all of this and still be able to say that the decision to end life voluntarily in certain cases may be moral if there is proportionate reason to do so.

The domino or wedge theory, however, may be presented in more subtle dress. It is inferred that if we allow exceptions even in the case of a mature adult who wishes his death in the face of unbearable alternatives, the logic of the dominoes will still obtain and send us cascading all the way to compulsory imposition of death. As G. K. Chesterton put it: "Some are proposing what is called euthanasia; at present only a proposal for killing those who are a nuisance to themselves; but soon to be applied to those who are a nuisance to other people" (quoted by Kamisar 1958). At the very least, it is argued, there will be as a result of this a general erosion of the respect for the sanctity of life. Those who object in this fashion do not see exceptions as the harbingers of a new Hitlerian *Reich* but as dangerous slarckenings in our already precarious grasp of the sacredness of life.

I respond to this version of the domino theory by distinguishing between the theory and the sociopsychological effects of exception making in the matter of death. Theoretically, the objection fails; psychologically, it has something going for it. At the level of theory, the objection is saying that if X is allowed, then Y and Z follow. If you grant X, you cannot draw a line before Y and Z. The assertion is theoretically gratuitous. It has been said that ethics like art is precisely a matter of knowing where to draw lines. Without the drawing of lines, there is no ethics or no art. More directly to the point, the cardinal fact here is that X *is* not Y, nor *is* it Z. And since they are different realities, they may merit a different moral judgment. Ethics is not just a matter of logical deduction from principle. It is also a matter of evaluating different empirical realities in their morally meaningful concreteness. For this reason a moral principle (like "Thou shalt not kill") is not like a balloon, which, if pierced at the point of X, deflates also at the points of Y and Z.

Psychologically, however, it should be granted that an impetus toward excess can be created when we make exceptions. There is a danger here that must not be minimized. The history of warfare proves it and after any war, there tends to be an increase in violent crime when the warriors return home. It seems hard for some to turn the killing off. The history of abortion in many countries indicates a similar psychological thrust toward excess. We can dissipate a principle in exceptions.

This reaction is especially likely when a taboo begins to crumble. Taboos forbid certain actions absolutely. Taboo is not open to reasonable exception. It simply forbids—by edict, as it were. When reason and light begin to pierce the province of a taboo, the situation is both promising and dangerous. It is promising because ethics by taboo is not ethics. Taboo does not give reasons; ethics must. Movement out of taboo then, intimates progress. It is dangerous, however, because a study of taboo shows that taboos, even those that seem silly at first blush, are rarely mindless or valueless. They often represent a primitive way to fence off a value by banning intrusion with no ifs, ands, buts, or unlessments. Taboo, therefore, represents one far swing of the pendulum. Reaction to taboo can swing you to the other extreme. The experience of liberation from taboo is exhilarating and a heady wine. It can lead to a binge of exceptions before the value experiences once encapsulated in unyielding taboo can become ensconced in a mature and discerning ethics.

This possibility of abuse might suggest two remedies: keep the taboo (on the grounds that where there are *no* exceptions there can be no *abusive* exceptions) or make the necessary distinctions where there are differences and strive to contain the possible abuses. There is an old Latin axiom that pertains to this problem: *abusus non tollit usum*, the fact that something can be abused does not mean that it should not be used. Rather, the use should be promoted if it is good, and the abuse curtailed by every means available.

To say that there is no possible way of curtailing abuse if we grant the morality of some voluntary, self-imposed (or assisted) acts of death by choice, and then to conclude that because of that impossibility, no such act can be moral, is an immense and unwarranted leap. Such an argument would not be accepted in other contexts. Suppose one were to argue that all investigatory or experimental medicine, even when performed on consenting subjects, is immoral on the grounds of the extreme danger of abuse. If one were to impose the logic of the domino, a similar case could be made. One could say that, theoretically, the domino or wedge theory does not hold, but given the nature of man, abuse will follow upon use, involuntary experimentation upon voluntary. To support such a case one could turn to Dr. Henry K. Beecher (1968), who reports on the kinds of experiments that go on. He is not selecting rare and extraordinary cases, but assures us that "examples can be found wherever experimentation in man occurs to any significant extent."

To cite a few of his randomly selected examples: 31 subjects, 29 of them black, were used in a study of cyclopropane. Toxic levels of carbon dioxide were achieved and maintained for considerable lengths of time, creating a condition that often leads to fatal fibrillation of the heart.

Whether or not the subjects gave consent, this type of experimentation is a sort of medical roulette. Without the consent of the subjects, the experiment would be gross in its immorality. With the consent, the case becomes open to discussion, but one wonders whether 31 subjects could be found to accept experiments at these stakes if they were really informed as to the nature of the stakes.

In another case, 22 human subjects were injected with live cancer cells. They were "merely told they would be receiving 'some cells.'" One of the investigators admitted that he would not have submitted to such a risky experiment himself.

In another case, a small piece of a patient's cancerous tumor was transplanted into her mother. The mother volunteered for the experiment. The purpose of those who reported the experiment was "the hope of gaining a little better understanding of cancer immunity and in the hope that the production of tumor antibodies might be helpful in the treatment of the cancer patient." The daughter died the following day. The mother died 450 days later from the cancer that had spread from the original transplant.

A final example concerns the treatment of patients suffering from acute streptococcic pharyngitis. For experimental reasons, penicillin was withheld from 525 men despite the investigator's avowed knowledge that "penicillin and other antibiotics will prevent the subsequent development of rheumatic fever." Dr. Beecher reports the result: "Thus, 25 men were crippled, perhaps for life." He adds the significant data that the subjects were not informed, did not consent, and were not aware that any kind of experiment was being performed.

Note well, Dr. Beecher is not detailing experiments conducted in Nazi Germany, but "practices found in industry, in the universities, and university hospitals and private hospitals, in the government, the army, the air force, the navy, the Public Health Service, the National Institutes of Health, and the Veterans Administration." He cites a salient and portentous motive for research experimentation by observing that, in recent years, few if any doctors achieved professorships until they proved themselves productive in investigatory research. From the patient's viewpoint, that introduces a conflict of interest. In spite of these gory examples, which Beecher says "are by no means rare" and which indicate not what might happen but what has happened, I would not see the domino theory as proving that all human experimentation is immoral. Neither do I find my colleagues in ethics rushing to that conclusion. A harsh judgment must be levied against abuses of investigatory medicine, and defenses against them must be mounted, but experimental medicine, under proper conditions, justified by proportionate reasons, may be morally good. The abuse does not make all use wrong.

The matter of experimentation is, I judge, especially useful because it shows the fallacy in the use of the domino or wedge theory used against death by choice. Whereas actual and very impressive abuses in experimentation (including death, mutilation, and deception) do not lead to the conclusion that all experimentation is immoral, the *potential* abuses of death by choice are offered to support the judgment that all death by choice is immoral. If it can be shown that the dangers inherent in death by choice are worse and unavoidable, the case against death by choice will stand. Short of that, this argument fails.

Those who use the domino theory to ground their assertion that each and every act of voluntary death by choice is immoral are trying to prove an immense thesis in terms of foreseeable effects alone. This is a species of what I have been calling one-rubric ethics. It is a simplistic and partial approach to the question. It furthermore does not prove that moral doomsday follows inevitably from the admission that some mercy killings appear justifiable. It simply presumes that we have no way of preventing abuses of this moral freedom.

Also, those who argue this way leave themselves open to the charge of the British philosopher Anthony Flew. Flew (1969) argues for voluntary euthanasia only. He does not argue the case for ending the lives of those who are not in a position to consent because they are permanently unconscious. Flew is impatient with those who respond to this argument by saying that they cannot countenance the involuntary euthanasia which presumably would follow from the voluntary kind. His retort: "Anyone, therefore, who dismisses what is in fact being contended on the gratuitously irrelevant grounds that he could not tolerate compulsory euthanasia, may very reasonably be construed as thereby tacitly admitting inability to meet and to overcome the case actually presented."

The domino or wedge theory warns us against the possible diminishment of respect for life that may flow from the acknowledgment of another exception to the principle that forbids killing. To this extent it is to be taken seriously. It focuses our attention on foreseeable effects, and good ethics requires this because effects *partially* constitute the moral object. The domino theory does not, however, prove that every single act of voluntary death by choice is immoral. To attempt to achieve so much so simplistically is to fall under the indictment of the ancient adage: *qui nimis probat, nihil probat.* He who proves too much, proves nothing. . . .

Playing God

In one form or other the objection is often heard that to take steps to end life is playing God, for it is God's prerogative to determine the end of life, not man's. To terminate a life is to violate the property rights of God. As the objection is often phrased, it sounds like a program of pure pacifism. Interrogation, however, usually reveals that the objector does not object to killing in war. There, apparently, we have a permit from God to go at it, using appropriate ethical calculations.

The objection is, at root, a kind of religious, biologistic determinism. Now that, admittedly, is a mouthful. In more kindly language, what the objection implies is that God's will is identified with the processes of man's physical and biological nature. When God wants you to die, your organs will fail or disease will overcome you. Organic collapse is the medium through which God's will is manifested. Positive action to accelerate death, however, would amount to wresting the matter out of God's hands and taking it into your own. It is a sin of arrogant presumption.

If this objection were taken literally, it would paralyze technological man. And this, of course, would mean that it would paralyze medicine. For if it is wrong to accelerate death, by what right do we delay it by ingenious cures and techniques? Is not medicine tampering with God's property rights by putting off the moment of death and thus frustrating God in his effort to reclaim his property?

Men who believe that God's will is manifested through the physical facts and events of life would have to sit back and await the good pleasure of Nature. All efforts to step in and take over by reshaping the earth in accord with our own designs would be blasphemous. We are here at the level of discourse expressible in the statement: if God wanted you to fly, he would have given you wings.

The mentality of this objection is utterly at odds with genuine Christian theology. According to the Christian view, man is created in the image of the creator God. He is thus himself commissioned to creativity, a co-creator with God destined to exercise fruitful and ingenious stewardship over the earth. He is not a pawn of the earth's forces, but a participator in God's providence, invited by his nature and his God to provide for himself and for others. This, of course, is not to say that Christian theology is committed to death by choice. It is, however, to say that the presuppositions of the "playing God" objection are not Christian even though Christians are among those who offer it.

Philosophically, there is in the "playing God" objection a problem with the idea of authority. Many people have difficulty believing that they have moral authority over their dying. One of the principal reasons why this question is opening up for reconsideration today is that the idea of authority is being rethought. This is due in no small part to technological man's new awareness of his abilities. Professor Diana Crane alludes to this when she says that there has been

> . . . a change in social attitudes toward human intervention at both the beginning and the end of life. Birth and Death are now viewed as events which need not be blindly accepted by human beings. . . . Suicide and euthanasia are being tolerated to a greater extent, or at least viewed differently. Consequently, we are in the midst of developing new ethics. (quoted by Morris 1970)

The natural course of events is less and less seen as normative. Unlike his ancestors, technological man is inclined to rise up, not lie down before fate. Obviously, he can overdo this, as our ecocatastrophe bears witness. But it is an apparently irreversible fact of our lives that we envision ourselves less as *homo actus* (man acted upon) and more as *homo agens* (man achieving).

The notion of moral authority is unavoidably affected by this major shift in self-consciousness. If we go back into the centuries, we find that the effort to explain unaccustomed exercises of moral freedom relied heavily on divine intervention. Thus Samson's pulling the house down on himself was seen as justifiable suicide. The justification, however, came from the fact that Samson was divinely inspired. Otherwise there would be no way of knowing that this was a good act. Likewise St. Apollonia saved her virtue by throwing herself into a fire. Her action, too, was deemed good because she was judged to be divinely inspired.

Thomas Aquinas even managed to justify acts of adultery and fornication by this notion of divine authority. He did this by saying that these acts of intercourse with someone who is not one's wife, were not really fornication or adultery when they were divinely mandated. Thomas puts it this way (in his *Summa Theologica*): "Consequently intercourse with any woman, by the command of God, is neither adultery nor fornication." (Clearly, a divine command in these matters is not easily come by, so Thomas was not being all that permissive.)

Thomas uses this same approach to justify the direct taking of innocent life. He considered the case of God's command to Abraham to kill his own son and concluded that whoever kills either the innocent or the unjust by divine command does not sin. Thus direct ending of innocent life is moral and good if God commands you to do it. Thomas is not saying that something is good just because God commands it. It is his position that God can only command that which is good. Thus, in these cases, Thomas is conceding that the direct taking of innocent life such as Abraham was ordered to do was a good moral action. The command of God *revealed* that it was good; it did not *make* it good. Thomas was a realist, not a nominalist. This meant that he believed that things are not good because commanded; they could only be commanded if they are good. For Thomas and his colleagues, given their cultural setting, suicide or direct ending of life could only be known to be good if God gave an explicit order. Authority was from on high. Thus, in effect, there could be no knowable exceptions to the self-killing principle without a mandate.

This thought is not very palatable to a twentieth-century mind for this reason: we have come to see that it is not through burning bushes but through thinking minds that God reveals the holy places of human freedom. The divine mandate is to think and feel and listen and do all of the things that make a moral being fully alive in all of his sensitivities. Moral man does not stand idly all day looking into the heavens awaiting a miracle of knowledge; the miracle is his own mind. And modern religious man is no less religious for so locating the miracle and for availing himself of it. Moral authority is seen now as coming, not from a mountaintop, but from within the struggling moral community, where men attempt to know the limits of their God-given moral freedom.

Notice, however, that we are not entirely parting company with the ancients on the issue of whether direct termination of life could be moral, but only on how we know that it can be moral. Moral authority is now seen as discoverable. Applied to the question of death by choice, we need not await a miraculous divine revelation of the sort that Abraham is said to have had, to assume this freedom. Rather we must probe and see whether there are proportionate and good reasons to recognize this moral dominion over our dying. To do this is not to play God but, if you will, to play man. It is to do what is proper to man as man, a being with power to deliberate and to act on his deliberations when that action appears to achieve what is good.

Christians and other religious persons who would oppose mercy killing must not pretend there is a divine edict against it. Father Bernard Häring (1973), who opposes euthanasia, puts it this way: "In earlier times, the general argument, "You may not choose when to fall into the arms of God who alone is Lord over life and death" seemed sufficient. Today however, it is not as simple as that because Christian Scientists and the Witnesses of Jehovah invoke this argument equally in proscribing blood transfusions." Häring might also have added that the same argument was used by Catholics and others against the control of birth as is now used against the control of death. When Häring goes on to argue against euthanasia, he does what he has to do. He tries to find reasons against it. The reasons that he offers (e.g., "the wedge reaction") I do not find compelling, but his manner of argumentation is correct. He is seeking reasons to support a position that is not self-evident one way or the other.

Consent or Despair?

We are considering the objections against death by choice when the patient makes the decision for himself. These cases are easier to judge morally than cases where the decision is made for someone else now unconscious. How can we judge that a person has made a free decision for death? Is the patient just undergoing a temporary period of depression? Or could it be something worse than depression—his relatives? Could those who care for him be tiring of the burden and communicating to him subtly that he avail himself of his moral freedom for death by choice? Could there be, as in the mystery stories, an eager band of relatives chafing at the bit in anticipation of a rich legacy? Though this is more of a danger when we speak of deciding for someone who has lapsed into coma, the desire for death could be prompted by the selfish needs of others.

It is, of course, a fact that a person suffering does have his moments of despair when he feels that his resources of patience are spent and he can endure no more. Then he says with Job (7:15): "Strangling I would welcome rather, and death itself, than these my sufferings!" However, Job did have better days. "After his trials, Job lived on until he was a hundred and forty years old, and saw his children and his children's children up to the fourth generation" (Job 42:16). Job's story of despair, then, had a happy ending. A terminal patient cannot perhaps expect as much, although there are remarkable cases of remission of the worst of illnesses. Still, the possibility for a premature wish for death is a real problem.

Dr. G. E. Schreiner (1966) of Georgetown University Hospital reports on a kidney patient who asked to be taken off dialysis. The result of this, of course, would be his death. Dr. Schreiner gave the patient a very thorough dialysis treatment to put him in excellent chemical shape and then asked him if he still wanted to discontinue. "Don't listen to me," he replied. "That's my uremia talking, not me. I want to stay in the program." Another patient, however, said the same thing and was given the same special treatment. He persisted in his desire to stop treatment, and so he withdrew and died. (Interestingly, Dr. Schreiner says, "We allowed him to withdraw," as though the decision were the doctors' and not the patient's, even though the patient was in full and reflective possession of his senses.)

In other illnesses, it is not possible to give a treatment that will provide such favorable physical conditions for a decision. The problem of temporary depression is more difficult in these cases. Some proposed euthanasia bills have tried to meet this problem. The Voluntary Euthanasia bill offered in 1969 in England proposed a 30-day waiting period after a person made a declaration for death by euthanasia. The declaration could be revoked at any time in that period. In some cases, this could leave a person in unrelievable pain for a longer period than he might wish, but it does represent an effort to guarantee real consent.

The ways in which relatives and/or medical personnel could suction the desire to live out of a patient are not easily warded off by legislation. At the level of morality, however, the sin of such persons is heinous. We spoke of the danger of making a sick person feel useless and therefore worthless as though our ability to be of use was the base of our human dignity. Likewise, uncomfortable as we tend to be with suffering and the approach of death, it is possible to insinuate some of our inability to cope with the fact of dying. This, too, could create a premature desire for the release of death.

Most important in this regard is an awareness that it may be the patient's uremia or something else that is requesting death. If the patient is open to it, good counseling can help him evaluate his situation. Sometimes, the closer you are to the patient, the less help you would be in this kind of a decision; other kinds of closeness can give a friend or relative better qualifications than a professional counselor. Overall, the problem of consent is not insuperable, but it is also not to be minimized.

Suppose a Cure is Found

In 1921, George R. Minot was found to have diabetes at the age of 36. For the next two years he fought a losing battle to control his disease by diet, the only means then available. In 1923, insulin became available and Dr. Minot's life was saved. After this, Minot went to work on a series of experiments that culminated in his 1927 report that large quantities of liver could bring about the regeneration of red cells in the bone marrow. This was an effective treatment of pernicious anemia and won for Minot the Nobel prize in 1934.

This story called dramatic attention to the possibility of a new cure being found to bring sudden and unexpected help for a disease that had been fatal. Many people use this as an argument against death by choice, the idea being that a cure might be just around the corner. Medical science has surprised us before.

The problem of what medicine might do is compounded by what medicine might not be able to do. I refer to the not very fine art of prognosis. Dr. Lasagna (1968) calls this art "an elusive one" and notes that "many an embarrassed doctor has failed to outlive the patient whose immediate doom he prophesied." There are also numerous cases of regression of a disease, including cancer, for no apparent reason. Dr. Lasagna writes: "Even where questionable cases are ruled out because of inadequate information, there are still a sizable number of patients considered by cancer experts to show spontaneous disappearance of what appears to be typical malignant disease."

Therefore, prognosis is fallible, diseases go into unaccountable remission, the power of life is unpredictable. How could we ever impose death—an irreversible condition—since, where there is life, there is hope?

In response, I would say that for all its fallibility, prognosis can enjoy a high degree of certainty. The percentage of correct diagnosis is exceptionally high in cancer cases, and these are the patients most likely to opt for death by choice. Other terminal conditions, especially in their later stages, are open to very precise prognosis. These are cases where there is life but no hope.

With regard to the possibility of a cure, there are advanced cases where death would remain a certainty even if a cure were to be found today, due to the extent of deterioration. Also, as Anthony Flew says: ". . . the advance of medicine has not reached a stage where all diseases are curable. And no one seriously thinks that it has. At most this continuing advance has suggested that we need never despair of finding cures *some day*."

This objection sins by abstraction. It tenders a vague hope for medical miracles as an argument against death by choice. In particular cases this vague hope can be dismissed by the concrete facts.

They Shoot Horses, Don't They?

Euthanasia is a bad word. It is bad for two reasons: first, it means too many different things to too many people. Secondly, it is bad because it connotes an attitude on suffering that is false.

As to its indefiniteness, Paul Ramsey (1970) says that in current usage it means direct killing and that efforts to use the term in some other way do not succeed. Yet, for example, lawyer Arval Morris (1970) uses it in another way when he says that Pius XII did not uniformly condemn euthanasia. As direct killing Pius certainly did condemn it. The Euthanasia Educational Fund uses the term in two senses and therefore must employ the modifiers active and passive. A *New York Times* editorial (July 3, 1973) speaks of the frequent practice of euthanasia in this country and abroad, and then explains that normally this takes the form of a cessation of extraordinary measures. Moralist Gerald Kelly (1950) has to point out that he is not using the term euthanasia to denote the mere giving of drugs to a dying patient to ease his pain, as some theologians do. Some (e.g., Silving 1954) use the qualifier "pure" euthanasia to describe the use of pain-killers which do not shorten life. Also, in some cases the term has been used to describe dangerous medical experiments performed on human beings. As a result of this confusion, many people sense the need to move away from that term and develop terms that do justice to the various and different ways of meeting death. And so we meet the terms orthothanasia, agathanasia, benemortasia, dysthanasia, antidysthanasia, and mercy killing.

Most often, however, the term euthanasia has reference to direct killing with an accent on relief of suffering. Thus a dictionary definition calls it "an act or method of causing death painlessly, so as to end suffering; advocated by some as a way to deal with the victims of incurable disease." The Voluntary Euthanasia bill of 1969 in England defined euthanasia as "the painless inducement of death." It is to this accent on painlessness that a false philosophy of suffering easily attaches. One of the bad arguments that persistently surfaces in the literature defending euthanasia is in reference to what we do for animals. As the argument goes, we see it as cruel and inhumane to leave an animal in hopeless pain and so we "put him to sleep." Could we do less for one of our own?

Because of this kind of argument, one of the arguments that is brought against any liberalization of the moral right to death by choice is that those who press such a right are infected by a crassly materialistic philosophy of suffering. Since a mistaken philosophy of suffering is reductively a mistaken philosophy of man, this objection is serious. In responding to it, I find myself responding to those who support death by choice with bad arguments (They shoot horses . . .) and to those who rely on those bad arguments to object to death by choice.

The philosophical error involved here is one that should be refutable by observation. Horses and men are different in some rather impressive ways. A horse can be relieved of his suffering but he does not have the human power to transcend that suffering by giving it meaning.

Man is a meaning seeker. Where he finds meaning he is fulfilled, and, by a remarkable alchemy, he can find meaning in the most unlikely experiences. Put in another way, man's consciousness, unlike that of the horse, is open to and geared to the pursuit of the possible that is latent in the actual. The human spirit has a divining power that can detect redemptive possibilities in a situation that would otherwise be crushing and destructive. Were Helen Keller a horse, born blind and deaf, it might have been best to shoot her. Being a person amid other persons, her exquisite possibilities could be and were realized.

Our suffering is human suffering and that means that it is suffering with possibilities. These possibilities may not always be realized, for though we be godly we are not gods. We experience limit. But still, the human capacity to transcend gives human suffering a qualitative distinctiveness.

There is no suggestion here that we return to the views of the past which gave suffering a per se value. Such a value suffering does not have, but rather assumes its meaning, value or disvalue, from the special circumstances of the sufferer. Christians see the crucifixion sufferings of Jesus as meaningful not because they have a sadistic love of crucifixions, but because the circumstances of this particular one lent it a special meaning. Only a sadomasochistic philosophy could see suffering as a value in itself. Of itself it is a disvalue to be alleviated if at all possible. Where no relief is possible, suffering at times can be made meaningfully redemptive through the creative spirit of the sufferer.

First of all, the suffering can be of benefit to the sufferer. As the British lawyer Norman St. John-Stevas put it: "The final stage of an incurable illness can be a wasteland, but it need not be. It can be a vital period in a person's life, reconciling him to life and to death and giving him an interior peace. This is the experience of people who have looked after the dying" (quoted in *America*, May 2, 1970). It should be noted, of course, that what is suggested here is something that *might* be achieved. It is also possible that it could not be and that a final agony will destroy peace rather than enhance it. In spite of all best efforts, the final stage of life may be a wasteland. It is then that the question of terminating that life takes on potential meaning, since death may be the only peace achievable.

There are possible ways also in which final suffering could be helpful to others. For one thing, the dying, while they still have sufficient consciousness, could help the living to come to a more realistic consciousness of death. Many of the dying have been doing this and Dr. Elizabeth Kübler-Ross (1970) has, in her writings, brought their teaching to a wide audience.

Also, terminally ill persons should feel free to cooperate in experiments that might help future sufferers from the same disease. We have noted earlier the suggestion of Mary Rose Barrington (1969) that a patient near the end of his life might arrange his death so as to permit an immediate transfer of a vital organ to a younger person. Given all the proper sensitivities of the medical profession about organ piracy or anything redolent thereof, it is not likely that this suggestion will get a hearing at this time. If the person to receive the vital organ were a relative or friend, the emotional effects of this generosity on the recipient could be anticipated to be such as to make the action morally unwise. There is also the medical problem of the value of the organs of a person dying of certain diseases. All the reality-revealing questions used in setting up the "moral object" would have to be focused on this case. It is not impossible, however, that all of the moral objections to such a procedure could be met in a particular case.

Aside from Barrington's suggestion of arranging death so as to make a vital organ available, there is also the possibility of donating a cornea or one of the other paired organs during a terminal illness. The operation for organ removal could be expected to hasten the dying process of the patient, but the benefits of the operation to someone else could easily be proportionate to the hastened death of the already dying donor. In fact, if a patient was anxious to bring on death sooner, the donation of an organ could be seen as a benevolent way of achieving this. The relevant moral questions would focus on medical feasibility, the mental state of the donor-patient, his relationship to the recipient, possible impact on the public acceptance of transplantation, etc.

Persons with a terminal illness who are still very alert of mind and imagination, or persons who have a serious illness such as kidney failure with a consequent need for dialysis, could see their illness as a platform from which to address the needs of their society. The sick could look for opportunities to help the well. With their unique credentials, and while their strength lasts, they could do more than they might realize. By working creatively with politicians and legislators, national health organizations, medical and legal societies, news media, writers, etc.—and in ways as yet unthought of which their healthy imaginations will bring forth—the lobby of the dying and the gravely ill could become a healing force in society. They could seek ways to address the sick priorities of our nation. They could call attention to the needs of the neglected poor of our land and of the third world. They could bear witness to the medical problems of the poor and to the need for better health insurance programs. They could educate legislators and others on the need for legislation to protect their right to die.

The words and feelings of those who stand at the brink of death have a special power. There is in literature a genre of "farewell addresses," real or imagined, but carefully preserved and attended to. The words of those who will soon leave us merit a natural and spontaneous esteem. We would have a healthier society if the dying found ways to speak to those who will survive them for a while.

While urging the positive possibilities of the suffering-dying, we cannot foreclose the sad possibility that a person's condition may be such that the value of terminating life might supersede all other values. There is such a thing as unbearable and undefeatable suffering of the sort that only death can end. In that event, it would be another mark of the distinctively human approach to death to procure the only relief imaginable. For the human person, unlike the horse, knows that he is going to die, knows that death can be a friend, and knows how to bring on death at a time when he can suffer no more. He has the capacity for death by choice; the horse does not.

Killing for the Sake of Life

Arthur J. Dyck (1973) of Harvard Divinity School opposes death by choice of the kind of which we have been speaking. He writes that "any act, insofar as it is an act of taking a human life, is wrong, that is to say, taking a human life is a wrong-making characteristic of actions." This, however, does not make Dyck an absolute pacifist. Some killing is good killing. Here is how he justifies that:

> To say, however, that killing is prima facie wrong does not mean that an act of killing may never be justified. For example, a person's effort to prevent someone's death may lead to the death of the attacker. However, we can morally justify that act of intervention only because it is an act of saving a life, not because it is an act of taking a life. If it were simply an act of taking a life, it would be wrong.

This particular argument of Dyck's has some basic weaknesses. First of all, most of the killing that is done in the self-defense situation of war, for example, is not done to save life in the physical sense of keeping someone alive. Most wars are fought to protect the quality of human life. They are fought because it is decided that a change in the quality of life is more important than submissive behavior that would probably let more people live but in conditions that are intolerable. Some wars, like the India-Pakistan war, can have the purported or even real purpose of ending an ongoing slaughter and therefore of "saving life." Other wars, such as wars of national independence, are waged for the same reason that tyrants are assassinated, to change the quality of life which had become intolerable under the reigning powers.

Obviously, war, tyrannicide, and killing in self-defense are different from death by choice in a medical context. In the latter case, however, the motive for imposing death is that the quality of this person's life, wracked as he may be by undefeatable and overwhelming pain, is intolerable. Obviously, in a narrow physical sense he is not "saving" his life by choosing to end it. He does, however, decide that he is saving himself by so choosing since the minimal requirements for personal existence have been obliterated by his condition. It would be sheer materialism to identify the patient's person and personal good with physical perdurance of life in any state.

Furthermore, as Dyck says, the mandate against killing derives from the perception that "no society can be indifferent about the taking of human life." Ending the life of a person who wants it ended because of unsupportable agony is the very opposite of indifference to life. The respect for human life in this case leads to a respect for human death. Ultimately it is the experience of the value of the person that leads to the recognition of the value of death as well as the value of life.

It can also be said in response to Dyck's position that, although he is working out of a Christian perspective, he seems to ignore the Christian belief in an afterlife. It is Christian belief that death does not end life; it merely changes its condition. The ancient preface for the Mass of the Dead says that "life is changed, not taken away" in death. For a Christian and for anyone who believes in an afterlife, to "terminate life" is not to terminate life, but to move on to a new life. With such a faith, death is not nearly so drastic. It has lost its sting of finality. This would seem to make it easier for a Christian to see death as a friend, especially when he has, through his illness, lost all ability to respond and react to the invitation of his God to join him in the building up of this earth. . . .

The Sense of Profanation

It might further be objected that there is something sacrosanct about a person's life, even his physical life. The proper attitude toward this life is awe, reverence, and support. Tampering with it, experimenting with it, or certainly ending it, is a profanation of the sacred. There is something jarring about the very idea. This, perhaps, is the reason why people have been so slow to accept the idea of mercy killing and why such killing is illegal in almost every land. This is a serious objection, based upon something (the sense of profanation) which I have presented as fundamental to good ethics.

In response, it can be said that the sense of profanation is a two-edged sword. It can, as I have mentioned, also be evoked by the sight of a person whose life is being agonizingly prolonged when truly personal living has become impossible because of unrelenting pain. In such a case, not to allow such a person the right to abbreviate his suffering could seem to subject this person to the dictates of his disease. Not being able to choose death when death is experienced as an essential benefit could easily seem degrading and profaning of personhood. Why should the disease have all the say, and the patient none? By succumbing to such moral determinism, is not the sacred power of deliberation and choice profaned?

It must be remembered, too, that the sense of profanation does not of itself constitute an independent argument. Ethics is wholistic. All the questions must be asked and all the evaluational capacities of the human spirit tapped before moral judgment is pronounced. Moral discourse must operate with a system of checks and balances. No one activity or faculty, whether it be *Gemüt*, the sense of profanation, the use of principle, etc., must be allowed an unquestioned hegemony.

In the second part of this objection, it was suggested that maybe the negative stance of most law regarding mercy killing constitutes an argument (based on group experience) against mercy killing. To this, it must be said that law is rarely a pioneer which stakes out new vistas for moral freedom. Law normally has deep historical roots which can be either an illuminating asset or a recalcitrant drag on moral progress. Law has the weaknesses as well as the strengths of the past. On the positive side we must trust it as the fruit of much experience. On the negative side we must reject its myopia when we come to see an issue better. That is why law must be open to reform, or it becomes demonic.

Thomas Jefferson is an eloquent witness to the stranglehold of inadequate law. In 1816 he wrote:

> I know also that laws and institutions must go hand in hand with the progress of the human mind. . . . As new discoveries are made, new truths disclosed, and manners and opinions change with the change of circumstances, institutions must advance also, and keep pace with the

times. We might as well require a man to wear still the coat which fitted him when a boy, as civilized society to remain ever under the regimen of their barbarous ancestors. (Padover 1939)

Before concluding that the voice of the law is the voice of God, it is well to look at the values and disvalues that the law has embodied in the past. Look how long law resisted the right of conscientious objection to war. With the greatest struggle and patience, the Quakers managed to win from government exemption to military service on conscientious grounds. And this was in 1802. For centuries this right, now generally seen as sacred, was denied by law. Long denied too was the right of women to vote and of black persons to be free. For the reasons offered in this book and for reasons that others offer, I judge that current laws are denying a human right when they inhibit the individual's right to death by choice. In this case, law is a tabernacle of taboo, and not a beacon of light.

The Hippocratic Oath

Hippocrates lived in the fifth century B.C. In his time, medicine was terribly intertwined with superstition and decadent religiosity. Hippocrates is generally credited with instituting a revolution that desacralized medicine. Morris H. Saffron (1970), the Archivist and Historian of the State Medical Society of New Jersey, says of Hippocrates: "To his majestic figure, subsequent generations of physicians turned as to a demigod, attributing to him many tracts written centuries after his death, so that the Hippocratic Corpus as it now stands, includes more than 70 works." Of all the works attributed to Hippocrates, there is no part more influential than his famous oath, which has guided physicians for centuries. The key passage relevant to death by choice is this: "I will neither give a deadly drug to anybody, if asked for, nor will I make a suggestion to this effect."

This passage is thought to show the influence of Pythgorean philosophy on Hippocratic thought. Pythagoras denied the right of an individual to take his own life. It is to these words of the oath that many people repair when contradicting the right to death by choice.

The prestige of this oath is enormous. Dr. H. Pitney van Dusen (1971), former president of Union Theological Seminary, says that he does not think "there is any other profession that is wedded to such an ancient document, not even the clerical profession with its Ten Commandments." Many physicians argue from this oath against death by choice as though they have an unwavering reliance on the self-sufficiency of this text that can only be compared to the attitude of a fundamentalist sectarian to his Bible. Undoubtedly, this attitude has been productive of much good, but it is again a one-rubric approach to the ethical issues involved and it has all the deficiencies that accrue to simplism in ethics.

In an effort to open the euthanasia issue to discussion, Joseph Fletcher has taken the tack of finding contradictions in the oath (a tactic also used against fundamentalist interpreters of the Bible). Fletcher (1954) notes that the oath promises two things: first, to relieve suffering, and, second, to prolong and protect life. Then he argues: "When the patient is in the grip of an agonizing and fatal disease, these two promises are incompatible. Two duties come into conflict. To prolong life is to violate the promise to relieve pain. To relieve the pain is to violate the promise to prolong and protect life."

More directly to the point, however, the oath has proved itself an invaluable encapsulation of some of the highest ideals in medical history. It is, however, not inspired by God, or by Apollo or Aesculapius, who are mentioned in the historical form of the oath. It is not a divine substitute for doing ethics. It is not oracular. Though it is good, it is perfectible. In fact, a modified form of the Hippocratic oath was adopted by the General Assembly of the World Medical Association meeting in Geneva in 1948. This form of the oath was also included in the International Code of Medical Ethics, which was adopted in 1949 and is used by physicians and medical schools. This version does not include the passage that swears against giving or counseling the use of something that would cause death. This omission did not constitute an endorsement of mercy killing in any form, but it does present a declaration that would admit of either a pro or con position on death by choice.

> Declaration of Geneva: I solemnly pledge myself to consecrate my life to the service of humanity. I will give to my teachers the respect and gratitude which is their due; I will practice my profession with conscience and dignity; the health of my patient will be my first consideration; I will respect the secrets which are confided in me; I will maintain by all means in my power the honor and noble traditions of the medical profession. My colleagues will be my brothers; I will not permit considerations of religion, nationality, race, party politics, or social standing to intervene between my duty and my patient. I will maintain the utmost respect for

human life from the time of conception; even under threat, I will not use my medical knowledge contrary to the laws of humanity. I make these promises solemnly, freely, and upon my honor. (quoted in Wolstenholme and O'Connor 1966)

One could maintain "the utmost respect for human life" and observe the "laws of humanity" by recognizing that the inducement of death when death is good and befitting is a reasonable and good service to human persons. The decision to do this, of course, would not be the doctor's, since he does not have the moral authority to make these decisions for anyone. His expertise does not in any way equip him to make moral decisions for his patients. He may be asked to administer the injection that causes death. In that case his conscience must guide his own response. The decision to initiate is not his; the decision to cooperate is.

Of Laws and Insurance Companies

Objection: if morality is based on reality, one of the realities of life is the law. In the United States, for example, it is illegal to induce one's own death or to help someone to end his life. Therefore, if all the arguments of ethics point to the fact that a particular act of termination might be moral, the arguments fail by reason of the illegality. It is not moral to act in a way that puts you and others at odds with the law. On top of that, insurance companies take a dim view of this sort of thing and will probably claim exemption from liability for the death. Thus your insurance is wiped out, and how could that be rational or moral?

These are practical objections. To spin out a theory that detaches from such concrete realities as law and insurance is hardly acceptable. And, indeed, it would not only make bad sense but bad ethics. First of all, then, the objection is heavy with overtones of that pernicious confusion that identifies legality and morality. In reply let it be said (again) that what is illegal may be moral, even heroically so. Of this, we have said enough previously.

Secondly, it is not illegal to kill yourself in all states. And modern law does not punish you by stripping you of your estate. However, in some jurisdictions, self-killing is a crime and those who aid or abet a person normally incur responsibility before the law in any jurisdiction. We have alluded to the Texas case *Sanders* v. *State*, where it was judged that aiding a person to kill himself is not a crime since self-killing is not a crime. This case, however, was later overruled in Texas in *Aven* v. *State,* which held that one who furnishes poison to another, knowing that the purpose of the latter is to commit suicide, and who assists in administering the poison which is the cause of death, is guilty of murder. Therefore, there can be no doubt about it. Death by choice does not enjoy the formal protection of the law. The tendency, as we have seen, is to treat these cases leniently, but this offers precarious promise at best. Anyone who attempts death by choice and succeeds obviously has little to fear from the law. Also, if he attempts and fails, he has little to fear even though in some states the attempt is an indictable offense. The hopes for leniency here are well founded. Assisting someone to die is, however, still legally perilous.

There are three options available in the face of this legal situation. Abstain from assisting in death by choice; assist and admit and hope for the best as Dr. Postma and Dr. Sander did; or assist clandestinely. The first course presents no legal problems. It could present moral problems if the patient's request for assistance is well considered and apparently justifiable. Then, it could be judged wrong not to give assistance such as making pills available. On the other hand, even if you felt that this person had a clear moral right to death by choice, it would be morally proper to weigh your consequent legal problems against his extended agony. Notice here again that omission is not an escape from moral choice. In such a case it is a moral choice and not necessarily a good one.

The second solution is the Postma-Sander solution. This requires considerable moral courage. Even though Dr. Postma escaped punishment in the form of a jail sentence, she must have been seriously punished by the trial and by the intense publicity visited upon her private sorrow.

Dr. Sander also had his ordeal even though he was found not guilty in the crowded, cheering courtroom. His right to practice medicine in New Hampshire was temporarily revoked and he was ousted by state and local medical societies. Reportedly, he was at one point reduced to plowing neighbors' fields for four dollars an hour. No one could be morally bound to endure what might have to be endured for assisting someone to die by positive means . . . no matter how deserving the case. Normally, we are not morally bound to heroic acts. We are here in the realm of what some moralists call ultraobligation. It could also, of course, be called the realm of moral opportunity.

Persons who do move ahead of the law here may, by their heroism, succeed in updating the law. Even within the conceptual inadequacies of the relevant American law, ingenious lawyers might be able to explore the possibility of defending this kind of action as being within the legitimate perimeters of religious freedom. Other defenses might also present themselves to the creative lawyer. The time might now be ripe for the development of precedents here.

The third course is the clandestine one. It has been suggested that there has been many an unrecorded use made of drugs such as bichloride of mercury, potassium, and some of the barbiturates. This may be, but how would one judge it morally? All of the reality-revealing questions would have to be asked, especially the question of who was making the decision. Only then could this course of action be judged. This clandestine course is not a priori wrong. Conscientious objection in the form of both overt and clandestine action is a necessary corrective for those situations where reality demands what the law forbids. Thus assisting a consenting person to achieve death by choice would not be wrong on the sole count of illegality.

But what of insurance? Insurance companies may protect themselves from liability by a suicide clause, at least at the beginning of a policy. The term suicide would include all forms of self-killing, whether the person was well or dying, sane or mentally ill. So someone planning to abbreviate the process of dying in which he finds himself, has to weigh the possibility of loss of coverage. In proportional calculus this might outweigh the gains of an earlier death . . . or it might not. But what of the morality of a person surreptitiously hastening his death in a way that allows him to keep his insurance coverage intact? Insurance companies presume that death occurs without human intervention, even though they often pay in cases of self-killing if the person has been a policyholder for a reasonably long period.

As a moralist, I would suggest that insurance companies should make distinctions where there are differences in the area of self-killing. Motive and other circumstances are, after all, reality-constituting factors. If a man who is repentant over being a poor provider takes out a policy to make his family beneficiaries, and then does himself in, in a way that makes his death look accidental, he is guilty of fraud. His generosity is at the expense of the company and other policyholders.

This is not the same as the case of a person who in extreme neurotic depression kills himself. In such a case, the darkness and terror of overwhelming emotions might plunge him into this act. This, it would seem, should be recognized as death from fatal illness. Uncontrollable depression can be fatal. It would seem wrong to punish this person posthumously by withholding payment on his policy. It can be said quite accurately that in such cases, death occurs because of illness. Normally, psychiatry will be able to attest to the active presence of serious illness preceding death in such a case. Obviously, if someone is emotionally ill when he takes out a policy, this should be revealed, since he has, by this reasoning, a potentially fatal illness. But if this kind of illness struck after the policy was taken out and while the policy is yet young, insurance coverage should not be lost any more than if the person had succumbed to rapidly developing cancer. To do otherwise reveals an archaic and cruel conception of mental illness.

There is also a difference between a person who, in ending his life, interrupts a healthy process and one who interrupts a dying process. A person dying of bone cancer who takes an overdose of barbiturates is not the same as the spurned lover who throws himself off a bridge. In the latter case, there might be good reasons to withhold payment on the policy. It may seem unromantic to suggest it, but this venal fact of life might be something of a deterrent to at least some frustrated lovers. Still, even here, such a desperate act is not calculated to be too frequent in our culture and insurance empires would not be likely to crumble if they covered such pathetic cases.

In the former case, involving the person dying of bone cancer, acceleration of this death should not in any way affect coverage. If it does, then the insurer is, in effect, punishing the insured for not holding the insurer's moral position on death by choice. There would seem to be something immoral and possibly unconstitutional about this. At any rate, the patient is, in this case, already in the dying process. The reasonable acceleration of that process should not be subject to financial punishment. . . .

References

Alexander, Leo. "Medical Science under Dictatorship." *New England Journal of Medicine* 241 (July 14, 1949): 39–47.

Barrington, Mary Rose. "Apologia for Suicide." In *Euthanasia and the Right to Death*, edited by A. B. Downing. Los Angeles: Nash Publishing, 1969.

Beecher, Henry K. "Medical Research and the Individual." In *Life or Death: Ethics and Options*, edited by Daniel Labby. Seattle: University of Washington Press, 1968.

Dyck, Arthur J. "An Alternative to the Ethic of Euthanasia." In *To Live or To Die:*

When, How, and Why?, edited by Robert H. Williams. New York: Springer-Verlag, 1973.

Fletcher, Joseph. *Morals and Medicine*. Princeton, N.J.: Princeton University Press, 1954.

Flew, Antony. "The Principle of Euthanasia." In *Euthanasia and the Right to Death*, edited by A. B. Downing. Los Angeles: Nash Publishing. 1969.

Häring, Bernard. *Medical Ethics*. Notre Dame, Ind.: Fides Publishers, 1973.

Kamisar, Yale. "Euthanasia Legislation: Some Non-Religious Objections." In *Euthanasia and the Right to Death*, edited by A. B. Downing. Los Angeles: Nash Publishing, 1969.

Kelly, Gerald. "The Duty of Using Artificial Means of Preserving Life." *Theological Studies* 11 (June 1950): 203–20.

Kübler-Ross, Elisabeth. *On Death and Dying*. New York: Macmillan, 1969.

Kutner, Luis. "Due Process of Euthanasia: The Living Will, A Proposal." *Indiana Law Journal* 44 (Summer 1969): 539–54.

Lasagna, Louis. *Life, Death, and the Doctor*. New York: Knopf, 1968.

Morris, Arval. "Voluntary Euthanasia." *Washington Law Review* 45 (April 1970): 239–71.

Padover, Saul K., ed. *Thomas Jefferson on Democracy*. New York: Mentor, 1939.

Ramsey, Paul. *The Patient as Person*. New Haven: Yale University Press, 1970.

Saffron, Morris H. "Euthanasia in the Greek Tradition." In *Attitudes toward Euthanasia*. New York: Euthanasia Educational Fund, 1970.

Silving, Helen. "Euthanasia: A Study of Comparative Criminal Law." *University of Pennsylvania Law Review* 103 (December 1954): 350–89.

van Dusen, Henry P. *The Right to Die with Dignity*. New York: Euthanasia Educational Fund, 1971.

Wolstenholme, G. E. W., and Maeve O'Connor, eds. *Ethics in Medical Progress*. Boston: Little, Brown, 1966.

23

Ethics and Euthanasia

Joseph Fletcher

IT is harder morally to justify letting somebody die a slow and ugly death, dehumanized, than it is to justify helping him to escape from such misery. This is the case at least in any code of ethics which is humanistic or personalistic, i.e., in any code of ethics which has a value system that puts humanness and personal integrity above biological life and function. It makes no difference whether such an ethics system is grounded in a theistic or a naturalistic philosophy. We may believe that God wills human happiness or that man's happiness is, as Protagoras thought, a self-validating standard of the good and the right. But what counts ethically is whether human needs come first—not whether the ultimate sanction is transcendental or secular.

What follows is a moral defense of euthanasia. Primarily I mean active or positive euthanasia, which helps the patient to die; not merely the passive or negative form of euthanasia which "lets the patient go" by simply withholding life-preserving treatments. The plain fact is that negative euthanasia is already a fait accompli in modern medicine. Every day in a hundred hospitals across the land decisions are made clinically that the line has been crossed from prolonging genuinely human life to only prolonging subhuman dying, and when that judgment is made respirators are turned off, life-

Reprinted from Robert H. Williams, ed., *To Live or To Die*, pp. 113–22, with the permission of Springer-Verlag, Inc. Copyright 1973 by Springer-Verlag, Inc.

perpetuating intravenous infusions stopped, proposed surgery canceled, and drugs countermanded. So-called Code 90 stickers are put on many record-jackets, indicating "Give no intensive care or resuscitation." Arguing pro and con about negative euthanasia is therefore merely flogging a dead horse. Ethically, the issue whether we may "let the patient go" is as dead as Queen Anne.

Straight across the board of religious traditions there is substantial agreement that we are not morally obliged to preserve life in all terminal cases. (The religious-ethical defense of negative ethuanasia is far more generally accepted by ministers and priests than medical people recognize or as yet even accept.) Humanist morality shows the same nonabsolutistic attitude about preserving life. Indeed, not only Protestant, Catholic, and Jewish teaching take this stance; but it is also true of Buddhist, Hindu, and Moslem ethics. In short, the claim that we ought always to do everything we can to preserve any patient's life as long as possible is now discredited. The last serious advocate of this unconditional provitalist doctrine was David Karnofsky—the great tumor research scientist of the Sloan-Kettering Institute in New York. The issue about negative euthanasia is settled ethically.

Given modern medicine's capabilities always to do what is technically possible to prolong life would be morally indefensible on any ground other than a vitalistic outlook; that is, the opinion that biological survival is the first-order value and that all other considerations, such as personality, dignity, well-being, and self-possession, necessarily take second place. Vestigial last-ditch provitalists still mumble threateningly about "what the Nazis did," but in fact the Nazis never engaged in euthanasia or mercy killing; what they did was merciless killing, either genocidal or for ruthless experimental purposes.

The Ethical and the Pre-ethical

One way of putting this is to say that the traditional ethics based on the sanctity of life—which was the classical doctrine of medical idealism in its prescientific phases—must give way to a code of ethics of the quality of life. This comes about for humane reasons. It is a result of modern medicine's successes, not failures. New occasions teach new duties, time makes ancient good uncouth, as Whittier said.

There are many pre-ethical or "metaethical" issues that are often overlooked in ethical discussions. People of equally good reasoning powers and a high respect for the rules of inference will still puzzle and even infuriate each other. This is because they fail to see that their moral judgments proceed from significantly different values, ideals, and starting points. If God's will (perhaps "specially revealed" in the Bible or "generally revealed" in his Creation) is against any responsible human initiative in the dying process, or if sheer life is believed to be, as such, more desirable than anything else, then those who hold these axioms will not find much merit in any case we might make for either kind of euthanasia—positive or negative. If, on the other hand, the highest good is personal integrity and human well-being, then euthanasia in either form could or might be the right thing to do, depending on the situation. This latter kind of ethics is the key to what will be said in this chapter.

Let's say it again, clearly, for the sake of truly serious ethical discourse. Many of us look upon living and dying as we do upon health and medical care, as person-centered. This is not a solely or basically biological understanding of what it means to be "alive" and to be "dead." It asserts that a so-called vegetable, the brain-damaged victim of an auto accident or a microcephalic newborn or a case of massive neurologic deficit and lost cerebral capacity, who nevertheless goes on breathing and whose midbrain or brainstem continues to support spontaneous organ functions, is in such a situation no longer a human being, no longer a person, no longer really alive. It is *personal* function that counts, not biological function. Humanness is understood as primarily rational, not physiological. This "doctrine of man" puts the *homo* and *ratio* before the *vita*. It holds that being human is more "valuable" than being alive.

All of this is said just to make it clear from the outset that biomedical progress is forcing us, whether we welcome it or not, to make fundamental conceptual changes as well as scientific and medical changes. Not only are the conditions of life and death changing, because of our greater control and in consequence our greater decision-making responsibility; our definitions of life and death also have to change to keep pace with the new realities.

These changes are signaled in a famous surgeon's remark recently: "When the brain is gone there is no point in keeping anything else going." What he meant was that with an end of cerebration, i.e., the function of the cerebral cortex, the person is gone (dead) no matter how many other spontaneous or artificially supported functions persist in the heart, lungs, and vascular system. Such noncerebral processes might as well be turned off, whether they are natural or artificial.

This conclusion is of great philosophical and religious interest because it reaffirms the ancient Christian-European belief that the core of humanness, of the humanum, lies in the ratio—man's rational faculty. It is not the loss of brain function in general but of cerebral function (the synthesizing "mind") in particular that establishes that death has ensued.

Using the old conventional conceptual apparatus, we naturally thought about both life and death as events, not as processes, which, of course, they are. We supposed that these events or episodes depended on the accidents of "nature" or on some kind of special providence. It is therefore no surprise to hear people grumbling that a lot of the decision making that has to be carried out in modern medical care is "playing God." And given that way of thinking the only possible answer to the charge is to accept it: "Yes, we are playing God." But the real question is: Which or whose God are we playing?

The old God who was believed to have a monopoly control of birth and death, allowing for no human responsibility in either initiating or terminating a life, was a primitive "God of the gaps"—a mysterious and awesome deity who filled in the gaps of our knowledge and of the control which our knowledge gives us. "He" was, so to speak, an hypothecation of human ignorance and helplessness.

In their growing up spiritually, men are now turning to a God who is the creative principle behind things, who is behind the test tube as much as the earthquake and volcano. This God can be believed in, but the old God's sacralistic inhibitions on human freedom and research can no longer be submitted to.

We must rid ourselves of that obsolete theodicy according to which God is not only the cause but also the builder of nature and its works, and not only the builder but even the manager. On this archaic basis it would be God himself who is the efficient as well as the final cause of earthquake and fire, of life and death, and by logical inference any "interference with nature" (which is exactly what medicine is) is "playing God." That God, seriously speaking, is dead.

Elective Death

Most of our major moral problems are posed by scientific discoveries and by the subsequent technical know-how we gain, in the control of life and health and death. Ethical questions jump out at us from every laboratory and clinic. May we exercise these controls at all, we wonder—and if so, then when, where, how? Every advance in medical capabilities is an increase in our moral responsibility, a widening of the range of our decision-making obligations.

Genetics, molecular biology, fetology, and obstetrics have developed to a point where we now have effective control over the start of human life's continuum. And therefore from now on it would be irresponsible to leave baby-making to mere chance and impulse, as we once had to do. Modern men are trying to face up in a mature way to our emerging needs of quality control—medically, ecologically, legally, socially.

What has taken place in birth control is equally imperative in death control. The whole armory of resuscitation and prolongation of life forces us to be responsible decision makers about death as much as about birth; there must be quality control in the terminating of life as in its initiating. It is ridiculous to give ethical approval to the positive ending of subhuman life in utero, as we do in therapeutic abortions for reasons of mercy and compassion, but refuse to approve of positively ending a subhuman life in extremis. If we are morally obliged to put an end to a pregnancy when an amniocentesis reveals a terribly defective fetus, we are equally obliged to put an end to a patient's hopeless misery when a brain scan reveals that a patient with cancer has advanced brain metastases.

Furthermore, as I shall shortly explain, it is morally evasive and disingenuous to suppose that we can condemn or disapprove positive acts of care and compassion but in spite of that approve negative strategies to achieve exactly the same purpose. This contradiction has equal force whether the euthanasia comes at the fetal point on life's spectrum or at some terminal point postnatally.

Only man is aware of death. Animals know pain, and fear it, but not death. Furthermore, in humans the ability to meet death and even to regard it sometimes as a friend is a sign of manliness. But in the new patterns of medicine and health care patients tend to die in a moribund or comatose state, so that death comes without the patient's knowledge. The Elizabethan litany's petition, ". . . from sudden death, good Lord, deliver us," has become irrelevant much if not most of the time.

It is because of this "incompetent" condition of so many of the dying that we cannot discuss the ethical issues of elective death only in the narrow terms of voluntary, patient-chosen euthanasia. A careful typology of elective death will distinguish at least *four* forms—ways of dying which are not merely willy-nilly matters of blind chance but of choice, purpose, and responsible freedom (historical ethics and moral theology are obviously major sources of suggestion for these distinctions):

1. Euthanasia, or a "good death," can be *voluntary and direct*, i.e., chosen and carried out by the patient. The most familiar way is the overdose left near at hand for the patient. It is a matter of simple request and of personal liberty. If it can be held in the abortion debate that compulsory pregnancy is unjust and that women should be free to control their own bodies when other's lives (fetuses) are at stake, do not the same moral claims apply to control of the lives and bodies of people too? In any particular case we might properly raise the question of the patient's competence, but to hold that euthanasia in this category is justifiable entails a rejection of the simplistic canard that all suicide victims are mentally disordered.

Voluntary euthanasia is, of course, a form of suicide. Presumably a related issue arises around the conventional notion of consent in medical ethics. The codes (American Medical Association, Helsinki, World Medical Association, Nuremberg) all contend that valid consent to any surgery or treatment requires a reasonable prospect of benefit to the patient. What, then, is benefit? Could death in some situations be a benefit? My own answer is in the affirmative.

2. Euthanasia can be *voluntary but indirect*. The choice might be made either in situ or long in advance of a terminal illness, e.g., by exacting a promise that if and when the "bare bodkin" or potion cannot be self-administered somebody will do it for the patient. In this case the patient gives to others—physicians, lawyers, family, friends—the discretion to end it all as and when the situation requires, if the patient becomes comatose or too dysfunctioned to make the decision pro forma. There is already a form called the Living Will, sent upon request to thousands by the Euthanasia Educational Fund (although its language appears to limit it to merely negative methods). This perfectly reasonable "insurance" device is being ex-

plored by more and more people, as medical prolongation of life tends to make them more afraid of senescence than of death.

Since both the common-law tradition and statute law are caught practically unequipped to deal with this medical-legal lag, the problem is being examined worriedly and behind the scenes by lawyers and legislators. They have little or no case law to work with. As things stand now the medieval outlook of the law treats self-administered euthanasia as suicide and when effected by a helping hand as murder.

3. Euthanasia may be *direct but involuntary*. This is the form in which a simple "mercy killing" is done on a patient's behalf without his present or past request. Instances would be when an idiot is given a fatal dose or the death of a child in the worst stages of Tay-Sachs disease is speeded up, or when a man trapped inextricably in a blazing fire is shot to end his suffering, or a shutdown is ordered on a patient deep in a mindless condition, irreversibly, perhaps due to an injury or an infection or some biological breakdown. It is in this form, as directly involuntary, that the problem has reached the courts in legal charges and indictments.

To my knowledge Uruguay is the only country that allows it. Article 37 of the *Codiga Penal* specifically states that although it is a "crime" the courts are authorized to forgo any penalty. In time the world will follow suit. Laws in Colombia and in the Soviet Union (Article 50 of the Code of Criminal Procedure) are similar to Uruguay's, but in their codes freedom from punishment is exceptional rather than normative. In Italy, Germany, and Switzerland the law provides for a reduction of penalties when it is done upon the patient's request.

The conflict and tension between the stubborn prohibitionism on the one hand and a humane compassion on the other may be seen in the legal history of the issue in the United States. Eleven cases of "mercy killing" have actually reached the courts: one was on a charge of voluntary manslaughter, with a conviction and penalty of three to six years in prison and a $500 fine; one was for first-degree murder, resulting in a conviction, which was promptly reduced to a penalty of six years in jail with immediate parole. All of the other nine cases were twisted into "temporary insanity" or no-proof judgments—in short, no convictions.

4. Finally, euthanasia might be *both indirect and involuntary*. This is the "letting the patient go" tactic which is taking place every day in our hospitals. Nothing is done for the patient positively to release him from his tragic

condition (other than "trying to make him comfortable"), and what is done negatively is decided for him rather than in response to his request.

As we all know, even this passive policy of compassion is a grudging one, done perforce. Even so, it remains at least theoretically vulnerable to malpractice suits under the lagging law—brought, possibly, by angry or venal members of the family or suit-happy lawyers. A sign of the times was the bill to give negative euthanasia a legal basis in Florida, introduced by a physician member of the legislature.

But *ethically* regarded, this indirect-involuntary form of euthanasia is manifestly superficial, morally timid, and evasive of the real issue. I repeat: it is harder morally to justify letting somebody die a slow and ugly death, dehumanized, than it is to justify *helping* him to avoid it.

Means and Ends

What, then, is the real issue? In a few words, it is whether we can morally justify taking it into our own hands to hasten death for ourselves (suicide) or for others (mercy killing) out of reasons of compassion. The answer to this in my view is clearly Yes, on both sides of it. Indeed, *to justify either one, suicide or mercy killing, is to justify the other.*

The heart of the matter analytically is the question of whether the end justifies the means. If the end sought is the patient's death as a release from pointless misery and dehumanization, then the requisite or appropriate means is justified. Immanuel Kant said that if we will the end we will the means. The old maxim of some moral theologians was *finis sanctificat media.* The point is that no act is anything but random and *meaningless* unless it is purposefully related to some end or object. To be moral an act must be seeking an end.

However, to hold that the end justifies the means does not entail the absurd notion that *any* means can be justified by *any* end. The priority of the end is paired with the principle of "proportionate good"; any disvalue in the means must be outweighed by the value gained in the end. In systems analysis, with its pragmatic approach, the language would be: the benefit must repay the cost or the trade-off is not justified. It comes down to this, that in some situations a morally good end can justify a relatively "bad" means, on the principle of proportionate good.

The really searching question of conscience is, therefore, whether we are right in believing that *the well-being of persons* is the highest good. If so, then it follows that either suicide or mercy killing could be the right thing to do in some exigent and tragic circumstances. This could be the case, for instance, when an incorrigible "human vegetable," whether spontaneously functioning or artificially supported, is progressively degraded while constantly eating up private or public financial resources in violation of the distributive justice owed to others. In such cases the patient is actually already departed and only his body is left, and the needs of others have a stronger claim upon us morally. The fair allocation of scarce resources is as profound an ethical obligation as any we can imagine in a civilized society, and it arises very practically at the clinical level when triage officers make their decisions at the expense of some patients' needs in favor of others.

Another way of putting this is to say that the crucial question is not whether the end justifies the means (what else could?) but *what justifies the end?* And this chapter's answer is, plainly and confidently, that human happiness and well-being is the highest good or *summum bonum*, and that therefore any ends or purposes which that standard or ideal validates are just, right, good. This is what humanistic medicine is all about; it is what the concepts of loving concern and social justice are built upon.

This position comes down to the belief that our moral acts, including suicide and mercy killing, are right or wrong depending on the consequences aimed at (we sometimes fail, of course, through ignorance or poor reasoning), and that the consequences are good or evil according to whether and how much they serve humane values. In the language of ethics this is called a "consequential" method of moral judgment.

I believe that this code of ethics is both implicit and explicit in the morality of medical care and biomedical research. Its reasoning is inductive, not deductive, and it proceeds empirically from the data of each actual case or problem, choosing the course that offers an optimum or maximum of desirable consequences. Medicine is not a-prioristic or *prejudiced* in its ethos and modalities, and therefore to proscribe either suicide or mercy killing is so blatantly nonconsequential that it calls for critical scrutiny. It fails to make sense. It is unclinical and doctrinaire.

The problem exists because there is another kind of ethics, radically different from consequential ethics. This other kind of ethics holds that our actions are right or wrong according to whether they follow universal rules of conduct and absolute norms: that we ought or ought not to do certain things no matter how good or bad the consequences might be foreseeably. Such rules are usually prohibitions or taboos, expressed as thou-shalt-nots. Whereas this chapter's ethics is teleological or end-oriented, the opposite approach is "deontological" (from the Greek *deonteis*, meaning duty); i.e., it is duty-ethics, not goal-ethics. Its advocates sometimes sneer at any determination of obligation in terms of consequences, calling it "a mere morality of goals."

In duty-ethics what is right is whatever act obeys or adheres to the rules, even though the foreseeable result will be inhumane. That is, its highest good is not human happiness and well-being but obedience to a rule—or what we might call a prejudiced or predetermined decision based not on the clinical variables but on some transcending generality.

For example, the sixth of the Ten Commandments, which prohibits killing, is a no-no rule for nonconsequentialists when it comes to killing in the service of humane values like mercy and compassion, and yet at the same time they ignore their "moral law" when it comes to self-defense. The egocentricity and solipsism in this moral posture, which is a very common one, never ceases to bemuse consequentialists. You may end your neighbor's life for your own sake but you may not do it for his sake! And you may end your own life for your neighbor's sake, as in an act of sacrificial heroism, but you may not end your life for your own sake. This is a veritable mare's nest of nonsense!

The plain hard logic of it is that the end or purpose of both negative and positive euthanasia is exactly the same: to contrive or bring about the patient's death. Acts of deliberate omission are morally not different from acts of commission. But in the Anglo-American *law*, it is a crime to push a blind man off the cliff. It is not, however, a crime to deliberately not lift a finger to prevent his walking over the edge. This is an unpleasant feature of legal reasoning which is alien to ethics and to a sensitive conscience. Ashamed of it, even the courts fall back on such legal fictions as "insanity" in euthanasia cases, and this has the predictable effect of undermining our respect for the law.

There is something obviously evasive when we rule motive out in charging people with the crime of mercy killing, but then bring it back in again for purposes of determining punishment! It is also a menacing delimitation of the concepts of culpability, responsibility, and negligence. No *ethically* disciplined decision maker could so blandly separate right and wrong from motives, foresight, and consequences. (Be it noted, however, that motive is taken into account in German and Swiss law, and that several European countries provide for recognition of "homicide when requested" as a special category.)

It is naïve and superficial to suppose that because we don't "do anything positively" to hasten a patient's death we have thereby avoided complicity in his death. Not doing anything is doing something; it is a decision to act every bit as much as deciding for any other deed. If I decide not to eat or drink any more, knowing what the consequence will be, I have committed suicide as surely as if I had used a gas oven. If physicians decide not to open an imperforate anus in a severely 21-trisomy newborn, they have committed mercy killing as surely as if they had used a poison pellet!

Let the reader at this point now ask himself if he is a consequentialist or an a priori decision maker; and again, let him ask himself if he is a humanist, religious or secular, or alternatively has something he holds to be better or more obliging than the well-being of the patient. (Thoughtless religious people will sometimes point out that we are required to love God as well as our neighbors, but can the two loves ever come into conflict? Actually, is there any way to love God other than through the neighbor? Only mystics imagine that they can love God directly and discretely.)

Occasionally I hear a physician say that he could not resort to positive euthanasia. That may be so. What anybody would do in such tragic situations is a problem in psychology, however, not in ethics. We are not asking what we would do but what we should do. Any of us who has an intimate knowledge of what happens in terminal illnesses can tell stories of rational people—both physicians and family—who were quite clear ethically about the rightness of an overdose or of "turning off the machine," and yet found themselves too inhibited to give the word or do the deed. That is a phenomenon of primary interest to psychology, but of only incidental interest to ethics.

Careful study of the best texts of the Hippocratic Oath shows that it says nothing at all about preserving life, as such. It says that "so far as power and discernment shall be mine, I will carry out regimen for the benefit of the sick and will keep them from harm and wrong." The case for euthanasia depends upon how we understand "benefit of the sick" and "harm" and "wrong." If we regard dehumanized and merely biological life as sometimes real harm and the opposite of benefit, to refuse to welcome or even introduce death would be quite wrong morally.

In most states in this country people can and do carry cards, legally established (by Anatomical Gift Acts), which explain the carrier's wish that when he dies his organs and tissue should be used for transplant when needed by the living. The day will come when people will also be able to carry a card, notarized and legally executed, which explains that they do not want to be kept alive beyond the *humanum* point, and authorizing the ending of their biological processes by any of the methods of euthanasia which seems appropriate. Suicide may or may not be the ultimate problem of philosophy, as Albert Camus thought it is, but in any case it is the ultimate problem of medical ethics.

FIVE
Suicide

24

Preventing Suicide

EDWIN S. SHNEIDMAN

IN almost every case of suicide, there are hints of the act to come, and physicians and nurses are in a special position to pick up the hints and to prevent the act. They come into contact, in many different settings, with many human beings at especially stressful times in their lives.

A suicide is an especially unhappy event for helping personnel. Although one can, in part, train and inure oneself to deal with the sick and even the dying patient, the abruptness and needlessness of a suicidal act leaves the nurse, the physician, and other survivors with many unanswered questions, many deeply troubling thoughts and feelings.

Currently, the major bottleneck in suicide prevention is not remediation, for there are fairly well-known and effective treatment procedures for many types of suicidal states; rather it is in diagnosis and identification (Farberow and Shneidman 1961).

Assumptions

A few straightforward assumptions are necessary in suicide prevention. Some of them:

Individuals who are intent on killing themselves still wish very much to be rescued or to have their deaths prevented. Suicide prevention consists essentially in recognizing that the potential victim is "in balance" between his wishes to live and his wishes to die, then throwing one's efforts on the side of life.

Suicide prevention depends on the active and forthright behavior of the potential rescuer.

Most individuals who are about to commit suicide are acutely conscious of their intention to do so. They may, of course, be very secretive and not communicate their intentions directly. On the other hand, the suicidally inclined person may actually be unaware of his own lethal potentialities, but nonetheless may give many indirect hints of his unconscious intentions.

Practically all suicidal behaviors stem from a sense of isolation and from feelings of some intolerable emotion on the part of the victim. By and large, suicide is an act to stop an intolerable existence. But each individual defines "intolerable" in his own way. Difficulties, stresses, or disappointments that might be easy for one individual to handle might very well be intolerable for someone else—in *his* frame of mind. In order to anticipate and prevent suicide one must understand what "intolerable" means to the other person. Thus, any "precipitating cause"—being neglected, fearing or having cancer (the fear and actuality can be equally lethal), feeling helpless or hopeless, feeling "boxed-in"—may be intolerable for *that* person.

Although committing suicide is certainly an all-or-none action, thinking about the act ahead of time is a complicated, undecided, internal debate. Many a black-or-white action is taken on a barely pass vote. Professor Henry Murray of Harvard University has written that "a personality is a full Congress" of the mind. In preventing suicide, one looks for any indications in the individual representing the dark side of his internal life-and-death debate. We are so often surprised at "unexpected" suicides because we fail to take into account just this principle that the suicidal action is a decision resulting from an internal debate of many voices, some for life and some for death. Thus we hear all sorts of postmortem statements like "He seemed in good spirits" or "He was looking forward to some event next week," not recognizing that these, in themselves, represent only one aspect of the total picture.

In almost every case, there are precursors to suicide, which are called "prodromal clues." In the "psychological autopsies" that have been done at the Suicide Prevention Center in Los Angeles—in which, by interview with survivors of questionable accident or suicide deaths, they attempt to reconstruct the intention of the deceased in relation to death—it was found that very few suicides occur without casting some shadows before them. The concept of prodromal clues for suicide is certainly an old idea; it is really not very different from what Robert Burton, over 300 years ago in 1652, in his famous *Anatomy of Melancholy*, called "the prognostics of melancholy, or signs of things to come." These prodromal clues typically exist for a few days to some weeks before the actual suicide. Recognition of these clues is a necessary first step to lifesaving.

Suicide prevention is like fire prevention. It is not the main mission of any hospital, nursing home, or other institution, but it is the minimum ever-present peripheral responsibility of each professional; and when the minimal signs of possible fire or suicide are seen, then there are no excuses for holding back on lifesaving measures. The difference between fire prevention and suicide prevention is that the prodromal clues for fire prevention have become an acceptable part of our commonsense folk knowledge; we must also make the clues for suicide a part of our general knowledge.

Clues to Potential Suicide

In general, the prodromal clues to suicide may be classified in terms of four broad types: verbal, behavioral, situational, and syndromatic.

Verbal

Among the verbal clues we can distinguish between the direct and the indirect. Examples of direct verbal communications would be such statements as "I'm going to commit suicide," "If such and such happens, I'll kill myself," "I'm going to end it all," "I want to die," and so on. Examples of indirect verbal communications would be such statements as "Goodbye," "Farewell," "I've had it," "I can't stand it any longer," "It's too much to put up with," "You'd be better off without me," and, in general, any statements that mirror the individual's intention to stop his intolerable existence.

Some indirect verbal communications can be somewhat more subtle. We all know that in human communication, our words tell only part of the story, and often the main "message" has to be decoded. Every parent or spouse learns to decode the language of loved ones and to understand what they really mean. In a similar vein, many presuicidal communications have to be decoded. An example might be a patient who says to a nurse who is leaving on her vacation, "Goodbye, Miss Jones, I won't be here when you come back." If some time afterward she, knowing that the patient is not scheduled to be transferred or discharged prior to her return, thinks about that conversation, she might do well to telephone her hospital.

Other examples are such statements as, "I won't be around much longer for you to put up with," "This is the last shot you'll ever give me" or "This is the last time I'll ever be here," a statement which reflects the patient's private knowledge of his decision to kill himself. Another example is, "How does one leave her body to the medical school?" The latter should never be answered with factual information until after one has found out why the question is being asked, and whose body is being talked about. Individuals often ask for suicide-prevention information for a "friend" or "relative" when they are actually inquiring about themselves.

Behavioral

Among the behavioral clues, we can distinguish the direct and the indirect. The clearest examples of direct behavioral communications of the intention to kill oneself is a "practice run," an actual suicide attempt of whatever seriousness. Any action which uses instruments which are conventionally associated with suicide (such as razors, ropes, pills, and the like), regardless of whether or not it could have any lethal outcome, must be interpreted as a direct behavioral "cry for help" and an indication that the person is putting us on our alert. Often, the nonlethal suicide attempt is meant to communicate deeper suicidal intentions. By and large, suicide attempts must be taken seriously as indications of personal crisis and of more severe suicide potentiality.

In general, indirect behavioral communications are such actions as taking a lengthy trip or putting affairs into order. Thus the making of a will under certain peculiar and special circumstances can be an indirect clue to suicidal intention. Buying a casket at the time of another's funeral should always be inquired after most carefully and, if necessary, prompt action (like hospitalization) taken. Giving away prized possessions like a watch, earrings, gold clubs, or heirlooms should be looked on as a possible prodromal clue to suicide.

Situational

On occasion the situation itself cries out for attention, especially when there is a variety of stresses. For example, when a patient is extremely anxious about surgery, or when he has been notified that he has a malignancy, when he is scheduled for mutilative surgery, when he is frightened by hospitalization itself, or when outside factors (like family discord, for example, or finances) are a problem—all these are situational. If the doctor or nurse is sensitive to the fact that the situation constitutes a "psychological emergency" for that patient, then he is in a key position to perform lifesaving work. His actions might take the form of sympathetic conversation, or special surveillance of that patient by keeping him with some specially assigned person, or by requesting consultation, or by moving him so that he does not have access to windows at lethal heights. At the least, the nurse should make notations of her behavioral observations in the chart.

To be a suicide diagnostician, one must combine separate symptoms and recognize *and label* a suicidal syndrome in a situation where no one symptom by itself would necessarily lead one to think of a possible suicide.

In this paper we shall highlight syndromatic clues for suicide in a medical and surgical hospital setting, although these clues may also be used in other settings. First, it can be said that patient status is stressful for many persons. Everyone who has ever been a patient knows the fantasies of anxiety, fear, and regression that are attendant on illness or surgery. For some in the patient role (especially in a hospital), as the outer world recedes, the fantasy life becomes more active; conflicts and inadequacies and fears may then begin to play a larger and disproportionate role. The point for suicide prevention is that one must try to be aware especially of those patients who are prone to be psychologically overreactive and, being so, are more apt to explode irrationally into suicidal behavior.

Syndromatic

What are the syndromes—the constellations of symptoms—for suicide? Labels for four of them could be: depressed, disoriented, defiant, and dependent-dissatisfied.

1. Depressed: The syndrome of depression is, by and large, made up of symptoms which reflect the shifting of the individual's psychological interests from aspects of his interpersonal life to aspects of his private psychological life, to some intrapsychic crisis within himself. For example, the individual is less interested in food, he loses his appetite, and thus loses weight. Or, his regular patterns of sleeping and waking become disrupted, so that he suffers from lack of energy in the daytime and then sleeplessness and early awakening. The habitual or regular patterns of social and sexual response

also tend to change, and the individual loses interest in others. His rate or pace or speed of talking, walking, and doing the activities of his everyday life slows down. At the same time there is increased preoccupation with internal (intrapsychic) conflicts and problems. The individual is withdrawn, apathetic, apprehensive and anxious, often "blue" and even tearful, somewhat unreachable and seemingly uncaring.

Depression can be seen too in an individual's decreased willingness to communicate. Talking comes harder, there are fewer spontaneous remarks, answers are shorter or even monosyllabic, the facial expressions are less lively, the posture is more drooped, gestures are less animated, the gait is less springy, and the individual's mind seems occupied and elsewhere.

An additional symptom of the syndrome of depression is detachment, or withdrawing from life. This might be evidenced by behavior which would reflect attitudes, such as "I don't care," "What does it matter," "It's no use anyway." If an individual feels helpless he is certainly frightened, although he may fight for some control or safety; but if he feels hopeless, then the heart is out of him, and life is a burden, and he is only a spectator to a dreary life which does not involve him.

First aid in suicide prevention is directed to counteracting the individual's feelings of hopelessness. Robert E. Litman (1963), chief psychiatrist of the Los Angeles Suicide Prevention Center, has said that "psychological support is transmitted by a firm and hopeful attitude. We convey the impression that the problem which seems to the patient to be overwhelming, dominating his entire personality, and completely insidious, is commonplace and quite familiar to us and we have seen many people make a complete recovery. Hope is a commodity of which we have plenty and we dispense it freely."

It is of course pointless to say "Cheer up" to a depressed person, inasmuch as the problem is that he simply cannot. On the other hand, the effectiveness of the "self-fulfilling prophecy" should never be underestimated. Often an integral part of anyone's climb out of a depression is his faith and the faith of individuals around him that he is going to make it. Just as hopelessness breeds hopelessness, hope—to some extent—breeds hope.

Oftentimes, the syndrome of depression does not seem especially difficult to diagnose. What may be more difficult—and very much related to suicide—is the apparent improvement after a severe depression, when the individual's pace of speech and action picks up a little. The tendency then is for everyone to think that he is cured and to relax vigilance. In reality the situation may be much more dangerous; the individual now has the psychic energy with which to kill himself that he may not have had when he was in the depths of his depression. By far, most suicides relating to depression occur within a short period (a few days to 3 months) after the individual has made an apparent turn for the better. A good rule is that any significant change in behavior, even if it looks like improvement, should be assessed as a possible prodromal index for suicide.

Although depression is the most important single prodromal syndrome for suicide—occurring to some degree in approximately one-third of all suicides—it is not the only one.

2. Disoriented: Disoriented people are apt to be delusional or hallucinatory, and the suicidal danger is that they may respond to commands or voices or experiences that other people cannot share. When a disoriented person expresses any suicidal notions, it is important to take him as a most serious suicidal risk, for he may be in constant danger of taking his own life, not only to cut out those parts of himself that he finds intolerable, but also to respond to the commands of hallucinated voices to kill himself. What makes such a person potentially explosive and particularly hard to predict is that the trigger mechanism may depend on a crazed thought, a hallucinated command, or a fleeting intense fear within a delusional system.

Disoriented states may be clearly organic, such as delirium tremens, certain toxic states, certain drug withdrawal states. Individuals with chronic brain syndromes and cerebral arteriosclerosis may become disoriented. On the other hand, there is the whole spectrum of schizophrenic and schizoaffective disorders, in which the role of organic factors is neither clearly established nor completely accepted. Nonetheless, professional personnel should especially note individuals who manifest some degree of nocturnal disorientation, but who have relative diurnal lucidity. Those physicians who see the patients only during the daytime are apt to miss these cases, particularly if they do not read nurses' notes.

Suicides in general hospitals have occurred among nonpsychiatric patients with subtle organic syndromes, especially those in which symptoms of disorientation are manifested. One should look, too, for the presence of bizarre behavior, fear of death, and clouding of the patient's understanding and awareness. The nurse might well be especially alert to any general hospital patient who has any previous neuropsychiatric history, especially where there are the signs of an acute brain syndrome. Although dyspnea is not a symptom in the syndrome related to disorientation, the presence of severe dyspnea, especially if it is unimproved by treatment in the hospital, has been found to correlate with suicide in hospitals.

When an individual is labeled psychotic, he is almost always disoriented in one sphere or another. Even if he knows where he is and what the date is, he may be off base about who he is, especially if one asks him more or less "philosophic" questions, like "What is the meaning of life?" His thinking processes will seem peculiar, and the words of his speech will have some special or idiosyncratic characteristics. In general, whether or not such patients are transferred to psychiatric wards or psychiatric hospitals, they should—in terms of suicide prevention—be given special care and surveillance, including consultation. Special physical arrangements should be made for them, such as removal of access to operable screens and windows, removal of objects of self-destruction, and the like.

3. Defiant: The Welsh poet, Dylan Thomas, wrote: "Do not go gentle into that good night/. . . . rage, rage against the dying of the light," Many of us remember, usually from high school literature, Henley's "Invictus," "I am the master of my fate/ I am the captain of my soul." The point is that many individuals, no matter how miserable their circumstances or how painful their lives, attempt to retain some shred of control over their own fate. Thus a man dying of cancer may, rather than passively capitulate to the disease, choose to play one last active role in his own life by picking the time of his death; so that even in a terminal state (when the staff may believe that he doesn't have the energy to get out of bed), he lifts a heavy window and throws himself out to his death. In this sense, he is willful or defiant.

This kind of individual is an "implementer" (Farberow et al. 1963). Such a person is described as one who has an active need to control his environment. Typically, he would never be fired from any job; he would quit. In a hospital he would attempt to control his environment by refusing some treatments, demanding others, requesting changes, insisting on privileges, and indulging in many other activities indicating some inner need to direct and control his life situation. These individuals are often seen as having low frustration tolerance, being fairly set and rigid in their ways, being somewhat arbitrary and, in general, showing a great oversensitivity to outside control. The last is probably a reflection of their own inability to handle their inner stresses.

Certainly, not every individual who poses ward-management problems needs to be seen as suicidal, but what personnel should look for is the somewhat agitated concern of a patient with controlling his own fate. Suicide is one way of "calling the shot." The nurse can play a lifesaving role with such a person by recognizing his psychological problems and by enduring his controlling (and irritating) behavior—indeed, by being the willing target of his berating and demanding behavior and thus permitting him to expend his energies in this way, rather than in suicidal activities. Her willingness to be a permissible target for these feelings and, more, her sympathetic behavior in giving attention and reassurance even in the face of difficult behavior are in the tradition of the nurturing nurse, even though this can be a difficult role continually to fulfill.

4. Dependent-dissatisfied: Imagine being married to someone on whom you are deeply emotionally dependent, in a situation in which you are terribly dissatisfied with your being dependent. It would be in many ways like being "painted into a corner"—there is no place to go.

This is the pattern we have labeled "dependent-dissatisfied" (Shneidman and Farberow 1962). Such an individual is very dependent on the hospital, realizing he is ill and depending on the hospital to help him; however, he is dissatisfied with being dependent and comes to feel that the hospital is not giving him the help he thinks he needs. Such patients become increasingly tense and depressed, with frequent expressions of guilt and inadequacy. They have emotional disturbances in relation to their illnesses and to their hospital care. Like the "implementer," they make demands and have great need for attention and reassurance. They have a number of somatic complaints, as well as complaints about the hospital. They threaten to leave the hospital against medical advice. They ask to see the doctor, the chaplain, the chief nurse. They request additional therapies of various kinds. They make statements like, "Nothing is being done for me" or "The doctors think I am making this up."

The reactions of irritability on the part of busy staff are not too surprising in view of the difficult behavior of such patients. Tensions in these patients may go up especially at the time of pending discharge from the hospital. Suicide prevention by hospital staff consists of responding to the emotional needs and giving emotional support to these individuals. With such patients the patience of Job is required. Any suicide threats or attempts on the part of such patients, no matter how "mild" or attention-getting, should be taken seriously. Their demand for attention may lead them to suicide. Hospital staff can often, by instituting some sort of new treatment procedure or medication, give this type of patient temporary relief or a feeling of improvement. But most of all, the sympathetic recognition on the part of hospital staff that the complaining, demanding, exasperating behavior of the dependent-dissatisfied patient is an expression of his own inner feelings of desperation may be the best route to preventing his suicide.

Coworkers, Family, Friends

Suicide is "democratic." It touches both patients and staff, unlettered and educated, rich and poor—almost proportionately. As for sex ratio, the statistics are interesting: Most studies have shown that in Western countries more men than women commit suicide, but a recent study (Eisenthal et al. 1966) indicates that in certain kinds of hospital settings like neuropsychiatric hospitals, a proportionately larger percentage of women kill themselves. The information in this paper is meant to apply not only to patients, but to colleagues, and even to members of our families as well. The point is that only by being free to see the possibility of suicidal potential in everybody can suicide prevention of anybody really become effective.

In our society, we are especially loath to suspect suicide in individuals of some stature or status. For example, of the physicians who commit suicide, some could easily be saved if they would be treated (hospitalized, for example) like ordinary citizens in distress. Needless to say, the point of view that appropriate treatment might cause him professional embarrassment should never be invoked in such a way so as to risk a life being lost.

In general, we should not "run scared" about suicide. In the last analysis, suicides are, fortunately, infrequent events. On the other hand, if we have even unclear suspicions of suicidal potential in another person, we do well to have "the courage of our own confusions" and take the appropriate steps.

These appropriate steps may include notifying others, obtaining consultation, alerting those concerned with the potentially suicidal person (including relatives and friends), getting the person to a sanctuary in a psychiatric ward or hospital. Certainly, we don't want to holler "Fire" unnecessarily, but we should be able to interpret the clues, erring, if necessary, on the "liberal" side. We may feel chagrined if we turn in a false alarm, but we would feel very much worse if we were too timid to pull that switch that might have prevented a real tragedy.

Earlier in this paper the role of the potential rescuer was mentioned. One implication of this is that professionals must be aware of their own reactions and their own personalities, especially in relation to certain patients. For example, does he have the insight to recognize his tendency to be irritated at a querulous and demanding patient and thus to ignore his presuicidal communications? Every rescue operation is a dialogue: Someone cries for help and someone else must be willing to hear him and be capable of responding to him. Otherwise the victim may die because of the potential rescuer's unresponsiveness.

We must develop in ourselves a special attitude for suicide prevention. Each individual can be a lifesaver, a one-person committee to prevent suicide. Happily, elaborate pieces of mechanical equipment are not needed; "all" that is required are sharp eyes and ears, good intuition, a pinch of wisdom, an ability to act appropriately, and a deep resolve.

References

Eisenthal, Sherman; N. L. Farberow; and Edwin Shneidman. "Follow-up of Neuropsychiatric Hospital Patients on Suicide Observation Status." *Public Health Reports* 81 (November 1966): 977–90.

Farberow, N. L., and Edwin Shneidman, eds. *The Cry for Help.* New York: McGraw-Hill, 1961.

Farberow, Norman L.; Edwin Shneidman; and Leonard Calista. *Suicide among General Medical and Surgical Hospital Patients with Malignant Neoplasms.* Washington, D.C.: Veterans' Administration, 1963.

Litman, Robert. "Emergency Response to Potential Suicide." *Journal of the Michigan Medical Society* 62 (1963): 68–72.

Shneidman, Edwin, and Norman Farberow. *Evaluation and Treatment of Suicidal Risk among Schizophrenic Patients in Psychiatric Hospitals.* Washington, D.C.: Veterans' Administration, 1962.

25

The Ethics of Suicide

Thomas S. Szasz

AN editorial in *The Journal of the American Medical Association* (March 6, 1967) declared that "the contemporary physician sees suicide as a manifestation of emotional illness. Rarely does he view it in a context other than that of psychiatry." It was thus implied, the emphasis being the stronger for not being articulated, that to view suicide in this way is at once scientifically accurate and morally uplifting. I submit that it is neither; that, instead, this perspective on suicide is both erroneous and evil: erroneous because it treats an act as if it were a happening; and evil, because it serves to legitimize psychiatric force and fraud by justifying it as medical care and treatment.

Before going further, I should like to distinguish three fundamentally different concepts and categories that are combined and confused in most discussions of suicide. They are: (1) suicide proper, or so-called successful suicide; (2) attempted, threatened, or so-called unsuccessful suicide; and (3) the attribution by someone (typically a psychiatrist) to someone else (now called a "patient") of serious (that is, probably successful) suicidal intent. The first two concepts refer to acts by an actually or ostensibly suicidal person; the third refers to the claim of an ostensibly normal person about someone else's suicide-proneness.

I believe that, generally speaking, the person who commits suicide in-

Reprinted from *The Antioch Review* 31 (Spring 1971): 7–17, with the permission of the author and publisher. Copyright 1971 by Thomas Szasz.

tends to die; whereas the one who threatens suicide or makes an unsuccessful attempt at it intends to improve his life, not to terminate it. (The person who makes claims about someone else's suicidal intent does so usually in order to justify his efforts to control that person.)

Put differently, successful suicide is generally an expression of an individual's desire for greater autonomy—in particular, for self-control over his own death; whereas unsuccessful suicide is generally an expression of an individual's desire for more control over others—in particular, for compelling persons close to him to comply with his wishes. Although in some cases there may be legitimate doubt about which of these conditions obtains, in the majority of instances where people speak of "suicide" or "attempted suicide," the act falls clearly into one or the other group.

In short, I believe that successful and unsuccessful suicide constitute radically different acts and categories, and hence cannot be discussed together. Accordingly, I have limited the scope of this essay to suicide proper, with occasional references to attributions of suicidal intent. (The ascription of suicidal intent is, of course, a very different sort of thing from either successful or unsuccessful suicide. Since psychiatrists use it as if it designated a potentially or probably fatal "condition," it is sometimes necessary to consider this concept together with the phenomenon of suicide proper.)

I

It is difficult to find "responsible" medical or psychiatric authority today that does not regard suicide as a medical, and specifically as a mental health, problem.

For example, Ilza Veith, the noted medical historian, writing in *Modern Medicine* (August 11, 1969), asserts that ". . . the act [of suicide] clearly represents an illness. . . ."

Bernard R. Shochet (1970), a psychiatrist at the University of Maryland, offers a precise description of the kind of illness it is. "Depression," he writes, "is a serious systemic disease, with both physiological and psychological concomitants, and suicide is a part of this syndrome." And he articulates the intervention he feels is implicit in this view: "If the patient's safety is in doubt, psychiatric hospitalization should be insisted on."

Harvey M. Schein and Alan A. Stone (1969), both psychiatrists at the Harvard Medical School, are even more explicit about the psychiatric coercion justified, in their judgment, by the threat of suicide. "Once the patient's suicidal thoughts are shared," they write,

> the therapist must take pains to make clear to the patient that he, the therapist, considers suicide to be a maladaptive action, irreversibly counter to the patient's sane interests and goals; that he, the therapist, will do *everything* he can to prevent it; and that the potential for such an action arises from the patient's illness. It is equally essential that the therapist believe in the professional stance; if he does not he should not be treating the patient within the delicate human framework of psychotherapy. (emphasis added)

Schein and Stone do not explain why the patient's confiding in his therapist to the extent of communicating his suicidal thoughts to him should *ipso facto* deprive the patient from being the arbiter of his own best interests. The thrust of their argument is prescriptive rather than logical. They seek to justify depriving the patient of a basic human freedom—the freedom to grant or withhold consent for treatment: "The therapist must insist that patient and physician—*together*—communicate the suicidal potential to important figures in the environment, both professional and family. . . . Suicidal intent must not be part of therapeutic confidentiality." And further on they write: "Obviously this kind of patient must be hospitalized. . . . The therapist must be prepared to step in with hospitalization, with security measures, and with medication. . . ."

Schein and Stone thus suggest that the "suicidal" patient should have the right to choose his therapist; and that he should have the right to agree with his therapist and follow the latter's therapeutic recommendation (say, for hospitalization). At the same time, they insist that if "suicidal" patient and therapist disagree on therapy, then the patient should *not* have the right to disengage himself from the first therapist and choose a second—say, one who would consider suicidal intent a part of therapeutic confidentiality.

Many other psychiatric authorities could be cited to illustrate the current unanimity on this view of suicide.

Lawyers and jurists have eagerly accepted the psychiatric perspective on suicide, as they have on nearly everything else. An article in the *American Bar Association Journal* (September 1968) by R. E. Schulman, who is both a lawyer and a psychologist, is illustrative.

Schulman begins with the premise that "No one in contemporary Western society would suggest that people be allowed to commit suicide as they please without some attempt to intervene or prevent such suicides. Even if a person does not value his own life, Western society does value everyone's life."

But I should like to suggest, as others have suggested before me, precisely what Schulman claims no one would suggest. Furthermore, if Schulman chooses to believe that Western society—which includes the United States with its history of slavery, Germany with its history of National Socialism, and Russia with its history of Communism—really "values everyone's life," so be it. But to accept this assertion as true is to fly in the face of the most obvious and brutal facts of history.

II

When a person decides to take his life, and when a physician decides to frustrate him in this action, the question arises: Why should the physician do so?

Conventional psychiatric wisdom answers: Because the suicidal person (now called "patient" for proper emphasis) suffers from a mental illness whose symptom is his desire to kill himself; it is the physician's duty to diagnose and treat illness: *ergo*, he must prevent the "patient" from killing himelf and, at the same time, must "treat" the underlying "disease" that "causes" the "patient" to wish doing away with himself. This looks like an ordinary medical diagnosis and intervention. But it is not. What is missing? Everything. This hypothetical, suicidal "patient" is not ill: he has no demonstrable bodily disorder (or if he does, it does not "cause" his suicide); he does not assume the sick role: he does not seek medical help. In short, the physician uses the rhetoric of illness and treatment to justify his forcible intervention in the life of a fellow human being—often in the face of explicit opposition from his so-called "patient."

I do not doubt that attempted or successful suicide may be exceedingly *disturbing* for persons related to, acquainted with, or caring for the ostensible "patient." But I reject the conclusion that the suicidal person is, *ipso facto*, disturbed, that being disturbed equals being *mentally ill*, and that being mentally ill *justifies* psychiatric hospitalization or treatment. I have developed my reasons for this elsewhere, and need not repeat them here (Szasz 1963; 1970). For the sake of emphasis, however, let me state that I consider counseling, persuasion, psychotherapy, or any other *voluntary measure*, especially for persons troubled by their own suicidal inclinations and seeking such help, unobjectionable, and indeed generally desirable, interventions. However, physicians and psychiatrists are usually not satisfied with limiting their help to such measures—and with good reason: from such assistance the individual may gain not only the desire to live, but also the strength to die.

But we still have not answered the question: Why should a physician frustrate an individual from killing himself? As we saw, some psychiatrists answer: Because the physician values the patient's life, at least when the patient is suicidal, more highly than does the patient himself. Let us examine this claim. Why should the physician, often a complete stranger to the suicidal patient, value the patient's life more highly than does the patient himself? He does not do so in medical practice. Why then should he do so in psychiatric practice, which he himself insists is a form of medical practice? Let us assume that a physician is confronted with an individual suffering from diabetes or heart failure who fails to take the drugs prescribed for his illness. We know that this often happens, and that when it does the patient may become disabled and die prematurely. Yet it would be absurd for a physician to consider, much less to attempt, taking over the conduct of such a patient's life, confining him in a hospital against his will in order to treat his disease. Indeed, any attempt to do so would bring the physician into conflict with both the civil and the criminal law. For, significantly, the law recognizes the medical patient's autonomy despite the fact that, unlike the suicidal individual, he suffers from a real disease; and despite the fact that, unlike the nonexistent disease of the suicidal individual, his illness is often easily controlled by simple and safe therapeutic procedures.

Nevertheless, the threat of alleged or real suicide, or so-called dangerousness to oneself, is everywhere considered a proper ground and justification for involuntary mental hospitalization and treatment. Why should this be so?

Let me suggest what I believe is likely to be the most important reason for the profound antisuicidal bias of the medical profession. Physicians are committed to saving lives. How, then, should they react to people who are committed to throwing away their lives? It is natural for people to dislike, indeed to hate, those who challenge their basic values. The physician thus reacts, perhaps "unconsciously" (in the sense that he does not articulate the problem in these terms), to the suicidal patient as if the patient had affronted, insulted, or attacked him: The physician strives valiantly, often at the cost of his own well-being, to save lives; and here comes a person who not only does not let the physician save him, but, *horribile dictu*, makes the physician an unwilling witness to that person's deliberate self-destruction. This is more than most physicians can take. Feeling assaulted in the very center of their spiritual identity, some take to flight, while others fight back.

Some nonpsychiatric physicians will thus have nothing to do with suicidal patients. This explains why many people who end up killing themselves have a record of having consulted a physician, often on the very day of their suicide. I surmise that these persons go in search of help, only to discover that the physician wants nothing to do with them. And, in a sense, it is right that it should be so. I do not blame the doctors. Nor do I advocate teaching them suicide prevention—whatever that might be. I contend that because physicians have a relatively blind faith in their lifesaving ideology—which, moreover, they often need to carry them through their daily work—they are the wrong people for listening and talking to individuals, intelligently and calmly, about suicide. So much for those physicians who, in the face of the existential attack which they feel the suicidal patient launches on them, run for *their* lives. Let us now look at those who stand and fight back.

Some physicians (and other mental health professionals) declare themselves not only ready and willing to help suicidal patients who seek assistance, but all persons who are, or are alleged to be, suicidal. Since they, too, seem to perceive suicide as a threat, not just to the suicidal person's physical survival but to their own value system, they strike back and strike back hard. This explains why psychiatrists and suicidologists resort, apparently with a perfectly clear conscience, to the vilest methods: they must believe that their lofty ends justify the basest means. Hence the prevalent use of force and fraud in suicide prevention. The consequence of this kind of interaction between physician and "patient" is a struggle for power. The patient is at least honest about what he wants: to gain control over his life *and* death—by being the agent of his own demise. But the (suicide-preventing) psychiatrist is completely dishonest about what he wants: he claims that he only wants to help his patient, while actually he wants to gain control over the patient's life in order to save himself from having to confront his doubts about the value of his own life. Suicide is medical heresy. Commitment and electroshock are the appropriate psychiatric-inquisitorial remedies for it.

III

In the West, opposition to suicide, like opposition to contraception and abortion, rests on religious grounds. According to both the Jewish and Christian religions, God created man, and man can use himself only in the ways permitted by God. Preventing conception, aborting a pregnancy, or killing oneself are, in this imagery, all sins: each is a violation of the laws laid down by God, or by theological authorities claiming to speak in His name.

But modern man is a revolutionary. Like all revolutionaries, he likes to take away from those who have and to give to those who have not, especially himself. He has thus taken Man from God and given him to the State (with which he often identifies more than he knows). This is why the State gives and takes away so many of our rights, and why we consider this arrangement so "natural."

But this arrangement leaves suicide in a peculiar moral and philosophical limbo. For if a man's life belongs to the State (as it formerly belonged to God), then surely suicide is the taking of a life that belongs not to the taker but to everyone else.

The dilemma of this simplistic transfer of body-ownership from God to State derives from the fundamental difference between a religious and secular world view, especially when the former entails a vivid conception of a life after death, whereas the latter does not (or even emphatically repudiates it). More particularly, the dilemma derives from the problem of how to punish successful suicide? Traditionally, the Roman Catholic Church punished it by depriving the suicide of burial in consecrated ground. As far as I know, this practice is now so rare in the United States as to be practically nonexistent. Suicides are given a Catholic burial, as they are routinely considered having taken their lives while insane.

The modern State, with psychiatry as its secular-religious ally, has no comparable sanction to offer. Could this be one of the reasons why it punishes so severely—so very much more severely than did the Church—the *unsuccessful* suicide? For I consider the psychiatric stigmatization of people as "suicidal risks" and their incarceration in psychiatric institutions a form of punishment, and a very severe one at that. Indeed, although I cannot support this claim with statistics, I believe that accepted psychiatric methods of suicide prevention often aggravate rather than ameliorate the suicidal person's problems. As one reads of the tragic encounters with psychiatry of people like James Forrestal, Marilyn Monroe, or Ernest Heming-way, one gains the impression that they felt demeaned and deeply hurt by the psychiatric indignities inflicted on them, and that, as a result of these ex-periences, they were even more desperately driven to suicide. In short, I am suggesting that coerced psychiatric interventions may increase, rather than diminish, the suicidal person's desire for self-destruction.

But there is another aspect of the moral and philosophical dimensions of suicide that must be mentioned here. I refer to the growing influence of the resurgent idea of self-determination, especially the conviction that men have certain inalienable rights. Some men have thus come to believe (or perhaps only to believe that they believe) that they have a right to life, liberty, and property. This makes for some interesting complications for the modern legal and psychiatric stand on suicide.

This individualistic position on suicide might be put thus: A man's life belongs to himself. Hence, he has a right to take his own life, that is, to commit suicide. To be sure, this view recognizes that a man may also have a moral responsibility to his family and others, and that, by killing himself, he reneges on these responsibilities. But these are moral wrongs that society, in its corporate capacity as the State, cannot properly punish. Hence the State must eschew attempts to regulate such behavior by means of formal sanctions, such as criminal or mental hygiene laws.

The analogy between life and other types of property lends further support to this line of argument. Having a right to property means that a person can dispose of it even if in so doing he injures himself and his family. A man may give away, or gamble away, his money. But significantly, he cannot—our linguistic conventions do not allow it—be said to *steal from himself.* The concept of theft requires at least two parties: one who steals and another from whom is stolen. There is no such thing as "self-theft." The term "suicide" blurs this very distinction. The etymology of this term implies that suicide is a type of homicide, one in which criminal and victim are one and the same person. Indeed, when a person wants to condemn suicide he calls it "self-murder." Schulman, for example, writes: "Surely, self-murder falls within the province of the law."

History does repeat itself. Until recently, psychiatrists castigated as sick and persecuted those who engaged in self-abuse (that is, masturbation); now they castigate as sick and persecute those who engage in self-murder (that is, suicide).

The suicidologist has a literally schizophrenic view of the suicidal person: He sees him as two persons in one, each at war with the other. One-half of the patient wants to die; the other half wants to live. The former, says the suicidologist, is wrong; the latter is right. And he proceeds to protect the latter by restraining the former. However, since these two people are, like Siamese twins, one, he can restrain the suicidal half only by restraining the whole person.

The absurdity of this medical-psychiatric position on suicide does not end here. It ends in extolling mental health and physical survival over every other value, particularly individual liberty.

In regarding the desire to live as a legitimate human aspiration, but not the desire to die, the suicidologist stands Patrick Henry's famous exclamation, "Give me liberty, or give me death!" on its head. In effect, he says: "*Give him* commitment, *give him* electroshock, *give him* lobotomy, *give him* life-long slavery, but *do not let him choose* death!" By so radically invalidating another person's (not his own!) wish to die, the suicide-preventer redefines the aspiration of the Other as not an aspiration at all: The wish to die thus becomes something an irrational, mentally diseased being displays, or something that happens to a lower form of life. The result is a far-reaching infantilization and dehumanization of the suicidal person.

For example, Phillip Solomon writes in the *Journal of the American Medical Association* (January 30, 1967), that "We [physicians] must protect the patient from his own [suicidal] wishes." While to Edwin Shneidman (1968), "Suicide prevention is like fire prevention. . . ." Solomon thus reduces the would-be suicide to the level of an unruly child, while Shneidman reduces him to the level of a tree! In short, the suicidologist uses his professional stance to illegitimize and punish the wish to die.

There is, of course, nothing new about any of this. Do-gooders have always opposed personal autonomy or self-determination. In "Amok," written in 1931, Stefan Zweig put these words into the mouth of his protagonist: "Ah, yes, 'It's one's duty to help.' That's your favorite maxim, isn't it? . . . Thank you for your good intentions, but I'd rather be left to myself. . . . So I won't trouble you to call, if you don't mind. Among the 'rights of man' there is a right which no one can take away, the right to croak when and where and how one pleases, without a 'helping hand.' "

But this is not the way the scientific psychiatrist and suicidologist sees the problem. He might agree (I suppose) that, in the abstract, man has the right

Zweig claimed for him. But, in practice, suicide (so he says) is the result of insanity, madness, mental illness. Furthermore, it makes no sense to say that one has a right to be mentally ill, especially if the illness is one that, like typhoid fever, threatens the health of other people as well. In short, the suicidologist's job is to try to convince people that wanting to die is a disease.

This is how Ari Kiev, director of the Cornell Program in Social Psychiatry and its suicide-prevention clinic, does it: "We say [to the patient], look, you have a disease, just like the Hong Kong flu. Maybe you've got the Hong Kong depression. First, you've got to realize you are emotionally ill. . . . Most of the patients have never admitted to themselves that they are sick . . ." (*New York Times*, February 9, 1969).

This pseudomedical perspective is then used to justify psychiatric deception and coercion of the crudest sort.

Here is how, according to the *Wall Street Journal* (March 6, 1969), the Los Angeles Suicide Prevention Center operates. A man calls and says he is about to shoot himself. The worker asks for his address. The man refuses to give it.

> 'If I pull it [the trigger] now I'll be dead,' he [the caller] said in a muffled voice. 'And that's what I want.' Silently but urgently, Mrs. Whitbook [the worker] has signalled a co-worker to begin tracing the call. And now she worked to keep the man talking. . . . An agonizing 40 minutes passed. Then she heard the voice of a policeman come on the phone to say the man was safe.

But surely, if this man was able to call the Suicide Prevention Center, he could have, had he wanted, called for a policeman himself. But he did not. He was thus deceived by the Center in the "service" he got.

I understand that this kind of deception is standard practice in suicide prevention centers, though it is often denied that it is. A report (*Medical World News*, July 28, 1967) about the Nassau County Suicide Prevention Service corroborates the impression that when the would-be suicide does not cooperate with the suicide-prevention authorities, he is confined involuntarily. "When a caller is obviously suicidal," we are told, "a Meadowbrook ambulance is sent out immediately to pick him up."

One more example of the sort of thing that goes on in the name of suicide prevention should suffice. It is a routine story from a Syracuse newspaper (Syracuse *Post Standard*, September 29, 1969). The gist of it is all in one sentence: "A 28-year-old Minoa [a Syracuse suburb] man was arrested last night on a charge of violation of the Mental Hygiene Law, after police authorities said they spent two hours looking for him in the Minoa woods." But this man has harmed no one; his only "offense" was that someone claimed he might harm himself. Why, then, should the police look for, much less arrest, him? Why not wait until he returns? Or why not look, offer help, but avoid arrest and coerced psychiatry?

These are rhetorical questions. For our answers to them depend on and reflect our concepts of what it means to be a human being.

IV

I submit, then, that the crucial contradiction about suicide viewed as an illness whose treatment is a medical responsibility is that suicide is an action but is treated as if it were a happening. As I showed elsewhere, this contradiction lies at the heart of all so-called mental illnesses or psychiatric problems (Szasz 1961). However, it poses a particularly acute dilemma for suicide, because suicide is the only fatal "mental illness."

Before concluding, I should like to restate briefly my views on the differences between diseases and desires, and show that by persisting in treating desires as diseases, we only end up treating man as a slave.

Let us take, as our paradigm case of illness, a skier who takes a bad spill and fractures an ankle. This fracture is something that has happened to him. He has not intended it to happen. (To be sure, he may have intended it; but that is another case.) Once it has happened, he will seek medical help and will cooperate with medical efforts to mend his broken bones. In short, the person and his fractured ankle are, as it were, two separate entities, the former acting on the latter.

Let us now consider the case of the suicidal person. Such a person may also look upon his own suicidal inclination as an undesired, almost alien, impulse and seek help to combat it. If so, the ensuing arrangement between him and his psychiatrist is readily assimilated to the standard medical model of treatment: the patient actively seeks and cooperates with professional efforts to remedy his "condition."

But as we have seen this is not the only way, nor perhaps the most important way, that the game of suicide prevention is played. It is accepted medical and psychiatric practice to treat persons for their suicidal desires against their will. And what exactly does this means? Something quite different from that to which it is often analogized, namely the involuntary (or nonvoluntary) treatment of a bodily illness. For a fractured ankle can be set whether or not a patient consents to its being set. That is because setting a fracture is a *mechanical act on the body*. But a threatened suicide cannot be prevented whether or not the "patient" consents to its being prevented. That is because, suicide being the result of human desire and action, suicide prevention is a *political act on the person*. In other words, since suicide is an exercise and expression of human freedom, it can be prevented only by curtailing human freedom. This is why deprivation of liberty becomes, in institutional psychiatry, a form of treatment.

In the final analysis, the would-be suicide is like the would-be emigrant: both want to leave where they are and move elsewhere. The suicide wants to leave life and embrace death. The emigrant wants to leave his homeland and settle in another country.

Let us take this analogy seriously. It is much more faithful to the facts than is the analogy between suicide and illness. A crucial characteristic that distinguishes open from closed societies is that people are free to leave the former but not the latter. The medical profession's stance toward suicide is thus like the Communists' toward emigration: the doctors insist that the would-be suicide survive, just as the Russians insist that the would-be emigrant stay home.

Whether those who so curtail other people's liberties act with complete sincerity, or with utter cynicism, hardly matters. What matters is what happens: the abridgement of individual liberty, justified, in the case of suicide prevention, by psychiatric rhetoric; and, in the case of emigration prevention, by political rhetoric.

In language and logic we are the prisoners of our premises, just as in politics and law we are the prisoners of our rulers. Hence we had better pick them well. For if suicide is an illness because it terminates in death, and if the prevention of death by any means necessary is the physician's therapeutic mandate, then the proper remedy for suicide is indeed liberticide.

References

Schein, Harvey M., and Alan A. Stone. "Psychotherapy Designed to Detect and Treat Suicidal Potential." *American Journal of Psychiatry* 125 (March 1969): 1247–51.

Shneidman, Edwin. "Preventing Suicide." *Bulletin of Suicidiology*, July 1968, pp. 19–25.
Shochet, Bernard. "Recognizing the Suicidal Patient." *Modern Medicine* 38 (May 1970): 114–23.
Szasz, Thomas S. *The Myth of Mental Illness*. New York: Harper and Row, 1961
———. *Law, Liberty and Psychiatry*. New York: Macmillan, 1963.
———. *Ideology and Insanity*. Garden City, N.Y.: Doubleday, 1970.

26

Philosophical and Ethical Considerations of Suicide Prevention

Paul W. Pretzel

THERE are times when the esoterics of philosophical and ethical theory emerge from the classroom and take their place as issues of social concern. There are several ways in which this has been happening of late.

Television network news specials have lately examined such topics as "The Pursuit of Pleasure," asking the question, "How much individual indulgence can society withstand before the cohesion of that society is destroyed?" Corollary to this is the ethical question of how much action a society is entitled to take to demand conformity from its members. Demanding too much conformity stifles creativity, produces stagnation, and runs the danger of fomenting revolution; too little control, on the other hand, results in anarchy and dissolution of the society. How much social dissent, then, are we to accept? How many do we permit to "turn on, tune in, and drop out"? How many do we permit to deviate from the social norm and in what ways?

This polarity between individual freedom and social cohesion is a social question, a religious question, a philosophical question, that has a long history which includes many different specific issues including birth control,

Reprinted from the *Bulletin of Suicidology*, July 1968, pp. 30–38, with the permission of the publisher. Some footnotes omitted.

capital punishment, abortion, euthanasia, and suicide and suicide prevention.

It is an unusual discussion on suicide in which someone does not pose the question, "But doesn't a person have the right to take his own life under certain circumstances?" Or, put more aggressively, "What right do you have interfering with the person's decision to take his own life?"

This is no problem, of course, in those cases where the patient himself calls for help, or where he is obviously too mentally disturbed to be entrusted with such a final decision. The question arises in the minority of cases where the suicidal person is apparently in full possession of his faculties and where the circumstances of his life appear to make such a decision a "rational" one. This may occur in some situations when hope seems literally beyond any reasonable expectation.

The individual right of a person to kill himself for any reason has been the object of philosophical discussion going back to the earliest roots of Greek philosophy and before.

Socrates, for example, saw suicide as an evil in most cases and asserted that "no man has a right to take his own life, but he must wait until God sends some necessity upon him, as he has now sent upon me." And as his own drinking of the hemlock indicates, there are such times of necessity.

Plato follows in this tradition, rigorously condemning the self-murder that takes place as a result of "slough or want of manliness" but tacitly approves of a suicide that takes place "under the compulsion of some painful and inevitable misfortune which has come upon him or because he has to suffer from irremediable and intolerable shame."

The second main tradition of Greek philosophy, that of the Epicureans, has a still more permissive stand in regard to the right of a person to take his own life. For the Epicureans death was not the terrifying object that it was to the other early Greeks. To them, death was simply the end of existence and an end that ought to be hastened whenever the individual wished it. Man is alive to enjoy life, was the Epicurean philosophy, and when life ceases to be enjoyable, there is no reason to continue to live. Lucretius, the Epicurean poet who himself died of suicide, expressed this point of view (Fedden 1938): "If, one day, as well may happen, life grows wearisome, there only remains to pour a libation to death and oblivion. A drop of subtle poison will gently close your eyes to the sun and waft you smiling into the eternal night whence everything comes and to which everything returns."

Perhaps the most famous quotation illustrating the Epicurean point of view is this one: "Above all things remember that the door is open. Be not more timid than boys at play. As they, when they cease to take pleasure in their games, declare they will no longer play, so do you; when all things begin to pull upon you, retire." For the Epicureans, then, the door is always open. Life will be lived as long as it is enjoyed, but when the hope for happiness dims, the door to death is always open.

The third major tradition of Greek philosophy, that of the Stoics, again endorses the right of the individual to take his life when he wishes it, providing the act is one of reason, will, and integrity. Suicide as a result of despair was weakness and represented failure, but a rational suicide was not uncommon among the Stoics and was endorsed by the community. The Stoic Seneca expressed it this way: "As I choose the ship in which I will sail and the house I will inhabit, so I will choose the death by which I leave life. In no matter more than in death should we act according to our own desire."

According to Stoic philosophy, it would be far better for one to choose death rather than to see that noble part of him be eaten away by old age or disease. Seneca says in another place:

I will not relinquish old age if it leaves my better part intact, but if it begins to shake my mind, if it destroys its faculties one by one, if it leaves me not life but death, I will depart from the putrid or tottering edifice. I will not escape by death and disease so long as it may be healed and leaves my mind unimpaired. I will not raise my hand against myself on account of pain, for so to die is to be conquered, but if I know I must suffer without hope of relief, I will depart, not through fear of pain itself but because it prevents all for which I would live.

Paul Tillich (1952) offers a good summary of the Stoic attitude toward suicide. "The Stoic recommendation of suicide is not directed to those who are conquered by life but to those who have conquered life and are able both to live and to die and can choose freely between them. Suicide as an escape dictated by fear contradicts the Stoic courage to be."

Perhaps Stoicism received its best contemporary expression in the person of Ernest Hemingway who saw man's decision in life as being one of choosing defeat or destruction. Hotchner (1966) catches Hemingway in a pensive mood on the occasion of the serious injury of a much-admired matador: "He's a brave man and a beautiful matador. Why the hell do the good and brave have to die before everyone else?" Hotchner explains that Hemingway did not mean die as in death, for Dominican was going to survive, but what was important is his living had died. I remember Ernest once telling me, "The worst death for anyone is to lose the center of his being, the thing he really is. Retirement is the filthiest word in the language. Whether by chance, or by fate, to retire from what you do—and what you do makes you what you are—is to back up into the grave."

These philosophical arguments defending man's right to kill himself under the "right circumstances" as expressed in the early Greek philosophy were reexamined and, in many cases, supported by the philosophers of the Enlightenment.

In his essay on suicide, Hume upheld man's freedom to do as he will with his own life. Along with Hume, Montaigne also affirmed the right of suicide on the grounds that life is a blessing and when it ceases to be desirable, one should be free to give it up. Voltaire, too, found the right of suicide in cases of extreme emergency to be an important individual right.

In our own time, writers such as James Hillman not only defend the right of the person to kill himself, but go on to argue that everyone who is so presumptuous as to try to prevent a suicide is depriving the patient of what might be the most significant decision of his life; even if that decision is to die, it does not necessarily mean there is a failure. Hillman (1964) holds that no one has ever proven that the soul perishes after death, and that the existential decision to kill oneself might be a necessary decision in terms of affirming the soul, in which case the analyst would be violating the right of his patient. Hillman: "Usually the death experience is in the psychological mode, but for some, organic death through actual suicide may be the only mode through which the death experience is possible."

But not all the philosophical thinkers of the past have been so vehement in defending the person's right to kill himself. One of the earliest Greek philosophers, the spokesman for the Orphic brotherhood, by the name of Pythagoras, saw suicide as an unmitigated evil. One of the important teachings of the Orphic brotherhood was that of the transmigrations of the soul, its purification in the wheel of births, and its final reunion with the divine. Jacques Choron (1963) describes this teaching:

> The soul is imprisoned in the body and leaves it at death, and after a period of purification, re-enters another body. This process repeats itself several times, but to make sure that with every new existence the soul

should retain its purity or become ever purer and better and thus come ever closer to the final stage where the reunion with the divine takes place, man must follow a certain discipline. Philosophy becomes with Pythagoras a way of life that assures salvation.

To Pythagoras, then, suicide is a rebellion against the gods. It is an action that stems from perturbation which is a pollution of the soul and is therefore an unworthy act.

Aristotle, too, condemned suicide on the grounds that it is always a cowardly act: "To seek death in order to escape from poverty or the pangs of love, or from pain or sorrow, is not the act of a courageous man but rather of a coward, for it is weakness to fly from troubles, and suicide does not endure death because it is noble to do so but to escape evil." But the main Aristotelian objection to suicide is on the basis that man is fundamentally the property of the state and he has no right to deprive the state of any of its property: "Therefore the suicide commits injustice but against whom? It seems to be against the state rather than against himself, for he suffers voluntarily. Nobody suffers injustice voluntarily. This is why the state exacts a penalty. Suicide is punished by certain marks of dishonor as being an offense against the state."

The period of the Enlightenment also had its philosophers which deny man's right to kill himself. Kant, for example, held that all human life was sacred and must be preserved at all costs. He stressed that suicide is inconsistent with reason and inconsistent with the categorical imperative by which every act should be judged. That is to say, the potential suicide should ask himself, "What would follow if everyone did what I am about to do?"

Schopenhauer was another philosopher who doubted the authenticity of the suicidal person's wish to die. Although Schopenhauer is famous for his pessimism, characteristically dwelling on the evils and ills in life, he discarded suicide as a possible answer to the problem. The suicidal person is not really desiring to reject life, Schopenhauer held. He is rejecting the conditions under which he has been forced to live. He is indeed expressing a will to live, in his rebellion against all the conditions of his life which limit his basic freedom to enjoy life. We might be struck by a similarity between Schopenhauer's position and our own orientation toward suicide, namely, that suicide can best be understood as an ambivalent cry for help.

In later times, William James (1904) also denied the individual's right to take his own life, holding that the human task is to find the religious meaning in our own individual human lives, and it is only when this religious search is taken seriously that human life becomes meaningful.

This brings us to the consideration of the stand which the major religions of our own culture have taken on the question of suicide. Judaism, which, according to most available statistics, has usually enjoyed a comparatively low suicide rate, holds to the traditional view of the sacredness of all human life which *was* ultimately the property of the Creator rather than the individual person. In the Old Testament, for example, God was very angry with Onan for spilling his own seed on the ground rather than using it for procreation. There are six accounts of suicide in the Old Testament, all of which are simply reported as historical facts without any judgment being attributed to them. In biblical times, then, there seems to have been no express law against suicide unless the commandment "Thou Shalt Not Kill" can be interpreted to include self-murder.

There is some indication that during some of the wars, suicide rather than capture by the enemy was accepted as a custom. Josephus put an end to this, however, by delivering a speech to his army which was considering suicide rather than capture during the siege of Jotaphata. Gathering his army before him, he delivered this stirring speech which he himself later recorded (Dublin and Bunzel 1933):

> Oh my friends, why are you so earnest to kill yourselves? Why do you set your soul and body which are such dear companions at such variance? It is a brave thing to die in war, but it should be by the hands of the enemy. It is a foolish thing to do that for ourselves which we quarrel with them for doing to us. It is a brave thing to die for liberty but still it should be in battle and by those who would take that liberty from us. He is equally a coward who will not die when he is obliged to die. What are we afraid of when we will not go and meet the Romans? Is it death? Why then inflict it on ourselves? Self-murder is a crime most remote from the common nature of all animals and an instance of impiety against God, our Creator.

This eloquent speech is possibly the first expression of what has come to be accepted as a traditional Jewish view of suicide.

Perhaps even more characteristic than this prohibition are the words of the Mishnah, part of the Talmud. Speaking of a suicide, Rabbi Elizer says: "Leave him not in the clothes in which he died. Honor him not nor damn him. One does not tear one's garments on his account or take off one's shoes, nor does one hold funeral rites for him, but one does comfort his family, for that is honoring the living."

Suicide, according to the Jewish tradition, implies freedom of choice and freedom of will. Almost by definition, a person who kills himself is not in control of his faculties, for it is not a rational act.

For several centuries, Christianity took no direct stand in regard to suicide. The New Testament makes no direct comment about it at all. There is some indication in its early years that certain suicidal deaths received the approval of the Christian community. Martyrdom, for example, was deemed a worthy act commenting as it did on the cruelty of the pagan world, the lack of fear of death, and the strength of faith. Saint Cyprian writes that the true Christians did not fear death and willingly gave their blood to escape from the cruel world. Tertullian, in defense of martyrdom, cites with approval some well-known suicides including those of Lucretia, Dido, and Cleopatra. Early Christian history is filled with stories of the faithful seeking out martyrdom as a sure means of eternal salvation.

In addition to the self-seeking martyrs, the early Christian community approved of those young women who took their own lives rather than lose their chastity. Saint Pelagia, a girl of 15, jumped from a roof to certain death to escape a Roman soldier and later was canonized for her action. Saint Ambrose said of her, "God was not offended by such a remedy and faith exalted it." Two other examples of such suicides include the death of Domena and her two daughters who accepted drowning in preference to loss of chastity, and Belsilla, a 20-year-old nun, who abused herself until she died and in so doing received the approval of Jerome.

The first clear statements against suicide in the Christian tradition came from the pen of Saint Augustine who, in the City of God, put forth the view that suicide is never justified. He supports his opinion on the basis of four reasons: (1) The Christian is never without hope as long as a possibility of repentance remains alive, but with suicide the possibility of repentance is gone; (2) suicide is homicide, and this is a forbidden act; (3) there is no sin worthy of death; and (4) suicide is a greater sin, at any choice. The Christian is better advised to make any choice other than killing himself, for he will be guilty of a lesser sin and still be alive to repent.

St. Augustine had to modify his position somewhat since the Church had already canonized some suicides such as that of St. Pelagia. Augustine handles this by assuming that she had received special divine revelation which sanctioned her act, and thus this exceptional case did not invalidate his reasoning.

St. Augustine's view prevailed in the Church, and beginning with the Council of Arles in 452, the Church issued a series of encyclicals defining their antisuicide position and designating a series of punishments for the act. As time went on, the punishments became more intense and more cruel, reaching their culmination in the eighteenth century when it was not uncommon for the body of a suicide to be dragged nude through the streets, be buried at the crossroads with a stake in its heart, being deprived of the rights of burial, and having the state confiscate all the deceased's property, thereby depriving the heirs of their inheritance.

The trend toward such cruel punishment began to be reversed with the publication of *Bianthanatos* by John Donne, Bishop of St. Pauls, in the mid-seventeenth century. His thesis was that the power of God is great enough that we are in error in assuming that all suicides are irremissible sins. It was the first plea for moderation and understanding, and as a result, both secular and church law against suicide began to be modified.

In our own time, those like Edwin Shneidman (1968), who would defend suicide-prevention activities as being ethical, even imperative, and based on solid philosophical convictions, have stressed three basic points: (1) the ambivalence that is always present in any human action, including that of suicide; (2) the fact that suicide is impulsive; and (3) the effect that such an action has upon the survivors, including the general community.

To those like Hillman who offer a mystical rationale defending the right of the individual to make this existential choice, other thinkers such as Robert E. Litman (1967) respond by pointing out that "from the medical point of view, questions of the soul and its destiny are rather irrelevant when confronted with a corpse. No matter how committed an analyst might be to the soul, it would seem his work, too, is stopped by physical death."

Litman goes on to observe that if philosophical and ethical theory are to be relevant to the work of the clinician, they cannot be developed apart from the clinical setting, or (to use Freud's image) they will be like the whale and the polar bear who cannot carry on meaningful conversation since each being confined to his own element, they cannot meet.

Hemingway's suicide, for example, cannot be attributed simply to his philosophy of life while the signs of his personality difficulties in the last year or so of his life are ignored.

What is needed, according to Litman, to provide a meeting ground for scientists, theorists, philosophers, and therapists who wish to discuss or argue suicide, is publication of the essential material of clinical psychology, a collection of detailed case reports on the lives and deaths of a variety of intensively studied individuals who committed suicide.

Perhaps we can begin here to focus on the relationship between the clinical and philosophical fields. Our society often endorses the following four types of suicides as being "rational" and in regard to which the ethics of intervention might be open to question:

1. those suicides carried out for the good of some cause, as in the case of religious martyrdom, military heroism, or dramatic social witness;
2. those carried out as a reaction to what appears to be a literally hopeless, painful, and debilitating situation, as in the case of lingering terminal illness;
3. those in which the circumstances are not desperate, but in which the individual is no longer receiving the pleasure from life that he wants and so makes the decision to go through the "open door" away from life;
4. the so-called love-pact suicide where the double death is seen as having some esthetic value, possibly being as expression of love, beauty, or dedication.

Let us examine some clinical illustrations of each of the categories. What we have designated as "suicide in support of a cause," Durkheim (1951) described in terms of the "altruistic suicide."

Such a suicide, according to Durkheim, takes place when a person is overintegrated into his society and subordinates his own desires to the will of the group. One example of this is that of a captain going down with his ship to certain death in obedience to the social tradition that expects such behavior. Another example is that of a case reported by the press in 1965 of a young man who died of self-immolation in Washington, D.C., as part of his protest against the war in Vietnam. Norman Morrison was 32 years old, married, and a father. He was a college graduate and also held a degree from a recognized theological seminary. People who knew him described him in terms of his capacity to be a close personal friend, profound in thinking, and sensitive to human suffering. They deny that he was eccentric or a fanatic. In fact they say

he was a normal person in that he was genuinely concerned with other human beings, those in Vietnam and those who were with him. He was flattering to others as a conversationalist because he took what one had to say as something very important. Norman wasn't just a good listener but was truly concerned about the concerns of others. He loved people not in the sense of polite liberal abstractions but in the sense that other people got inside and affected him. He enjoyed carpentry around the house, gardening, softball, ice hockey, the things we all find normal. He was not a pious saint attempting some kind of fanatical purity. (statement at memorial service)

Morrison was a Quaker, and as such believed in a concerned and loving God, the sacredness of human life, and he shared the traditional Quaker abhorrence of war. We have available to us, then, a rather clear picture of Morrison's philosophical orientation, and a clear rationale for the act of self-destruction that he performed. If this were all that there was to say, Morrison could be cited as one of the rational suicides which comes about through dedication to some cause. What is missing, however, is a complete write-up of Morrison's personality development and a thorough appraisal of any psychiatric symptoms that might have been appearing in the last few years. What is needed, then, before any kind of accurate judgment might be made about the rationality of this type of suicide, is more complete data so that a more accurate evaluation can be made from several points of view.

The second type of suicide which our society may consider to be rational and ethical is that which stems from what appears to be an apparently hopeless situation. The prototype for this type is the elderly person who is suffering from a chronic, painful, and terminal disease. What is surprising to most people is that suicide among this population is as rare as it is. One case which might serve as an example is that of Joan Smith, a 24-year-old, attractive girl who has been suffering from Hodgkin's disease since the age of 12. The progress of the disease has been slowed down but yet continues with no real hope of a cure. Joan has been married for four years to a man by whom she had become pregnant prior to the marriage and who has continued since the marriage to have numerous affairs of which she was aware. She feels unloved by him and describes her home situation as being intolerable. Joan feels affectionate toward their 3½-year-old son, but she also feels that he deserves a mother who will be alive throughout his childhood and adolescence. She has strong feelings of self-depreciation and feels that anyone with whom she is closely involved is somehow going to be infected by her. She has thought about terminating her very unsatisfactory marriage but feels that her son deserves a father, even one as inadequate as this, and does not know what she would do if she did divorce him. She feels it would be unfair of her to consider marriage to any man.

In addition to her husband and her son, she has a mother, a stepfather, and a sister. The stepfather pays very little attention to her. Her mother, on the other hand, is a very "sweet" woman, long-suffering and double-binding. Joan has strong dependency feelings toward her mother and feels trapped and unable to cope with the kinds of demands that her mother subtly puts on her. Her sister is widowed and struggles to support herself and her three children. Joan and her sister have a fairly good relationship, but Joan feels guilty about accepting any help from this sister who has problems of her own. Joan has been suicidal for several years, and has made two very serious attempts in the last six months, both of which required hospitalization. She feels that she is nothing but a burden to these people who are near her and feels helpless and hopeless about ever attaining any significant degree of self-sufficiency and independence. The world, in general, and her son, in particular, would be better off if she were to die immediately and not burden everyone with several more years of emotional and financial stress. Her fantasy is that if she were to kill herself, her husband soon would remarry and her son would have a better mother almost regardless of whom the husband married.

In this case, as in the case of many such "hopeless" situations, the hopelessness, it later became clear, was more a function of Joan's emotional attitude than it was a function of the philosophical reality of the situation. As a result of her repeated suicide attempts, Joan was placed in therapy and with the help and support of the therapist was able to make certain decisions which changed the complexion of her life entirely. She left her husband, moved in with her sister, and began to reorientate her life around finding satisfactions for herself. She made appropriate and realistic plans for her own social life, accepted certain financial and social responsibilities that gave her a feeling of self-sufficiency and ability, and was able to continue functioning effectively as a member of the family and of society. To be sure, it might be expected that Joan will come across future crises in which she will seriously consider suicide, but if this happens, it will be the result of her emotional situation rather than a rational decision.

The third type of suicide which some consider rational concerns the exit through the "open door" of the Epicureans when life has failed to provide sufficient satisfaction to justify continuation of life, even though there is no overt or physical, hopeless situation. One example of such a type may be that of Ernest Hemingway referred to earlier. Another example is that of Jim Johnson, a 60-year-old man whose wife had passed away several months earlier from cancer. The Johnsons had been married for some 35 years and although the marriage was childless, it was described by Jim as being a very close and a very happy marriage. Jim was steadily employed at one of the large manufacturing firms in the area where he held the position of skilled laborer. Four months prior to Mrs. Johnson's death they were told she had cancer and was given six months to a year. At that time Jim retired from his position at the manufacturing plant in order to be able to be at home and to nurse his ailing wife. When she died two months later he found himself without a job and without his wife—without his two main reasons for living. Being unable to tolerate the feelings he experienced in the house in which they had lived for many years, he sold it and purchased a trailer in a senior citizens' park.

Jim himself was in excellent physical health, had some interests, some hobbies, and was even able to formulate some plans for how he would spend his remaining years. He had no other family left, but had a close relationship with his wife's family. The problem was, as he put it, that he found no pleasure in anything anymore. He was chronically depressed and was unable to work through his grief. Life was flat and meaningless, and although there was no physical or mental agony, neither was there any pleasure or satisfaction in life. He began ruminating about suicide, considering several different plans. One night he came to the decision that life for him was no longer worth living, that he could no longer receive any satisfaction or pleasure from life, and so he killed himself.

To the Epicurean, this suicide might be seen as a rational act of a man who walked through the "open door," no longer willing to continue a life without satisfaction. To the clinician, however, the situation would seem quite different. The clinician would see an unresolved-grief reaction with difficulty in tolerating the depression which realistically follows such significant and important losses. The clinician's hope would be that although Jim would experience a residual sadness for the rest of his life, once the grief reaction had been dealt with, he would be able once again to experience satisfactions in certain aspects of living and that suicide was, for him, not the answer.

The fourth category of so-called rational suicide is that which we have called the love-pact suicide in which the double death is seen as having some esthetic value. Although not uncommon in romantic literature, such suicides are relatively rare in Western culture. They are more common in Far Eastern literature which characteristically portrays a pattern involving

a young merchant or craftsman and a young girl. Because of economic difficulties, problems preventing their marriage, such as their parents' or spouses' objections, poor living conditions such as pending criminal proceedings or inadaptability to rapid social change, one night in spring or summer of the Tokyo-Osaka area toward dawn, they stab themselves (occasionally hang or drown themselves) and almost never survive. (Ohara and Reynolds)

The actual love-pact suicides in Japan, however, do not follow this romantic picture. According to Dr. Ohara's study, these suicides are characterized by unstable job situations, unsatisfying sexual relationships, social, economic, and emotional difficulties. Far from being a high expression of beauty or dedication, they can be described more accurately as desperate and unhappy resolutions of painful conflicts. Parties to a love-pact suicide are not dissimilar to people who commit suicide under less romantic circumstances.

One type of love-pact suicide is the murder-suicide pact where one party seeks to take a loved one into death with him. One such case involved an attractive 35-year-old mother who shot her 10-year-old son and then killed herself, after writing a 22-page suicide note expressing her fears for herself and her son and explaining at some length that this seemed to her to be the kindest thing to do and the only way to resolve the conflicts that life offered. But again, clinical investigation into the life of this person reveals increasing and intensifying symptoms of schizophrenia, terrible confusion and fear, paranoid ideation, and suspicion that had its climax in a double tragedy.

This, then, is the kind of investigation that needs to take place as the philosophical and ethical considerations of suicide and suicide prevention are being considered. The investigation must have the double focus of philosophical ideas and metaphysical continuity along with clinical evaluation of what is happening within the life of the person who would perceive his act as being rational and *justifiable*.

For the person who is working in the field of suicide and suicide prevention, as well as for the person who is confronted with a suicidal situation, the question is when, if ever, is the clinician willing to say: "Yes, I agree. It is the best thing for you to do, and I have no right to interfere, so I won't." Where does he stop trying? How long does society desire to force continuation of life? Where is the point, if indeed there is one at all, at which the ambivalence inherent in any human action, including that of suicidal behavior, shades into self-determination? How far does the community want to go in forcing other people to adhere to life?

The purpose of this paper has been the limited one of attempting to set forth some of the basic considerations that should be weighed as the issue is being met.

References

Choron, Jacques. *Death and Western Thought*. New York: Collier Books, 1963.

Dublin, Louis, and Bessie Bunzel. *To Be or Not to Be*. New York: H. Smith and R. Haas, 1933.

Durkheim, Emil. *Suicide*. Glencoe, Ill.: Free Press, 1951.

Fedden, Henry Romily. *Suicide, A Social and Historical Study*. London: Peter Davies, 1938.

Hillman, James. *Suicide and the Soul*. New York: Harper & Row, 1964.

Hotchner, A. E. *Papa Hemingway*. New York: Random House, 1966.

James, William. *The Will to Believe*. New York: Longmans, 1904.

Litman, Robert. "Review of James Hillman's *Suicide and the Soul*." *Contemporary Psychology* 12 (1967): 449–50.

Ohara, K., and D. Reynolds. "Love Pact Suicide." Unpublished study.

Tillich, Paul. *The Courage to Be*. New Haven: Yale University Press, 1952.

Index

International Code of Medical Ethics, 342, 353

Internists, 14

Irreversible coma, 82-89

Isoelectric EEG, 95, 101, 104, 121, 227, 239

I-thou, 29

James, William, 391

Jehovah's Witnesses, 241-48, 331

John F. Kennedy Memorial Hospital v. Heston, 244

Johns Hopkins Hospital, xvi, 136, 145, 174, 292

Josephus, 392

Judeo-Christian tradition, 31, 47, 68, 77, 167, 172, 178-83, 193, 255, 275, 282-96, 301-7, 320-40, 380, 392-94

Justice, 152-54

Kamisar, Yale, 266

Kansas statute on death, xv, 99, 103, 117-19, 122-23

Kant, Immanuel, xiv, 41, 217, 391

Karnofsky, David A., 212, 222

Kass, Leon, xv, 70-81, 103-24

Kelly, Gerald, 180, 196, 199-204, 334

Kelly, William, xv, 3-8

Kennedy, Ian, 109

Kennedy Center for Bioethics, 176

Kiev, Ari, 383

Kirb, K. E., 39

Kübler-Ross, Elisabeth, 77, 336

Lasagna, Louis, 139, 141, 333

Law, xiii, xviii; and determination of death, 85-88, 97, 105-23; and allowing to die, 146, 160-61, 226-40, 243-52, 256-69; and euthanasia, 297-307, 340-41, 343-46, 354, 357-58; and suicide, 376, 381

Law and Equity Court (Richmond), 125

Legalization of euthanasia, xix-xx, 267-68, 281, 297-307, 321-33

Legislative bills, xvii, xix, 99-100, 111-14, 119-23

Lee, H. M., 125

Life-prolonging procedures, xv, xvii, 177, 189-91, 226, 271-73

Litman, Robert E., 368, 394

Logical truth, 30

Lower, Richard, 109, 125

Lucretius, 388

McCormick, Richard, xvii, 173-84

Maguire, Daniel, xx, 320-46

Maine Medical Center, 173, 185

Maine Medical Center v. Houle, xvii, 185-86

Mansson, Helge, xx, 308-19

"Meaningful life," 174-84

Meaning of death, xiii, xv, 57-69, 70-71, 112-14

Meaning of Right and Wrong, The (Cabot), 32

Means, 27, 64, 200-201, 217, 355-59

Medawar, Peter, 71

Medical College of Virginia, 109, 125

Medical technology, xv, 75-76, 80, 90-91, 104, 113, 120, 134, 177, 226, 275

Medicine, xiii, xvi, 25, 78, 356; and determination of death, 82-89, 92-101; and intensive-care nurseries, 133-43; and allowing to die, 173-84, 191; and euthanasia, 333-34, 341-43

Meningomyelocele, 140-41

Mental illness, xx, 363-65, 369-72, 374-85

"Mercy murder," 298, 301, 306

Meyer, Bernard, xv, 42-56

Michael Reese Hospital, 10

Milgram, Stanley, 308, 316-17

Minot, George, 333

Model statute on death, 119-23

Mondale, Walter, 107

Mongolism, 145-72

Montemarano, Vincent, xix

Moral truth, 30

Morison, Robert, xv, 57-69, 70-81, 286

Morris, Arval, 334

Morrison, Norman, 395-96

Muir, Robert, 273

Murray, Henry, 364

National Academy of Sciences, 107

National Advisory Commission on Health Science and Society (proposed), 107

National Institute of Neurological Diseases and Stroke, 95

National Institutes of Health, 107

Natural law, 68, 299, 301

Nazi Germany, 139, 292, 321-28, 349
Neocortex, 100-1
Neocortical death, 121
Neonatal mortality, 133
Neurologists, 95, 101
Neurosurgeons, 95
New York General Assembly, xix
Niebuhr, H. Richard, 294-95
Niebuhr, Reinhold, 299
Nolan, Kieran, 218
Nurses, 147, 163-64

Obligation, 28, 31, 39
O'Donnell, Thomas, 181, 208
Oken, Donald, xv, 9-25, 303
Olshansky, Simon, 139
"On the Supposed Right to Lie from Altruistic Motives" (Kant), xiv, 40
"Ordinary" means, xvii, 64, 88, 162, 192-211, 276
Otto, Rudolf, xi

Pain-relieving drugs, xviii, 201, 215, 284
Parens patriae doctrine, 243, 259-60
Patient questionnaire, 4
Patient rights, 26-41
Paul of Tarsus, 33, 36, 172, 320
Peabody, Francis, 28
Pediatricians, 140
Peter Bent Brigham Hospital, 30
Physician questionnaire, 11-14
Physicians, xiii-xiv, 91, 99, 105-106, 141, 146, 259, 266-67, 272, 341-43, 358, 377-78; and truthtelling, 9-25, 27, 42-56; motivation, 22; obligation to patients, 28, 230-31, 238-39, 272-73; and euthanasia, 80, 284, 289, 293; and determination of death, 85-88, 91, 99, 114; and allowing to die, 154-61, 173, 219-24, 226-40, 259
Pickett, Lawrence K., 174
Pius XII, 88, 97, 179, 183, 334
Placebo, 35
Plato, 388
Potter, Charles Francis, 300
Pretzel, Paul, xxi, 387-400
"Prolongation of Life, The" (Pius XII), 88
Psychiatrists, xxi, 9; and truthtelling, 35-36, 40; and suicide, 363-85, 374-84
Pythagoras, 390

Quality of life, 63-66, 177-83, 282
Quinlan, Karen, xiv, xvii, 271-77

Rahner, Karl, 179
Ramsey, Paul, xvii-xviii, 78, 189-225, 335
Religious freedom, 242-49, 258
Respirators, xv, xviii, 65, 83, 85, 113, 189, 229-32, 271-77, 283
Right of privacy, 274-77
Right to life, 145-72, 186, 273
Rilke, Rainer Maria, 189
Roberts, David G., 175, 186
Robey, William, 37
Roman Catholic tradition, xvii, xx, 162, 289, 301-307, 380
Rule of "double effect," xviii, 215, 219, 289
Rutstein, David, 104
Rynearson, Edward, 191

Saffron, Morris H., 341
St. John-Stevas, Norman, 336
Sanctity of life, 133, 253-54, 274, 316
Sanctity of Life and the Criminal Law, The (Williams), 299
Sander, Herman, xvii, 344
Sanders v. State, 343
Sartre, Jean-Paul, 309
Schein, Harvey, 375-76
Schmerber v. California, 250
Schopenhauer, Arthur, 391
Schreiner, G. E., 332
Self-destruction, xx-xxi, 384-85, 388-95
Self-determination, xx-xxi, 29, 242, 248, 267, 269, 276, 384-85
Seneca, xx, 389
Sewell, David H., 125
Shakespeare, William, 59
Shaw, Anthony, 175
Shneidman, Edwin, xxi, 363-373, 382, 394
Shochet, Bernard R., 375
Shurtleff, D. B., 140
Sixth Commandment, 255, 287, 357, 392
Slater, Eliot, 133
Smith, Joan, 396
Smith v. Smith, 86
Socrates, 388
Solomon, Philip, 382
Stanley v. Georgia, 250-51

Stevens, Wallace, 164
Stoicism, 285-91, 294, 389
Stone, Alan A., 375-76
Sudnow, David, 141
Suffering, xvii, xix, 28, 284
Suicidal behavior, xiv, 365-72
Suicide, xiii, xx-xxi, 20, 68, 79, 242, 255-56, 262-66, 284-85, 355, 359, 363-400; attempted suicide, 263, 374-75, 380; suicidal clues, 365-372; and mental illness, 363-65, 369-72, 374-85; rational, 384-85, 395-99
Suicide prevention, xxi, 363-73, 380-85, 387-400
Suicide Prevention Center (Los Angeles), 364, 368, 383
Suicide Prevention Service (Nassau County), 383
Superior Court of Maine, 185-86
Superior Court of New Jersey, xvii, 271-73
Supreme Court of Arkansas, 86-87
Supreme Court of Illinois, 245
Supreme Court of New Jersey, xiv, xvii, 244, 274-77
Szasz, Thomas, 374-85

Task Force on Death and Dying (Institute of Society, Ethics, and the Life Sciences), xv, 90-102
Taylor, Jeremy, 40
Teleology, 357
Terminal patients, xviii, 52, 189-225, 227
"Thirteen Ways of Looking at a Blackbird" (Stevens), 164
Thomas, Dylan, 370
Thomas v. Anderson, 85
Tillich, Paul, 291, 389

Toch, Rudolf, 212
Triage, 192
Truthtelling, xiii, 3-55; attitudes of patients, 3-8; attitudes of physicians, 9-25; relatives, 15; and education, 16-17, 24; and experience, 17-18; and emotion, 17-20, 25; and suicide, 20-21
Tucker, Bruce O., 125-28
Tucker v. Lower, xiv, xvi, 109, 125-28
Tucker, William E., 109, 125

"Unfit" members of society, xix, 309-17
Uniform Anatomical Gift Act, 112, 114, 122
United States Supreme Court, 247-49

van Dusen, Dr. and Mrs. Henry, xx, 341
Veith, Ilza, 375
Virginia Death by Wrongful Act Statute, 127
Voight, Jorgen, 194

Wasserman, H. P., 205
"Wedge" argument, xx, 321-28
Whitehead, Alfred N., 57
Williams, Glanville, 266, 299
Wisconsin v. Yoder, 249, 261
Withhold information, 13, 23, 34
Withhold/withdraw treatment, xvii, 72, 142, 191, 271-77, 348
Worcester, Alfred, 36
Wright, J. Skelly, 243

Yale-New Haven Hospital, 134, 174

Zachary, R. B., 140
Zalba, M., 180
Zweig, Stefan, 382